AF835211

Hi Betsy,

This has been a wonderful trip for me down memory lane. I hope you enjoy sharing my memories.

Grace Terry

With Faith and a Marketbasket

With Faith and a Marketbasket

The Story of St. Barnabas
The First Hospital in Minneapolis, Minnesota
1871-1991

By Grace Terry, RN, MEd

DeForest Press
Elk River, Minnesota

Permission gratefully acknowledged for the following:

Quotations from issues of the *Voice of St. Barnabas, Dimensions of Metropolitan Medical Center, Scope,* MMC Annual Report, Board of Trustees minutes, miscellaneous papers and programs, as well as photos, from the Metropolitan Medical Center Historical Library.

Portions of articles appearing on pages 340-341, copyright 2005 Star Tribune. Republished with permission of Star Tribune, Minneapolis-St. Paul. No further republication or redistribution is permitted without the written consent of Star Tribune.

Brief quotations from *History of Minnesota* by William Watts Folwell, published 1930 by Minnesota Historical Society Press, St. Paul, Minnesota.

Published by:
DeForest Press
P.O. Box 154
Elk River, MN 55330 USA
www.DeForestPress.com
Toll-free: 877-441-9733
Richard DeForest Erickson, Publisher
Shane Groth, Editor in Chief
Cover design by Linda Walters, Optima Graphics, Appleton, WI

ISBN 1-930374-14-3
Printed in the United States of America
09 08 07 06 05 5 4 3 2 1

Library of Congress Cataloging-in-Publication Data

Terry, Grace, 1929-
With faith and a marketbasket : the story of St. Barnabas, the first hospital in Minneapolis, Minnesota, 1871-1991 / by Grace Terry.
p. ; cm.
ISBN 1-930374-14-3
1. St. Barnabas Hospital (Minneapolis, Minn.) 2. Hospitals--Minnesota--Minneapolis--History. 3. Nursing schools--Minnesota--Minneapolis--History. 4. Medical care--Minnesota--Minneapolis--History.
[DNLM: 1. St. Barnabas Hospital (Minneapolis, Minn.) 2. Hospitals--history--Minnesota. 3. Delivery of Health Care--history--Minnesota. 4. History of Nursing--Minnesota. 5. History, 19th Century--Minnesota. 6. History, 20th Century--Minnesota. WX 28 AM6 T329w 2005] I. Title: Story of St. Barnabas, the first hospital in Minneapolis, Minnesota, 1871-1991. II. Title.
RA982.M62S838 2005
362.11'09776579--dc22

2005008291

To Gilma Joy Prestemon and Margery Stone Bischoff,

both members of the Class of 1951.

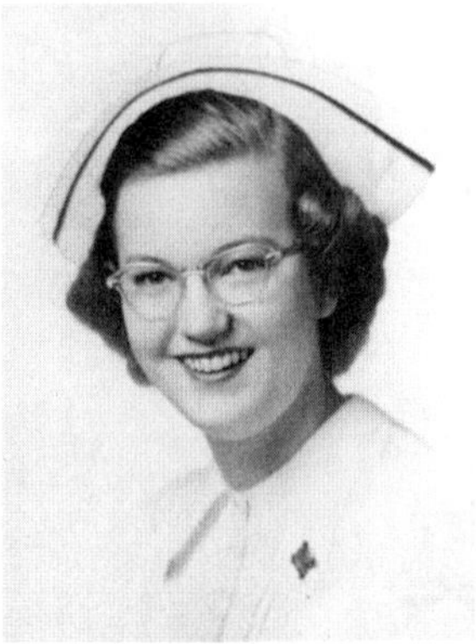

Gilma Joy Prestemon

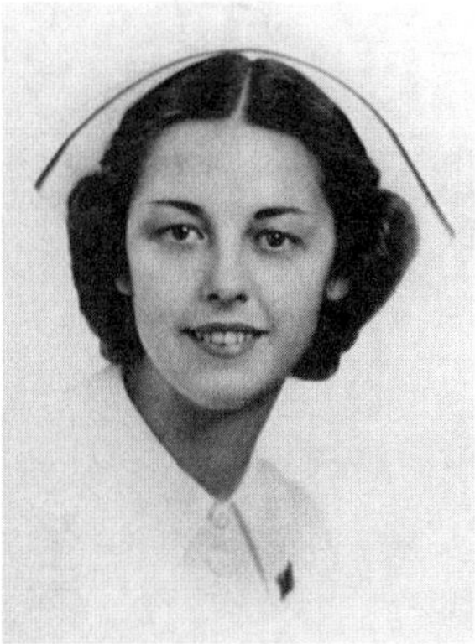

Margery Stone Bischoff

Two of the best nurses St. Barnabas ever produced.

The St. Barnabas Nursing School Pin

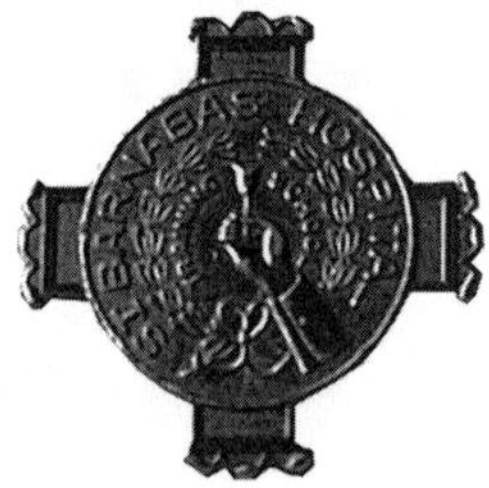

The pin given to each nurse at graduation was distinctive to the school. It was crafted of sterling silver. The design was done at Tiffany's in New York and pins were ordered from there at first. Later, Hudson's in Minneapolis carried the pins, making it much easier for the unlucky graduate who had to replace a lost pin to do so. The pin was in the shape of a Greek cross, signifying the religious origins of the school. Superimposed on the Greek cross was a disk, making the pin resemble the Celtic cross so common in churches in the British Isles, reflecting the Episcopal origins of the school. On the disk was a laurel wreath, the Greek symbol of honor, surrounding an up-stretched hand that held a communion cup, referring again to the religious origins of the school as well as to the honor of serving fellow men. Each nurse's name was engraved on the back of the pin.

Contents

Acknowledgments

The inspiration to write this book came to me in 2001 when I visited Minnesota for the fiftieth anniversary of our graduation from St. Barnabas Hospital School of Nursing. Our class celebration coincided with the alumnae banquet for that year and in addition, we planned other events for just our class members. At the banquet there was discussion of having each class write recollections of their associations with St. Barnabas. The following day our class visited the Historical Library and Museum containing old St. Barnabas artifacts and information. It became clear to me that no definitive history of St. Barnabas had ever been written, though the story was one that needed to be told for posterity. In my estimation, the early efforts of the Reverend Knickerbacker and his volunteers were the purest examples of Christian charity in action that I have ever encountered. This, alone, would be reason enough to document the history. But all the more so because St. Barnabas was the very first hospital in the young city of Minneapolis. Its story is also a piece of the story of the city. It needed to be told and I felt compelled to try my best to tell that story.

As in every undertaking like this, more people are involved than just the author who gets to add her name to the finished product. Following are several people who helped along the way. Gilma Joy Prestemon spent her entire professional life at St. Barnabas. Like me, she was an inveterate pack rat and I knew she had lots of St. Barnabas memorabilia stashed away, so she was the first person to whom I wrote about my intention to write the book. She was within weeks of her death then, but left instructions that on her death the information she had should be given to Marge Bischoff who would see that I received it. She even marked her instructions, "THIS IS VERY IMPORTANT." Gilma died in November 2001. On December 24, 2001, Marge and her husband, Kerm Bischoff, were at my home in McAlester and they brought me all of the things Gilma had earmarked for me. Little did the three of us realize that day would be the last day we three would be together. Marge died suddenly in July of 2002. At the beginning of this book is a dedication to these two beloved classmates. I mean it with all my heart when I described them as "two of the best."

The Hennepin County Service League through the Historical Library and Museum provided much information to me and all of the pictures included in this book. Helen Whiting, librarian at the Historical Library and Museum, and her three stalwart volunteers, Elma Ann, Carol and Mavis, have provided inestimable help to me. I had not met either Helen or Mavis prior to writing this book, but I am proud to call them friends now. Elma Ann and I have a history together dating back to 1959 when we worked together in the school. She was a wonderful help to me then and continues to be so to this day. And my relationship with Carol extends back much further, to my student days. She was a relatively new young RN and I a student—on nights together, as I recall. She was always a positive role model to me then and still is.

At the 2002 alumnae banquet I invited anyone present to send to me anecdotes to be included in the book. Several members responded by sending their own remembrances, or in one case, a story she wrote about an evening as an intensive care nurse. All of those are included in Chapter 16 with identification of the individual who sent the contribution. Thanks to each of you for your participation in this project.

I got addresses for Helen Hayden and Dorothy Merrell Engle from Elma Ann, and so I wrote to them to tell them of my plan and to solicit their help. Both ladies are in their venerable years now (aren't we all!) but both were gracious in responding to my letters. Both were outstanding leaders during their years at St. Barnabas and I am proud to have known them.

Bev Weber of the St. Barnabas Alumnae has also been a great encourager during the years I have been writing this book. Our alumnae have been well served by her willing service over several years. Thanks, so much, Bev.

Another alumnae member to whom I owe thanks is Dale Byson Elliott. Dale alerted me to the new project to be housed in the old Pavilion building by sending me a clipping from the *Star Tribune*. Thanks Dale.

The Reverend Anthony Holder, Rector of St. Michael's Episcopal Church in O'Fallon, Illinois, is a family friend who read part of the manuscript and made helpful comments regarding it. Thanks to Father Tony.

Quotations from other published works are included in several places. Permission to use these quotations was received from the Minnesota Medical Association, Hennepin Medical Society, the University of Minnesota Press and the Minnesota State Historical Society.

An Oklahoma friend who is deserving of thanks is Deborah Hackler, not just a friend, but an attorney who provided legal advice along the way. Thank you Deborah.

And last of all is another Oklahoma friend, Juanita Proctor, whom God sent to me just when I needed someone like her. She is a retired RN, former Director of Nursing at Presbyterian Hospital in Oklahoma City and at Methodist Hospital in the same city. She also served several years on the faculty of the nursing program at Oklahoma Baptist University. She retired while I was writing this book and moved to McAlester where she has family. Juanita read every chapter of the book as I wrote it. She made notes, then we would discuss her impressions chapter by chapter. Her rich background of experience was most helpful. Thanks to you, Juanita.

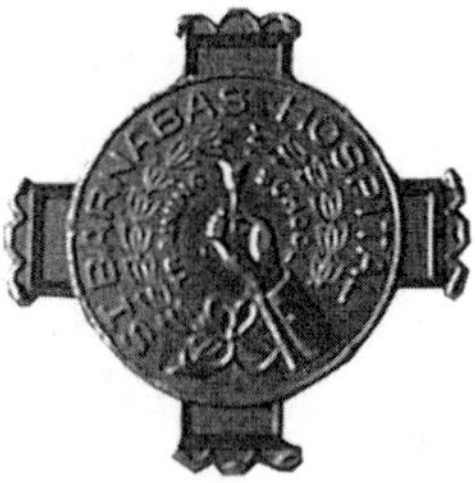

Chapter 1

Two Bishops and the First Hospital in the City

In 1856, a young man arrived in the small community of Minneapolis. He came from New York and had been assigned by the Protestant Episcopal Church to become the first rector of Gethsemane Episcopal Church, today known as the Church of Gethsemane. Minneapolis in 1856 was a rowdy, boisterous lumber town, with a two-class society. There were the entrepreneurs who had come to establish businesses in the town such as John Sargent Pillsbury, who had arrived just the year before the young rector. Pillsbury came to Minneapolis from Concord, New Hampshire, and set up a hardware store in the young community. Ultimately, that store failed, possibly because the population of only 200 at the time was not sufficient to support that kind of business. Later, he would establish a wholesale hardware company that flourished. By 1869, he had been joined by his brother, George, and nephew, Charles A.

Pillsbury, also emigrants from New Hampshire. Together, John, George and Charles formed a partnership, and in 1870 they opened Charles A. Pillsbury and Company, forerunner of Pillsbury Mills. It is likely the Pillsburys were among the flock at Gethsemane Church.

The other class of society in Minneapolis at the time consisted of lumberjacks employed to work in the sawmills built at the Falls of St. Anthony on the Mississippi River. On the east side of the river was a community that had existed in the area as a town since 1838. In 1855, it was incorporated as the City of St. Anthony. Its first mayor was Henry T. Welles, who will figure in the St. Barnabas story some years later.

Richard A. Chute owned a mill on the east side of the river. Chute's ancestry included several Presbyterian clergymen and when he died in 1893, his funeral was at St. Andrew's Presbyterian Church. Years later, in the mid twentieth century, St. Andrew's and St. Barnabas will share a common interest.

On March 1, 1856, the town of Minneapolis was incorporated on the west side of the river. It is said the Minneapolitans were irked by the fact that their community was labeled just a town while their rival on the east side of the river was known as a city. Dorilus Morrison had a sawmill at the falls on the west side of the river. He served as the first mayor of Minneapolis and he, too, will become a part of the St. Barnabas story at a later time.

Both Chute and Morrison were involved in platting communities north of St. Anthony Falls where there were vast stands of white pine growing along the Rum River, a tributary of the Mississippi. Logs that were felled along the Rum were floated down to its mouth near the present day city of Anoka and then down the Mississippi to the sawmills waiting at St. Anthony Falls. Both Chute and Morrison profited handsomely from their businesses at the Falls of St. Anthony. The supplies of timber along the Rum River were considered inexhaustible in the foreseeable future when the area was platted in the mid 1850s, but like many predictions, that was not true. After less than 70 years the vast stands of pine were gone. But, as the twentieth century dawned, Minneapolis had become the greatest lumber-producing center in the United States. The Minneapolis production of timber in 1900 alone totaled more than $12,250,000.00. But let us return to that young rector at Gethsemane Church, the Reverend Mr. Knickerbacker. He was only 23 years old when he came to Minneapolis and just 24 when he was

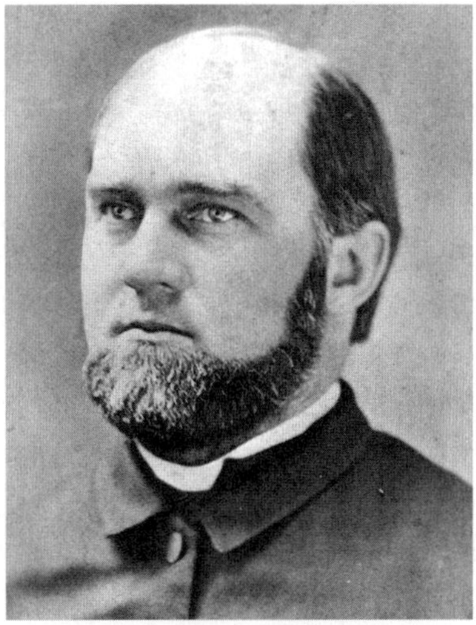

The Rev. David Buell Knickerbacker, Founder of St. Barnabas

made a priest of the Protestant Episcopal Church. David Buell Knickerbocker was born in Schaghticoke, Renssalaer County, New York. He was the youngest son of Hermon Knickerbocker, who was known in his home area as Prince Knickerbocker. References to the family appear in the writings of Washington Irving. When the spelling of the name was changed from Knickerbocker to Knickerbacker is not known, but it is the same family as those who were seventeenth century immigrants in New Amsterdam from Holland. When he was seventeen years old, David entered Trinity College in Hartford, Connecticut, graduating in 1853 when he was only 20 years old. He entered General Theological Seminary in New York City, from which he graduated in 1856 and was ordained a deacon of the church in June of 1856.

His first assignment from the church was as a missionary to the new community of Minneapolis, Minnesota. A year after his arrival in Minneapolis, on July 13, 1857, he was advanced to the priesthood in a ceremony at Gethsemane. There is no reference to a wife or children in the surviving records about the Reverend Knickerbacker, so it may be assumed that he was one of the Episcopal clergy to elect a celibate lifestyle and to devote his entire life to his ministry. That he could identify with the lumberjacks in the lower end of the social strata seems indisputable even though his parishioners at Gethsemane included many of the wealthier entrepreneurs of the town.

By 1870, the little community of only 200 to which the Reverend Mr. Knickerbacker had been assigned, had grown to 13,600. Even more astonishing is that in the decade ending in 1880 it grew to 46,887 and with almost exponential growth to 129,200 by 1885. With this remarkable growth came a broadening of the industrial base of the city. A new industry had developed at the Falls of St. Anthony, taking advantage of the power generated by the falls. Whereas the timberlands north of Minneapolis fed the sawmills, it was the farms in southern Minnesota that brought on the next industrial boom. The railroad had come to the Rochester-Winona area and farmers, on their fertile acreages, found it profitable to raise large fields of wheat, selling what they could locally as they had always done, but being able also, because of the railroads, to ship their grain to other destinations.

An early Minneapolis flour miller who played a key role in the wheat boom was George H. Christian. He was operating a flour mill in the city prior to 1870. The wheat used to make the best grade of flour in those days was winter wheat, a variety which did not grow well in Minnesota. Flour made from spring wheat, which could be grown in Minnesota, was darker in color than the winter wheat variety and in world markets it did not command premium prices as the winter wheat flour did. To make flour white, it had to be separated in the milling process from the bran of the wheat grain and a substance called "middlings." In spring wheat, the most nutritious part of the grain was in the middlings. Separating middlings from the flour made a whiter end product, but when the color of spring wheat flour was made to equal that of winter wheat flour, the end product lacked the nutrition of the winter wheat flour.

George H. Christian understood the problem and was studying ways of treating the middlings to improve the color while retaining the nutrients. Such a process was in use in French flour mills of the time. In 1870, Christian had in his employ a French immigrant who built an apparatus similar to that used in France to carry out the desired result. Over the next few years they were able to perfect the middlings purifier, paving the way for spring wheat to become king in Minnesota and placing Minneapolis flour in a competitive world position with winter wheat flour. George H. Christian would soon play a key role in the St. Barnabas story and his influence at St. Barnabas would be felt years later well into the twentieth century.

In Minneapolis at the last quarter of the nineteenth century some of the sawmill operators and owners saw the opportunity waiting at their southern door and switched production from lumber to flour milling. As lumber had made Minneapolis the greatest lumber-producing center in the country, so "the milling revolution" would make Minneapolis the milling capital of the world.

The earliest incursion into flour milling came in 1850 when John Eastman built a flour mill at St. Anthony Falls. But it would still be several years into the future before the flour milling boom days. In 1866, Cadwallader Colden Washburn, a transplanted New Englander living at that time in nearby Wisconsin, built at the Falls of St. Anthony the largest mill west of Buffalo. It was six stories tall, a gigantic height for that era, and it was capable of producing 840 barrels of flour each day. Washburn was on his way as a tycoon in the milling industry.

Both Washburn and his rival in the flour milling trade, Charles Pillsbury, learned of improved methods of milling being employed in Hungarian flour mills and both went off to Budapest during the 1870s to learn more about the European methods. The Hungarian innovation, the use of steel rollers, rather than large flat stones to grind the wheat, actually began in Switzerland and spread east to Hungary where the whole idea was refined. When Washburn returned to Minneapolis, he changed his plant to incorporate steel rollers in place of the old grindstones. Pillsbury, on his return in 1881, built a six-story mill of his own on the east side of the river and in it steel rollers were installed from the very beginning. The capacity of his mill reached 5,000 barrels per day.

As the twentieth century rolled around for the flour milling industry, Minneapolis was not only producing flour at one of the highest rates in the world, but their flour was also known as the world's best quality. With such fantastic industrial growth came a price to be paid in the hazards to which the workers in these industries were exposed. The Reverend Mr. Knickerbacker, identifying as he did with the workers, became acutely aware of the hazards. A catastrophe that occurred on October 4, 1869 may have made him more aware than ever of the hazards.

On that day, the falls of St. Anthony collapsed, destroying three mills in the process. It turns out there had been a tunneling project beneath the falls which it was hoped would allow for the capture of some of the power being lost at the surface. The tunnelers apparently didn't realize that the edge of the falls was only a thin crust. Beneath that crust was soft sandstone that the river quickly washed away after the tunnel operation began. Once the underlying sandstone washed away, the crust crumbled.

The disaster drove home the vulnerability of the young workers in the mills. The Reverend Mr. Knickerbacker knew that many of these young men had nowhere to go nor anyone to care for them if they were injured on the job. Many were single men living in boarding houses. Other boarders were men who were married, but had left families elsewhere to wait while they went to the city to earn their fortunes.

Not only were there dangers from the sawmills and flour mills, but infectious diseases and diseases related to poor nutrition were rampant. Basically, by eastern standards, the air and climate in Minnesota were considered "very healthy." As a matter of fact, more than one Easterner, suffering from respiratory disorders, came to Minnesota and found they were cured by the change in climate. But living spaces of that era were poorly heated and drafty. Not only that, sanitation was poor and the relationship between poor sanitation and infectious disease was not yet clearly understood. The need to keep food under refrigeration was also not understood and even when it was, facilities were lacking, so people frequently ate foods that were tainted and should have been discarded. Typhoid fever, scarlet fever, diphtheria, croup, pneumonia, tuberculosis and smallpox were around constantly and the men working at the mills, usually in close proximity to one another, were exposed to all of these ills as well as the accidents common on the job.

In early 1871, the Reverend Mr. Knickerbacker appealed to the City Council to establish a charity hospital to care for the sick and injured. He specified a charity hospital because the wealthy of the community did not face the same problems as the workers did. When they were ill, they had servants to care for them in their own homes and family members around them who could also provide care. But the young man living in a boarding house had none of this. The good rector's petition to the City Council fell on deaf ears, so he went about meeting the need on his own.

At Gethsemane, he had organized the men into a group known as the Gethsemane Brotherhood. He enlisted their aid in his cause. But they hadn't the needed funds and equipment to do the job alone. On March 3, 1871, the Reverend Mr. Knickerbacker made the following appeal in the *Minneapolis Daily Tribune*: "The Brotherhood, believing that the time has come when in a population of 18,000 souls, largely a manufacturing community and liable to frequent accidents, there should be a hospital where the sick who have no homes may be properly cared for...they have determined to make a venture of faith and have rented a building containing twelve rooms...The cost of furnishing the building, is estimated, will be five hundred dollars...For the maintenance of the home and its inmates after it is fairly inaugurated we shall trust simply to the loving hand of charity."

In addition to the Reverend Mr. Knickerbacker, the following members of the Brotherhood of Gethsemane also signed the article: Judge Beebe, W. H. Chamberlain, Dr. A. E. Ames, O. F. Tuttle, Al Robertson and S. B. Cowdry. And so began the first hospital in Minneapolis. Their resources were the vision of a young rector, his faith and that of his Gethsemane Brotherhood and the marketbasket which he carried on his arm as he made his daily rounds to all the businessmen in town begging for anything they could give that might be useful in the hospital.

The article in the newspaper was followed by a lecture at the opera house on the need for the proposed hospital. The response to the article and to the presentation at the opera house was good and the young rector and his Gethsemane Brotherhood received enough donations, and promises of more, to equip and open the hospital. The Masonic Order pledged to furnish one room while the employees of the Milwaukee Road Railroad pledged they would also furnish one room. And so the house at Washington Avenue North and Ninth Street became the first hospital in Minneapolis. It was named the Cottage Hospital, a name it would keep for twelve years until the new institution was dedicated to St. Barnabas.

The young rector had great visions for the new hospital. He saw in his mind a time when the rented facility would be too small to meet the growing need for a hospital. He even dreamed of a medical school being established at the young University of Minnesota and that his hospital might provide clinical facilities for training the student doctors enrolled in that medical school.

In those days medical education was still evolving. There were many small, actually inadequate medical education programs around, and there were still doctors learning on the job by being apprenticed to practicing physicians. The Mayo brothers in southern Minnesota understood the need for more academic preparation and were pushing for the development of a medical school in an academic setting. Obviously, the good rector also recognized this need. Though St. Barnabas was not a part of the picture, in 1887, largely through the efforts of Dr. Perry Millard, the College of Medicine was opened at the University of Minnesota.

The Cottage Hospital opened in 1871 very soon after the newspaper article and the presentation at the opera house. The first patient was admitted on March 14, 1871. He was an eighteen year-old newsboy on the

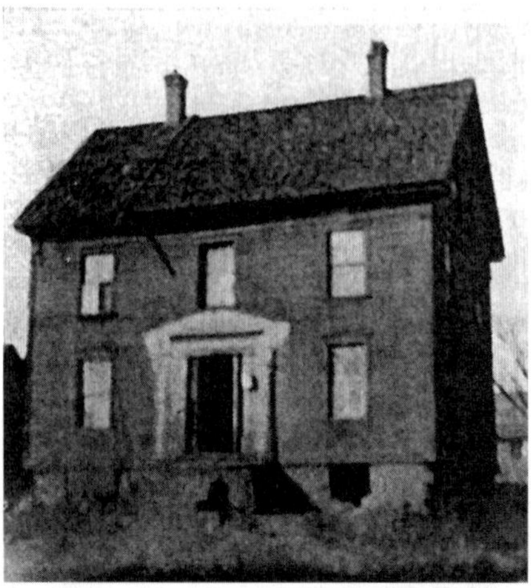
Cottage Hospital, the first hospital in Minneapolis, later named St. Barnabas. Opened March 1, 1871.

Pacific Railroad. Records of the time indicate that he was of German parentage, but orphaned at the time of his illness, a respiratory infection. The second patient came two days later. The record states he was a Swede, a Milwaukee railroad employee who had suffered an accident resulting in amputation of his leg. And still a third patient was listed as a Norwegian suffering from pneumonia. The newspaper published its first report from the new hospital on April 2, 1871, with the observation that seven males and one female had been admitted to the hospital. Of this number, four had been discharged, one had died and two others remained in the hospital.

It seems curious to us today that these early patients were identified by nationality, but this was during the era of European immigration to the area and it is quite probable that none of the three identified as German, Swedish and Norwegian, spoke English. Imagine the problems associated with diagnosing and caring for three patients who all spoke different foreign languages. The record doesn't give us a hint of how the problem was handled, but the good ladies of Gethsemane and the volunteer Dr. Ames must have known what to do. Some time in those early years, the hospital bought lots at Lakewood Cemetery for the burial of indigent patients.

Though they had the funds necessary to equip the hospital to receive patients, they still lacked funds to meet daily expenses. True to his word, the Reverend Mr. Knickerbacker turned to charity for operating funds. And so began his daily excursions through the business community with his marketbasket on his arm. When time permitted, he expanded his route to homes of the wealthy as well. Keenly aware of his responsibility as a steward of donated funds and materials, he kept scrupulous records of each donation. His journal included such entries in the Gifts Received section: "November

6, received two nightshirts, pieced; November 17, received reading material; November 23, two turkeys, three chickens and cranberries."

The gifts were varied, but he didn't turn anything down that might be put to use in the hospital. And donations were not restricted to material things. One man, a barber by trade, donated one day per week to shaving patients at the hospital. Other wealthier men contributed cash.

For staff, the rector turned to lady volunteers from Gethsemane. There were no trained nurses available to care for the patients. The first nursing school west of the Mississippi was still 12 years in the future. Northwestern Hospital in Minneapolis, not even in existence in 1871, would open that first nursing school in 1883. A matron was hired to provide coordination and supervision of the volunteers. The care given was comparable to what would be given at home by a family member: assisting with feeding, washing patients, changing and straightening linens and so on. But for the young man with no family around to care for him, this was more than he expected.

The work went on in the rented house on Washington until 1874. Except for the poor who needed its services and the people from Gethsemane who provided the support for the hospital, it is likely that few people in town were even aware of its existence. The daily census ranged from five to ten patients.

Although he was grateful for the start of the institution, the young rector realized that a more suitable location in a more permanent building was needed and he was ever alert for possibilities which might lead to something more permanent. In 1873 he learned of a large, unoccupied house sitting on the riverbank not far from one of the nicest living areas in the city. The house, known as Garland House, had recently come into the possession of C. C. Washburn, who a short time before had contributed to the hospital one city lot on South Sixth Street. In 1874 the men of Gethsemane raised money and bought another lot adjacent to the one on Sixth Street.

With his usual persuasive manner, the rector convinced Mr. Washburn not only to give the house to the hospital, but to pay for having it moved to the Sixth Street site.

The land owned by the hospital at that time on that site totaled about half an acre. The interior of the house was remodeled to make it suitable for hospital purposes.

The hospital on the site known to most present day Minneapolitans as St. Barnabas Hospital thus had its beginning, although this new building would still carry the Cottage Hospital name for another nine years. For their part, the indebtedness which the Brotherhood had incurred to buy the second lot was erased in only two years.

The area around the new hospital was at that time a choice living area and the residents who owned homes there were less than enchanted with the idea of having a hospital in their neighborhood. A vestige of the grandness of the neighborhood stood until the 1950s on the corner of Ninth Avenue South and Seventh Street. It was purchased by the hospital in 1944 and housed research labs and a medical photography lab for approximately ten years before it was razed in 1957 to make way for the new St. Barnabas.

According to an article written for the *Voice of St. Barnabas* (February-March 1957), Helen Hayden described Smith House as follows: "Called 'Smith House' because it was owned by Professor Lee Irwin Smith in the late 1930s. It was originally known as the 'Butter's Residence,' after its builder and first owner, Fred Butters. The house, built about 1868, was then a home of substance in a fine residential area of the city."

Helen describes how the once fine and beautiful residence fell into decay as the people in the area moved out to more distant sites on the city's edge and their fine homes were replaced with apartment houses, themselves decaying relics by the 1940s when the hospital came into possession of Smith House. She describes one feature of the house in these terms: "The home was built in an era when sawmills were never too far away and lumber was not so dear as today. Sawdust had no place in industry then as it now does in the manufacture of pressed woods. Sawdust was to the sawmill what liver was to the butcher in those days—something to be given away! Mr. Butters decided to make use of it as insulation material and between the studs it was packed so tightly that until the day of the building's demise it is said that every time a picture was hung or a nail pulled from the wall there was a fluttering of sawdust."

Smith House even had a greenhouse attached to its first floor, though that was gone by the time the house had come into the possession of St. Barnabas. Mr. Fred Butters, original owner of the house, was a botany professor at the University of Minnesota and he loved to putter in his own greenhouse during off duty time.

Near the end of her article on Smith House, Helen refers to the preparation for the new St. Barnabas of the block between Chicago Avenue and Ninth Avenue and Seventh and Eighth Streets: "The recent events of destruction of Smith House and the ancient apartment buildings on Chicago Avenue give promise of constructive things to come and dreams once dreamed give promise of being a reality. We hope soon to see a new St. Barnabas arising like a Phoenix bird from the ashes of the old buildings of a bygone era."

But let us return to 1874 and plans for moving to the new facility on Sixth and Ninth. Residents of this upscale area were vocal in their opposition to locating a hospital in their neighborhood. The Reverend Mr. Knickerbacker knew full well the ire to be aroused if he moved patients to the new house. He faced the problem squarely, and instead of retreating, he arranged that the transfer of patients would take place quietly in the dead of night. People tended not to be out on the streets at night, but to be closed up in their safe homes, so he thought the move could be accomplished with a minimum of opposition and disruption. Patients were dressed warmly and cautioned to be very quiet. The move went off as planned and when residents awoke the next day, having a hospital in their midst was an accomplished fact. Gradually, opposition ceased and the hospital remained at that site for the next seventy-six years.

The formal dedication of the new building was on April 14, 1874. Making the dedication was the other bishop about whom this chapter is written, Bishop Henry Whipple. Bishop Henry Benjamin Whipple came to Minnesota in 1859 as the first bishop of the Protestant Episcopal Church. Statehood had come to Minnesota the previous year and there were a number of Episcopal churches in the southern part of the state which had their beginnings during territorial days. Bishop Whipple and the Reverend Mr. Knickerbacker (not yet a bishop at that time) were approximately the same age, Bishop Whipple being the elder by a few months. But their charges were different. The Reverend Mr. Knickerbacker had been assigned to Minneapolis to develop a new parish there. The era of foreign immigration had not yet come to Minnesota in 1856 and a good many of the residents in the young city of Minneapolis had come from New York and New England where there had been a strong presence of the Episcopal Church. The first Christian church in the young city was an outgrowth of the Presbyterian mission established at Fort Snelling. But the mission field was fertile enough to sustain the growth of both denominations. Both were familiar to New Yorkers and New Englanders.

So one of Bishop Whipple's charges was administrative, providing leadership to the Episcopal churches in Minnesota. The other charge was a missionary charge, to be an advocate for the Indian tribes in Minnesota, most notably the Dakota in the southern half of the state and the Ojibway in the northern part of the state.

William Watts Folwell describes Bishop Whipple as "descended from distinguished Revolutionary stock" (*History of Minnesota* [St. Paul: MHS Press, 1960], Vol. 2, 206). By all accounts, Bishop Whipple was a handsome and very intelligent man, though he had suffered ill health during his childhood and so did not receive the usual classical education that his contemporaries at his station in society received. He worked in the family business for some time during which he had a mentor in the person of William Dexter Wilson, a professor of theology of great renown at the time. William Dexter Wilson would become one of the founders of Cornell University.

Folwell goes on to write, "If ever a man was fitted for the time and place, Bishop Whipple was. Tall and strongly built, gracious, but not patronizing in manner, he easily won the good will of men of every class and creed. His enthusiasm was tempered by a saving common sense and an abounding humor. He magnified his office, but only to do the greater service to those to whom he was called to minister. He loved all men; he feared no man" (ibid, 206).

Bishop Whipple took his second charge very seriously and was only in the territory for two weeks when he made a trip to Fort Ripley and Gull Lake to inspect the conditions there for the Ojibway people. Years before that James Lloyd Breck had established ministry to the Ojibway on Gull Lake. By the time of the arrival of Bishop Whipple, that ministry had been suspended and Dr. Breck was living and teaching in Faribault. Apparently the Ojibway had been introduced to the white man's "fire water." This and the breaking by the Europeans of treaties made with the Ojibway in 1854 and 1855 made the red men too unruly to manage by 1857 when the mission was suspended. The plight of the Ojibway impressed the bishop deeply and for the rest of his life he was an undying advocate for these people.

Bishop Whipple settled in Faribault, largely because of the influence of Dr. Breck, who after his move to Faribault following the suspension of his mission at Gull Lake became pastor of the Church of the Good Shepherd in Faribault. Dr. Breck wanted Bishop Whipple to establish a church in Faribault that would be his see or base of operations. As part of the incentive to entice Whipple to settle in Faribault, Breck raised $4,000 and persuaded Alexander Faribault, a Roman Catholic, to donate seven acres of land for Bishop Whipple's use. In 1862, work began on the Cathedral of Our Merciful Saviour, the first cathedral to be built as a cathedral by the Episcopal Church in America. Work continued on the cathedral for seven years before it was completed in 1869. Bishop Whipple said, "when we had means, we worked; when we had none, we waited on God in prayer" (ibid, 206).

This strong faith in God's help and guidance was the same kind of faith young Mr. Knickerbacker was about to demonstrate in Minneapolis.

Just a further word about Dr. James Breck, before proceeding with the St. Barnabas story. Before Bishop Whipple's arrival, Dr. Breck had already established a school at Good Shepherd Church that later evolved into Shattuck Grammar School and still later into Shattuck Academy. Shattuck served the educational needs of the boys of the area, but there was no counterpart for girls. After the arrival of Bishop Whipple, the Whipples established a school for girls in their home. Later that school became St. Mary's Hall. Today the two schools have combined, are thriving as a coed boarding school and occupy a beautiful campus on the east side of town.

Back in Minneapolis, by 1875 the hospital in the remodeled Garland house had outgrown its quarters on Sixth and Ninth. In 1896, Judge Isaac Atwater gave an address commemorating the 25th Anniversary of establishment of the hospital. He reviewed the growth of the hospital over that twenty-five years, citing the building of a fever ward to accommodate twenty patients. Typhoid, diphtheria, small pox and scarlet fever were common diseases at that time and so the fever ward was kept full most of the time. He also described another brick veneer structure built fronting on Sixth Street. It cost over two thousand dollars to build, thirteen hundred dollars of which had been donated by the Honorable H. T. Welles.

The erection of this building added sixteen beds to the hospital. The same year, the Honorable Henry T. Welles built and gave to the hospital a new frame building which would house six patients. It was designated exclusively for surgical patients and was named the Welles Pavilion. Antiseptic surgery had been developed at that point. Obviously, the danger of mixing infectious patients with surgical patients had also been identified. The Cottage Hospital had been accepted by the people of Minneapolis and its future seemed assured.

Another disaster on May 2, 1878, termed "the great mill disaster," showed the Reverend Mr. Knickerbacker and his colleagues that even the expanded Cottage Hospital was not sufficient to meet the needs of the growing city. In the mill disaster, the Washburn A Mill, that behemoth built 12 years previously by Cadwallader C. Washburn, exploded. Eighteen men were killed and many injured. The blast was so great that windows were blown out of homes on Summit Avenue in St. Paul. Two other mills near the Washburn mill were also destroyed. It turns out the cause of the fire was a problem which was always a bane to millers everywhere. The dust created by the milling process hung in the air and just a small spark was enough to ignite it as if it were dynamite.

Without realizing it, Cadwallader C. Washburn made a contribution to the milling industry that day. Following that great explosion, the combustibility of dust in the air was more clearly understood and dust collectors were developed and installed in all flour mills. A conscientious mill owner would also be particular about housekeeping in the area of the mills to reduce the dust hazard.

Through all these years, the Reverend Mr. Knickerbacker remained in charge of the hospital. It was a project near and dear to his heart and he was able to convey his enthusiasm for it to the many friends he had made in Minneapolis. The hospital grew and flourished. In 1883, the good man was called to become the bishop of Indiana. Wanting to assure the future of the hospital, he made arrangements before his departure to have the hospital incorporated and tied to the Episcopal Church. The Articles of Incorporation provided for a Board of Trustees of twelve members to be chosen from the different Episcopal parishes in the city of Minneapolis. The charter stated, "The hospital shall be permanently maintained as a church hospital, and its doors shall be open to all, irrespective of color, race or creed."

The constitution of the new corporation stated further, "The general purpose shall be in the Name of Jesus Christ and through His Church to relieve the sick, wounded, disabled, irrespective of sex, nationality, color or religious creed by providing a place for the care of such persons with medical attendants, nursing, food and clothing."

In keeping with the philosophy that anyone in need could be treated at the hospital, he chose the name "St. Barnabas Hospital" for the institution. As Bible scholars know, Barnabas was a contemporary of the apostle Paul. He was in charge of the Christian Church at Antioch. One of the keynotes of Paul's ministry was his great belief that Jesus Christ was the Messiah for all people, not just for the Jews. He used his ministry to carry the gospel of Jesus Christ not only to Jews, but also to Gentile people in all the known world at that time. The church at Antioch, Syria, was one of those Gentile churches. Barnabas believed as Paul did that the church must reach out to people in need without regard to ethnic background. The nickname given to Barnabas by his contemporaries meant "Son of Encouragement" or "Son of Consolation." Certainly no more appropriate name could have been found for the kind of hospital the Reverend Mr. Knickerbacker had established in Minneapolis.

Two years after the Reverend Mr. Knickerbacker's departure for Indiana, there was a fire at the hospital on August 27, 1885. Damages totaled $3,500. It was estimated it would take $15,000 to repair the damage and bring the hospital up to standards of other hospitals being built at that time. The Board of Trustees faced a dilemma. Basically, it came down to a question regarding the wisdom of investing $15,000 in repairing buildings which even then were not up to standards of the day for hospitals. Also at issue was how the daily hospital operations were to be financed. Two members of the board, Richard Martin and the Honorable Isaac Atwater, placed their own honor on the line by submitting their resignations in protest to the apparent lack of interest in the hospital shown by the churches represented on its board.

Later, Richard Martin apparently was asked to come back to the Board of Trustees. His response to Mr. LeRoy Robertson, Secretary of the board indicated he would not be interested in returning to the board unless changes were made. He was tired and frustrated at the way things were going and would only return to the board if the Episcopal churches in the city would assume their responsibility in placing the hospital on a sound financial footing. He held out an incentive to them by offering an undisclosed amount of money to the hospital, to be given only if and when the churches raised the money needed to provide the financial foundation he felt necessary for the hospital.

Obviously, with the departure of the Reverend Mr. Knickerbacker and his persuasive ways, the hospital had fallen on hard times and another man of the Reverend Mr. Knickerbacker's ilk was needed. It appears that when Richard Martin stood firmly on his principles, the churches finally heard the message. A hospital building was built on October 27, 1886. All but $1000 of the building cost was raised by subscription.

From time to time, varying amounts of money were donated to the hospital by individuals. For example, in 1875 $200 was given to the hospital by Mr. Joel B. Bassett. Mr. Bassett was a city councilman who had opposed increasing salaries of members of the city council. When the measure passed in spite of his opposition, he gave the amount of his annual salary increase, $200, to the hospital by way of protest. In 1876, $1000 came from a lady from Buffalo, New York, whose son had been treated at Cottage Hospital early in the decade. She raised the money by recruiting her friends to help her sew items they could sell. When she died in 1876, she had accumulated by this means the $1000 which came to the hospital under terms of her will. Through gifts such as these, small and large, the hospital was able, financially, to survive the lean times.

The building projects of the seventies and eighties did not meet the needs of the growing hospital for very long. The frame buildings were falling into decay and even with repair, wouldn't meet the standards for care which had developed since they were built. On December 30, 1893, John I. Black, the president of the Board of Trustees, wrote a report summarizing the activities and progress of the hospital from its beginnings through 1893. The basic question before the board at the time was "Do we repair and update or do we build new?"

Ultimately the decision was made to close the hospital on September 1, 1893, to demolish the old buildings in order to clear the site for a new building. Actually, demolition did not begin until November 16. Laying of the cornerstone for the new building took place on December 30—remarkable progress in a period of only six weeks. The cost of the new building was $32,000 in addition to architects' fees which were not specified. Richard Martin had made a bequest of $30,000 which made feasible the building of the completely new structure.

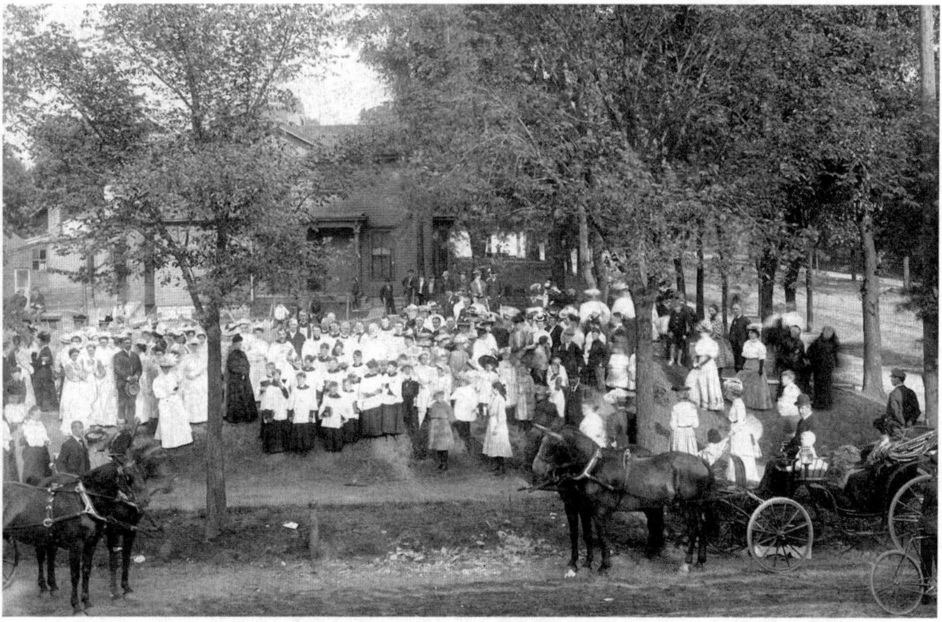

Ground breaking for the Martin building, 1893.

Leck and McLeod were the general contractors chosen; Tunstead and Moore did the heating and ventilating and H. Kelly and Company were the plumbers. The new, three story brick building was completed in 1894, the same year the hospital admitted its first nurses to the new nursing school. Since a bequest from Richard Martin made construction of the new building possible, it was decided the new building should be named for him. It continued to be known as the Martin building until it was torn down in 1962.

Just a few words about this remarkable Mr. Martin, board member and philanthropist who earlier had placed his name and honor on the line for the good of the hospital. He came from New York originally. He was born in Duchess County, New York, on November 16, 1821. In 1854, at the age of 33 years, he came to St. Anthony Falls where he was engaged in banking and real estate. He was brought up in the Lutheran Reformed Church, but after coming to Minnesota, he joined Gethsemane parish, although in later years he attended a parish nearer to his home. He had a physical deformity which resulted from having been dropped in infancy by his nurse. Though frail and deformed physically, he had acute mental faculties. In his early adult years in New York, he became a bookkeeper, a profession at which he was most successful. His health failed him after a few years, and as so many had done before him, he relocated to Minnesota with the anticipation of restoring his health. His hope for restoration of his health was fulfilled and he practiced his craft of bookkeeping successfully for many years in Minnesota. He earned the respect of others in the business community because of his good judgment, his sense of honor, his high standards of conduct and his big heart.

He admired and became a close friend of the Reverend Dr. Knickerbacker and the work he was doing with the Cottage Hospital. In 1883, Mr. Martin began arrangements which would insure that part of his estate, upon his death, would go to the hospital. He was a member of the board for five years, from 1883-1888. In January 1890, he died in Florida. He had willed property to the hospital which yielded $108,000 when it was sold.

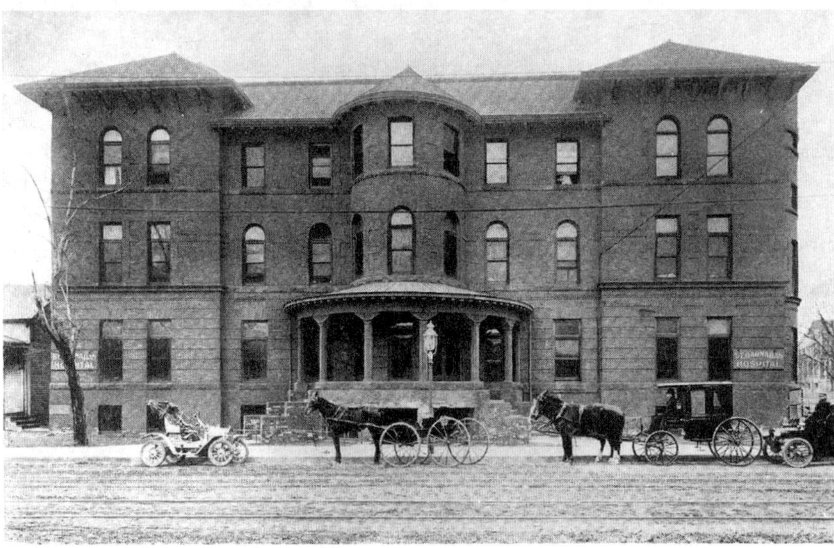

The Martin building, late nineteenth century.

The superintendent of the hospital in 1894 described the new building named for Richard Martin in these terms:

> The greater advantages secured by this handsome structure for increased and more successful work were beyond computation and will be realized more and more as the years go by. The halls and

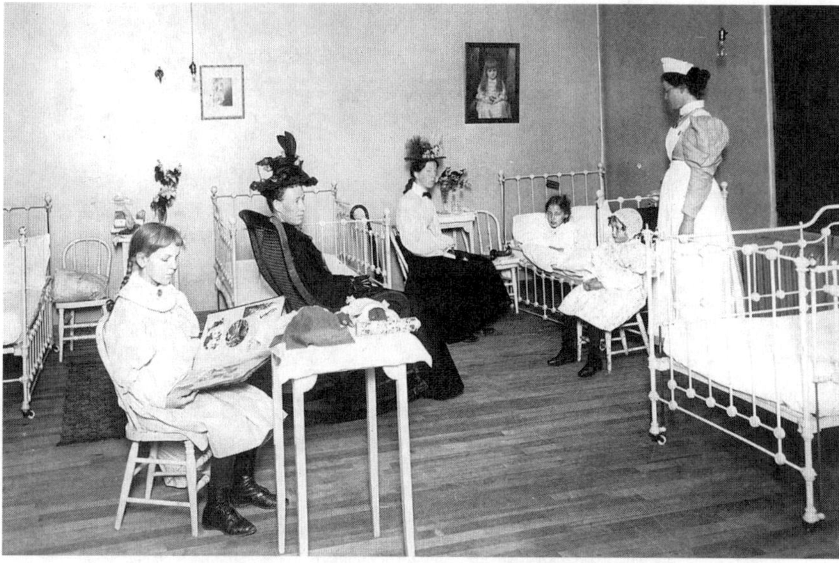

Children's ward, ground floor of the Martin Building, early twentieth century.

rooms are lighted and capacious with high ceilings and a perfect system of fan ventilation. The operating room is a model in the perfection and completeness of its equipment, it being furnished with an abundance of light in all modern appliances. In the opinion of prominent medical men, there is not a better appointed operating room in the West than that of St. Barnabas Hospital. The kitchen is on the top floor and in the rear of the structure so that no odors from cooking can penetrate in the rooms of patients and in all its arrangements neatness and convenience are its striking features.

For those who remember old 4 Martin, the operating room was at the west end of the hall, the circular room with many windows all around. Apparently the kitchen, to which reference is made, was in the area of the nursing station we all would have known. A few years later, when the corridor building was added, the kitchen was moved and expanded on the top floor of that wing. Nursing students lived on the top floor for a time, probably in the rooms at the east end of the Martin building, opposite the operating room on the west end. Later, when those rooms were needed for patients, students were housed in private homes in the area until Wellesmere residence was built early in the twentieth century. Minnie Paterson,

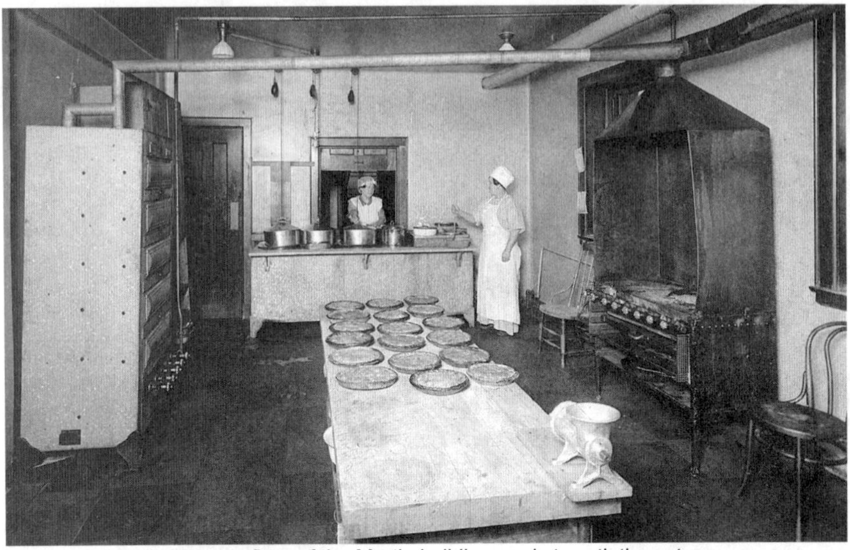

Kitchen, top floor of the Martin building, early twentieth century.

the first graduate of the school related how inconvenient it was to have to travel to the hospital to bathe since there was no bathroom in the home in which she lived.

It was most appropriate that Bishop Knickerbacker return to dedicate the new Martin building in late 1894. He lived only a few weeks after that trip to Minneapolis. His obituary states he died of pneumonia on January 3, 1895. He was 62 years old at the time, not a great age by today's standards, but for 1895, that was considered old age.

Perhaps the strain of the trip from Indiana and back again was too much or perhaps he took a chill on the drafty train during the midwinter trip. The obituary does not tell us that, just that he died of pneumonia. But we believe he died a fulfilled man. He was able to see tangible and impressive results of the efforts he and his Gethsemane Brotherhood had put forth so many years earlier to bring a hospital to Minneapolis.

A memorial service was held for Bishop Knickerbacker on January 20, 1895, in the little chapel on the first floor of the Martin building. The following was included in the Eulogy at that service: "He labored in season and out of season. It was by his personal efforts the first money and the first provisions in kind were brought to the Cottage Hospital. His hands carried many a basket laden with the necessities of maintenance and his personal solicitations from many a housewife brought for the bed furnishings."

Another speaker added to the memorial service, "It was with feelings of satisfaction we had among us at the opening of the new hospital the honored and revered Founder, whose blessing upon this institution was his last official act in the city of his early life work, and who more fitting to his own works of mercy than by giving it his fatherly blessing."

The following year, the hospital celebrated the twenty-fifth anniversary of its founding. Included in the address he gave on that occasion, Judge Isaac Atwater compared the early efforts of the good rector to those of an order in the Catholic Church. He said:

> There is an order in the Catholic Church in the city of New York, called the order of the 'Divine Compassion.' How sublime, how all embracing the idea of that quality of God, which these words represent. And it was an emanation from the Divine Compassion, which inspired and animated the heart of the first rector of this parish, the Reverend David B. Knickerbacker, as a pioneer in the city to engage this earnestness and zeal in this great work of building a hospital which has now assumed the proportions we witness. His name is indelibly connected with its origin and prosecution to the time of his election as Bishop of Indiana. As the name of the Saintly Muhlenburg stood in relation to the great St. Luke's Hospital in New York City, so does his stand in relation to St. Barnabas.

Flowery words to describe a great man. Curiously, it took 47 more years before the hospital board got around to naming a building in the Bishop's memory. When the old Asbury Hospital was purchased in 1943 and remodeled to become a residence for students, it was named Knickerbacker Residence.

Bishop Whipple outlived Bishop Knickerbacker by only seven years. He, too, accomplished great things during his years in Minnesota. He became an acknowledged authority on the Indians of Minnesota, acting as their advocate with several different presidential administrations. President Lincoln said the following after a visit with Bishop Whipple: "He came here the other day and talked with me about the rascality of this Indian business until I felt it down to my boots" (Folwell, *History*, 206, 208).

Folwell gives high praise to Bishop Whipple for his courage as an advocate for the Ojibway and Dakota people and his tireless efforts to bring about reform of government policy with regard to the Indian tribes.

Bishop Whipple knew the Indians probably better than most of the Indian agents did. The story went around that a Sioux Indian once asked Bishop Whipple if the Jesus of whom he preached to them was the same talked to by the white men at the agency when they were drunk!

The philosophy of the bishop with regard to the Indians can best be summed up in these suggestions included in a memo he sent to President Cleveland in 1885: "1) No almshouses for able-bodied men to graduate to savage paupers; 2) All funds except for aged, infirm and sick, widows and children to be expended as rewards for labor; 3) Provision for schools in each settlement; 4) Lands to be given on actual settlement in severalty and inalienable; 5) Provision for police administration of law; 6) White Earth Reservation to be kept for their inheritance forever" (ibid., Vol. 4, 201, 202).

Folwell relates that the commissioners of Indian affairs disapproved the principles and that was the end of it. Folwell concludes by saying, "The bishop's plan may have been the wiser one" (ibid., 204).

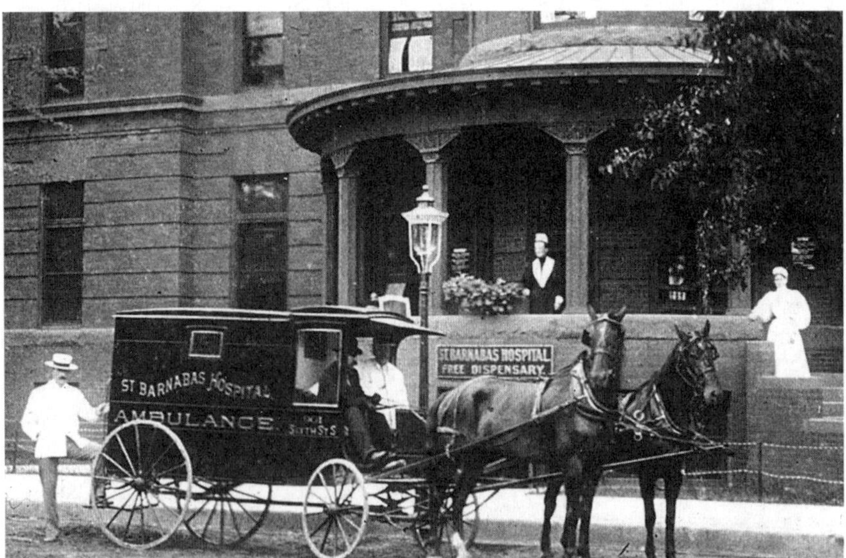

St. Barnabas Ambulance, early twentieth century.

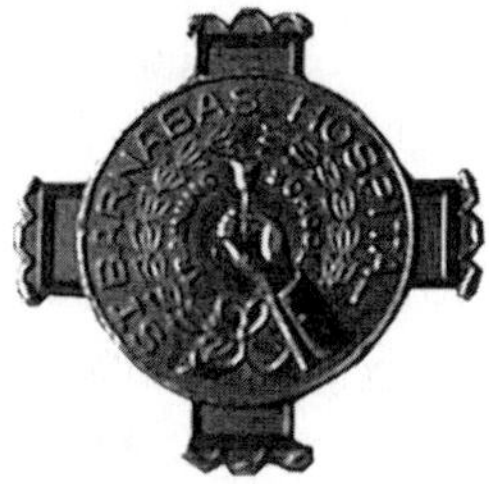

Chapter 2

Volunteers Through the Years

For the first 23 years of St. Barnabas Hospital—first in the Cottage Hospital and later in the buildings on Sixth Street and Ninth Avenue South—the nursing provided was of a rudimentary type, much as one family member with no medical or nursing training would give to another family member. Trained nurses anywhere in those days were in short supply, but particularly so in Minneapolis where, prior to the opening of the Cottage Hospital, there were no hospitals in which nurses could be trained. Northwestern Hospital opened the first nursing school west of the Mississippi, but that wasn't until 1883, so the women of Gethsemane Church, utilizing innate nurturing skills, were called upon to provide the hands-on help needed at the hospital. The Reverend Mr. Knickerbacker had organized the men of his parish into the Brotherhood of Gethsemane. They recruited support for the hospital, but it fell to their sisters and wives to provide services. These women brought food to the hospital, made beds, fed and washed patients and provided other comfort measures as needed. They often brought their maids from home and together helped to keep the hospital clean.

In the beginning, the volunteers were recruited by the Reverend Mr. Knickerbacker and members of the Brotherhood of Gethsemane. At the hospital, supervision was provided by the matron or perhaps at times also by the Reverend Mr. Knickerbacker. How much time the good rector spent at the hospital isn't known. We do know that he made his rounds each day and that he also still had day-to-day responsibilities as the rector at Gethsemane.

In 1889, Catherine Welles organized a group of ladies as the Guild at St. Mark's. They met at the church every Monday from October through May. Their prime function was to sew patient gowns for the hospital. The group continued to meet for years and by 1952, their goal was to make 500 gowns each year. Several long-time members of this dedicated group were Mrs. John Plum, Mrs. Ward Benton, Mrs. Edith Hutching, Mrs. George Perry, Mrs. Jerry Horn, Mrs. Herchiner and Mrs. S. M. Kitchen.

After the nursing school was opened at St. Barnabas in 1894, care of patients became the responsibility of the student nurses. Graduate staff, as we know it in modern hospitals, was a development of a later time. Hospitals established nursing programs in order to have a supply of student nurses to care for patients. Even after the opening of the nursing school, there was much left which could be done by volunteers. Women interested in promoting the work of the hospital found many other ways besides direct patient care to make their contributions to the work of the hospital. By 1893, the time had come to organize the volunteers into a group that could work more efficiently with the administration of the hospital. On St. Barnabas Day, June 11, 1893, a board of Women Directors was elected by the trustees of the hospital. Like the Board of Trustees, these women, twenty of them, represented all the Episcopal parishes in the city.

The organizational meeting of the new Board of Women Directors was held on January 27, 1894. Two officers were elected, Mrs. J. W. Lawrence to serve as president and a Miss H. Rollet to serve as secretary-treasurer. They also elected one member from the Board of Trustees to serve ex-officio. One of their first actions was the organization of a group of women who called themselves the "Thimble Bees." They were seamstresses and they made patient gowns for the hospital. In 1898, the name of the organization was changed from Board of Women Directors to the Woman's Auxiliary. The membership qualifications, namely that the twenty women be drawn from all the Episcopal parishes in the city, remained the same. Years later, under the presidency on the Board of Trustees of Charles Bolles Rogers, a Women's Board was organized which co-existed with the auxiliary.

One of the early projects of the Woman's Auxiliary was the building of a residence for nurses and nursing students. It was to become the first such residence for a nursing school in the city. The cornerstone was laid on June 11, 1906, and the residence was named Wellesmere in honor of three Welles women, Catherine, her sister and their mother, Mrs. Henry T. Welles. Henry Thomas Welles was an early benefactor and trustee of the hospital. The Welles ladies, particularly Catherine, or Kate as many knew her, worked tirelessly in supporting all kinds of projects for the hospital. A project similar to the building of Wellesmere was taken on by the auxiliary when the Pavilion building was opened in February of 1911. It was the auxiliary that worked to raise $4,788.20 (a sizable sum in 1911) used to buy furnishings for patient rooms in the new building.

In 1959, Robert Bachmeyer wrote an article for the *Bulletin Of The Hennepin County Medical Society* in which he reviewed the history of the use of volunteers at the Cottage Hospital and later St. Barnabas. He gave high praise to the volunteers who had served so well over so many years. He expressed the idea that without the help of the volunteers, work at the early St. Barnabas could not have proceeded.

In March of 1933, wives of staff doctors were organized to form the St. Barnabas Staff Auxiliary. Their first president was Mrs. W. B. Holt, who after her husband's early death, would become a longtime employee at the hospital. Her story is included in the chapter entitled, "The Greatest Resource St. Barnabas Had." The Staff Auxiliary met for eleven years. Initially, their objective was fellowship, getting to know each other and learning more about the hospital. As time went on, they identified services they could provide to the hospital including sewing and mending hospital garments, making linen and surgical bands, layettes and curtains, and donating time and money to the Red Cross, the Cancer Society and the Christmas Seal Campaign. A benefit card party in 1938 was a fund-raiser for their projects.

They also wrote letters and sent gifts to staff doctors who served in the armed forces during World War II. In 1942, they assisted with the opening of a new pediatric department at the hospital. The group disbanded in 1944.

On March 17, 1953, the Staff Auxiliary was reorganized. The function of the new organization was mainly fundraising to finance various projects for which they identified a need. Their first fund-raiser was a Waltz Night at the Minnikada Club on May 1, 1953, at which they raised $1,600 to start their fund for purchase of pieces of equipment needed by the hospital.

In March of 1941, the Women's Board opened a coffee shop on the ground floor of the Pavilion building between the hospital cafeteria and the entrance to the Wellesmere tunnel. The coffee shop, and later a small gift shop, were located in that area for 17 years until the move to the new hospital in 1958. In the beginning, the coffee shop was operated solely by volunteers, but later a paid manager was hired to coordinate the business of the shop. Volunteers continued to assist in the shop through the Women's Board Coffee Shop Committee. Though the shop was opened initially as a service to hospital personnel and visitors, it soon became a moneymaker for the board. The relaxed, pleasant atmosphere of the shop and the delicious homemade cakes, doughnuts and lunch entrees made it a favorite spot for hospital personnel, ambulatory patients and visitors.

In 1957, a volunteer director was hired to manage the volunteer program. This was not an innovation of itself, for other hospitals had on their payrolls a person hired to manage their volunteer programs. The difference at St. Barnabas was that the new director was hired by the auxiliary and her salary was paid by the auxiliary. Mrs. H. B. (Julie) Stoker was the first volunteer director. She was assisted by Mrs. Morgan Aldrich. The two presided over an office in one of the sunrooms of Wellesmere Residence. They coordinated the volunteer program by assigning volunteers according to their special talents, to all the places in the hospital where there was need for their services. When the auxiliary was reorganized in 1959, Julie Stoker was its first president. She and her husband had come to Minneapolis from Duluth in 1951. They were active members of the Cathedral Church of St. Mark. In Duluth, Julie had been active in the American Cancer Society, a member of the Junior League and on the board of the Duluth Children's Home. In addition, she was a volunteer at St. Luke's Hospital, so she brought a wealth of experiences to her position as volunteer director. In 1958, she chaired the moving day activities for volunteers as the move was made to the new hospital.

Mrs. Stoker and Mrs. Aldrich stepped down in 1959 and Mrs. Isabel Lugsdin became the new volunteer director. Like Mrs. Stoker, Mrs. Lugsdin brought a wealth of previous experience to her position. She had served as chairman of volunteers in several different organizations, most notably among them the Red Cross Grey Ladies. When Mrs. Lugsdin came on board, there were 102 hospital volunteers who had given 847 hours of service during the previous year. The volunteers were quick to stress that they never supplanted paid staff, but only complemented what was already being done by paid staff. Mrs. Lugsdin handled the position of volunteer director capably for five years, until her retirement in 1964. Mrs. Mary Witt replaced her and she, too, worked in that position for five years. But she longed to escape the cold Minnesota winters, so she resigned after five years and was replaced in 1970 by Mrs. Janet Moran.

By 1958, there were four different organizations whose membership came from similar but different, constituencies. All of them provided some kind of volunteer support for the hospital, but all were governed by different boards and directions. The four organizations were the Women's Board, the Junior Board, the Associate Board and the Medical Staff Auxiliary. The efforts of the four groups sometimes duplicated one another, and anyone outside these organizations who wanted to communicate an idea or a need found it difficult to know to which one they should turn. Under the able administration of Robert Bachmeyer, the four groups voted to dissolve and reorganize as just one organization, the St. Barnabas Auxiliary, with membership open to anyone interested in the welfare of the hospital and the school. Having just one auxiliary facilitated a closer relationship between the auxiliary and the administration of the hospital. In remarks he made at the 1959 annual meeting of the auxiliary (*Voice*, April-May 1959) Mr. Bachmeyer commented, "It is my opinion that one women's auxiliary will provide more and better service to patients." The reorganization eliminated the duplication of effort and it became easier to fill gaps in service which had existed in some areas.

Among the many services the auxiliary provided to the hospital, the nursing school and nursing students, were the staffing of a reception/information desk in the hospital lobby, distribution of mail to patients, delivery

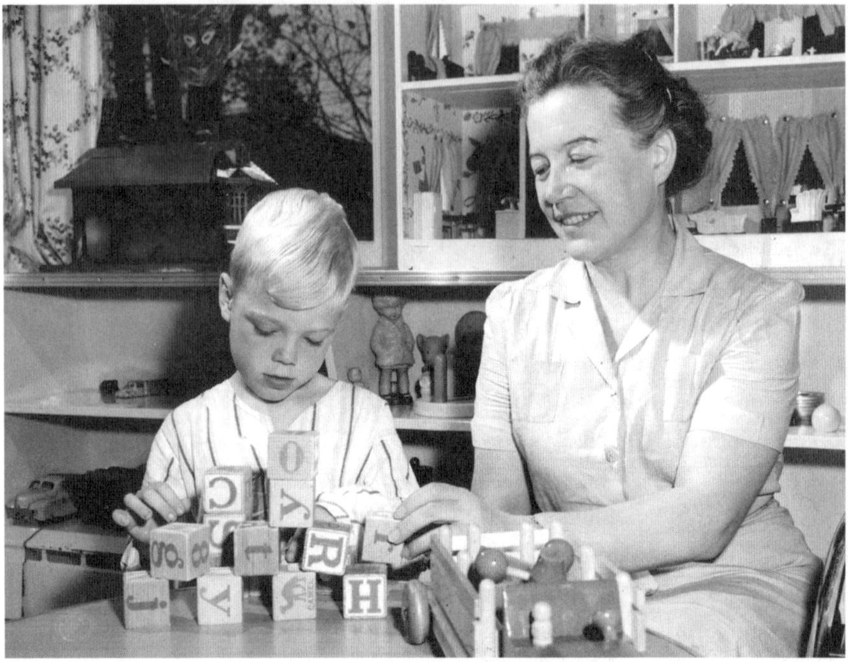

Gertrude Alana, Pediatric Playlady, and a young patient, 1950s.

of flowers to patient rooms and on occasion, when time permitted, changing water on flowers the patient already had in his or her room.

The Pink Lady program was theirs. The Pink Ladies were so named because they wore distinctive pink smocks whenever they were on duty in the hospital. They collected paperback books from their members and others and took these around to the nursing stations for patients to read as they felt up to it. They also took a cart filled with items from the Gift Shop which patients might wish to purchase. At Christmas time, they brought a cart of Christmas edible treats and beverages around to patient rooms, providing as much Christmas cheer as they could to people who had be hospitalized and away from family at the holiday season. They bought a special camera for the Newborn Nursery so that nurses could take a picture of each new born in its first days of life. They recruited seamstresses from their churches to make Pinky the Puppet. Pinky was a soft puppet given to each child on admission to pediatrics. In 1964, at the suggestion of Juta Mahaker, Playlady, Pinky was replaced with a red terrycloth Barney. The change to Barney came about because Barney was easier to make than Pinky and with the great demand for the puppet, this was a significant factor. In the early

1950s, new bassinets for the Newborn Nursery and two new incubators for the Premature Nursery were purchased by the Women's Board.

The auxiliary paid the salary of the Play Lady on Pediatrics and provided funds forneeded equipment and supplies in the playroom. The first Playlady was Gertrude Alania, hired in August 1951.

One auxiliary member, Mary Kerker, was married to a staff member at Tonka Toys. Through her efforts and those of her husband, a large shipment of Tonka toys was given to the playroom. It was the auxiliary that produced and financed the printing of a coloring book for pediatric patients which was not only a play activity, but a patient information tool as well. When the Teen-Adult Unit was added to Pediatrics in 1964, the auxiliary furnished the lounge for teen patients and their visitors.

They gave various pieces of hospital equipment to the hospital, often scheduling additional fundraisers to buy needed equipment. In 1954 they installed bedside radios for all patients. In 1958 they guided 5,000 visitors through the new hospital during the last three days prior to its opening. A portable respirator was given to the Anesthesia Department in 1966 and the next year they provided an EKG machine to the new Coronary Care Unit. Some of the members provided assistance as needed in the chaplaincy program. They took on the responsibility of providing fresh flowers in the hospital chapel.

They helped to fund research projects after the establishment of a research program at the hospital. Some examples of their donations to research were an award of $1,600 to Dr. Lawrence O. Pilgeram for arteriosclerosis research in 1957. Dr. Pilgeram's project continued to be a recipient of funds in other years following 1957. Also in 1957 they gave $7,500 to the St. Barnabas Research Foundation. In 1963, $1,500 went to Dr. Lyle Hay for the establishment of a Tumor Registry.

In 1957 the auxiliary redecorated a "catch-all" area at St. Andrew's and made it into an attractive lounge for women employees, a facility which had been lacking at St. Andrew's. In a similar project in 1966 at St. Barnabas, they furnished a Family Lounge and Waiting Area for the newly expanded Special Care Unit on third floor. In 1963 they prepared a booklet to be given to patients outlining the services available to them through the auxiliary and its volunteers. For several years, babies born during the Christmas holidays were sent home in large red or white Christmas stockings made by church seamstresses and donated by the auxiliary.

The relationship between the Women's Board, later the auxiliary, and the nursing school was always a close one. This is understandable considering women volunteers had carried on the nursing functions in the early days before the nursing school was established. After the opening of the school, they continued to have an interest in those who were providing the nursing care at the hospital. The Women's Board president, and later the auxiliary president, participated in every nursing school graduation for many years, pinning the distinctive silver pin on each new graduate. They also provided a corsage, usually of red roses, for each graduate. And they assumed full responsibility for the reception held following the Commencement Service. They provided a similar reception at the conclusion of each Capping Service, though they did not participate in those ceremonies.

Earlier on in this chapter, we indicated the key role the Women's Board played in the building of Wellesmere Residence. When Knickerbacker Residence was opened in 1943, they helped to furnish it and they were back at Knickerbacker a few years later to redecorate and furnish the lounge on the ground floor. The distinctive red sectional sofas which they purchased for Knicker were moved to the Whitney building when that became the home of the nursing school and all its students in 1960.

The Nurses Committee of the Women's Board had as its objective the provision of recreational activities for nursing students. In 1948 or 1949 they hired an instructor to give bridge lessons to all interested students. After that, a favorite leisure time activity for students was the almost perpetual bridge game played on the second floor of Knicker. One wag said that students coming off duty became so skilled at dealing cards that they could change clothes with one hand while dealing a hand of bridge with the other, even managing to light a cigarette before the first hand was played! An annual swim party and picnic was held for students at the Lake Minnetonka home of the Sweatts and later the home of the Newell Weeds. In 1954, they rented a cottage at Lake Minnetonka which was available all summer for groups of off duty students. For several years, they sponsored formal dances which were open to all hospital staff, but in fact the majority of those in attendance were nursing students and their escorts. At Christmas time, they sponsored a Christmas dinner for students and faculty. The Faculty assisted with program planning and in making little favors for all in attendance, but it was the auxiliary that paid for the event, considered by many to be the highlight of the Christmas season at St. Barnabas.

Each year, students held a Christmas party for children from Washington school. Members of the Student Government Association did the planning and were hostesses for the children, but again, the auxiliary picked up the tab for the party.

In 1953 the Episcopal women of the Minneapolis deanery formed an organization they called the "Friends of St. Barnabas." Their purpose was to provide an annual scholarship of $500 for a student in the nursing school. Members of Friends of St. Barnabas paid annual dues of $1.00 from which the scholarship was derived. For payment of $2.00 a member not only was contributing to the scholarship but would receive a subscription to the *Voice of St. Barnabas* as well. Though the Friends was a group separate from the Women's Board and later the Combined Auxiliary, their activity was coordinated through a chairman who was a member of the Women's Board.

When the Video Nursing Education program was begun in 1962, the TV sets in the classroom were donated by the auxiliary. Also in 1962, the auxiliary presented the nursing school with a check for $10,000 to be used to establish a revolving student loan fund. Prior to that time, the auxiliary had been furnishing a scholarship each year, but the loan fund made it possible to offer assistance to a greater number of students at one time during an era when costs for attending school had increased.

During the 1960s the auxiliary established the Volunteen or Candystriper program, so named because the teens participating in the program wore distinctive red and white striped pinafores while on duty. They recruited 100 high school students, all girls, to work the summer in this volunteer program. In order to qualify, the students had to be at least 14 years old at the beginning of the summer. If they were to work on a nursing station, they had to be 15 years old at the beginning of the summer. They were required to go through interviews and screening before being accepted into the program. Once accepted, they went through a training program, then were assigned to duties such as working in the Coffee Shop, making surgical dressings, assisting the Playlady in the pediatric play room and delivering mail and flowers to patients. When school started in the fall, many stayed on to work after school or on weekends or at holiday time. It not only provided needed service to the hospital, but gave students with possible interests in becoming nurses an opportunity to see life in the hospital setting up close. A similar program was started with the boys at Breck School (not yet a coed school at that time). The Breck boys worked on Saturdays assisting orderlies in Physical Therapy and X-ray. Later the same opportunity was opened to the boys from Blake School.

In 1962 the auxiliary instituted an awards program for recognition of volunteers. Previously, an annual recognition tea had been held for the volunteers, but with the new program they also received something tangible to keep in recognition for the hours of service given. Certificates were given to each volunteer who worked 100 hours or more over a three-year period. The next step up in recognition was the presentation of a gold charm in the shape of a bee. The charm was awarded for 300 hours of service or more over a three-year period. Those who gave 1,000 hours or more received ruby eyes in the gold bee. Though the motivation for service was generally not for the recognition, it was a nice bonus to provide to those who gave so much. Mary Witt reported that in 1964 volunteers gave a total of 19,570 hours of service, an increase of 100 hours over 1963. Put in other terms, it would have taken ten employees working almost full time to equal the amount of service donated to the hospital by volunteers.

The list given here of the projects of the auxiliary is not an exhaustive list. There are undoubtedly projects not mentioned, but the list does give an idea of the breadth of activities in which auxiliary members were involved in making life easier for patients and hospital staff and less costly for the hospital. It is easy to see why Mr. Bachmeyer viewed their contributions as significant to the operation of the hospital.

In order to pay for all these projects, members of the auxiliary were constantly on the lookout for fundraisers which they might sponsor. Again the list of fundraisers is almost as broad and varied as the activities funded by them. One of the events sponsored, in addition to the hospital Gift Shop and Coffee Shot, was Bridgerama–a marathon Bridge tournament for which participants paid an entrance fee, but received no prize save the satisfaction of winning since all proceeds went to the auxiliary. This was an annual fundraiser beginning in 1960. In 1962 they made $2,262 with just one bridgerama. The proceeds bought new equipment for the hospital.

There was also an annual gift fair in the hospital lobby. Usually this was held just before the Christmas season and many people, hospital staff, visitors and auxiliary members, used the opportunity to buy unusual Christmas gifts. They showed gift items which were for sale on the spot, or would be available after the fair in the Gift Shop. Year-round there were seasonal displays of Gift Shop items for sale.

In 1965 they sponsored the opening night of the Shipstad and Johnson Ice Follies. There were dinner dances and formal dances held as fundraisers. A fondue party was a fundraiser in 1970. In 1964, there was an artist who was a member of the auxiliary, Mrs. Deforest (Kip) Spencer Jr. She designed cards which were sold in the Gift Shop with proceeds going to the auxiliary. In 1965, she designed a Christmas card featuring a drawing of the Reverend Mr. Knickerbacker with marketbasket at his elbow, walking in front of the old Cottage Hospital. Another Christmas card design featured Garland House decked out for Christmas. She also designed notepapers which were sold that year. In October 1970 the Gift Shop had a garage sale, partly to clear out items that had been overstocked, but also an additional fundraiser for that year.

In the hospital before 1958, the gift and coffee shops were on the ground floor of the Pavilion building. In the new 1958 hospital they were just off the main lobby of the hospital on the north side of the building.

A member of the auxiliary from 1939 on through the 1940s and 1950s was Mrs. Amy Jaffray. Her experience as a buyer for J. B. Hudson made her a valuable asset to the Gift Shop. Because of her, the shop provided a variety of interesting and attractive gift items from jewelry to baby gifts, including some collectibles such as Danish Christmas plates, popular in Minneapolis in the 1940s and 1950s.

Florence Fritz was the manager of the Gift Shop from 1958 until her death in 1962. She guided the move from the old shop to the new and organized everything in the new building. The Gift Shop was staffed with volunteers from the auxiliary year round, augmented during the summer months and some after school hours by the Volunteens.

Mrs. William A. Williams was an early manager of the Coffee Shop who helped to establish the fine reputation the shop had for the quality of its food. Beginning in 1964, Sally Cook became the manager of the Coffee Shop. As with the Gift Shop, her staff consisted of Auxiliary members and Volunteens.

After 1970, when St. Barnabas and Swedish merged to become Metropolitan Medical Center (MMC) the auxiliaries of both hospitals continued to provide volunteer services working in a cooperative relationship, but as separate organizations. In May of 1978, the St. Barnabas Auxiliary changed its name, becoming the Metropolitan Medical Center Services Associates. The new name better described the service orientation of the group and it also facilitated the incorporation of male members who were interested in joining in the work of the organization. The Service Associates continued to operate side by side with the Swedish Auxiliary until December 19, 1983, when the two groups merged to become the Metropolitan Medical Center Service Guild, Inc. The guild operated one gift shop, The Bee Hive, and one coffee shop, The Kaffee Stugan. In May 1989 the name of the organization was changed again to reflect the merger of MMC with Mount Sinai Hospital. At that time it became the Metropolitan Mount Sinai Medical Center Service Guild, Inc. The Guild was dissolved on July 19, 1991, after the closure of the Medical Center. A long, varied and productive era had come to an end with the closure of the institution that had begun as the first hospital in Minneapolis.

Chapter 3

Beginning of a Modern Hospital Structure

With the completion of the Martin building and with scientific advances in medical and surgical arts, offering more services to aid in the diagnosis and treatment of patients became necessary. As the complexity of hospital care increased, the need for a well-trained, fulltime administrator for the hospital became apparent. Gone were the days when nursing care was provided almost entirely by well meaning volunteers from the local churches. Florence Nightingale in England had raised the clarion call for educational programs which would train nurses to effectively and safely care for the sick and injured. All over the United States nurse training programs patterned after the Nightingale model were being established. The Mayo brothers in a small town south of the Twin Cities were doing everything possible to elevate the standards of doctors. They recognized that on the job apprenticeships which had been used in years past to prepare the country's doctors were no longer adequate for the practice of medicine and surgery in the twentieth century.

The Reverend Dr. Knickerbacker had directed the operation of the Cottage Hospital as an extra-curricular activity of his ministry at Gethsemane Church. His replacement at the hospital was the man who replaced him at Gethsemane, the Reverend Mr. Cummings. He served for one year without pay, then resigned. It appears that the Reverend Dr. Knickerbacker also had served without pay from the hospital during the years he spent there. It wasn't too many years after the Reverend Mr. Cumming's service to the hospital that the board recognized the need for a fulltime director or administrator, though it would still be several years in the future before a director trained in hospital administration was available.

The problem of financing the hospital continued even after incorporation of the hospital. Late nineteenth century annual reports for the hospital indicated the final cost of the Martin building was $38,155.48. As of June 30, 1897. $16,000.00 came from the bequest of Richard Martin. Tied to that bequest was a provision that the hospital would get the balance of Mr. Martin's estate if the board raised half of the cost of the building from subscriptions of donors. Half of the mortgage was raised and with the remainder of the Martin bequest the mortgage was paid off.

To establish a charity fund, which had been from the beginning the dream of the Reverend Dr. Kickerbacker, the board used $100,000 from the sale of the Keegan lake farm that had been a part of the Martin bequest.

By the turn of the twentieth century, the hospital was already outgrowing even the commodius Martin building. Accordingly, plans were developed for construction of a three-story corridor building to be attached to the south side of the Martin building. Authorization to build that structure came from the board in July 1902. To finance the project, the board turned to the Women's Auxiliary which loaned the hospital $3,500 it had been saving to build a residence for nurses. The home for nurses was put on hold in favor of adding this much needed wing to the hospital. Actual cost of the Corridor building was $5,064.26.

Some records from the early part of the twentieth century appear to have been lost. For example there is no record of the administrative team from 1890-1907. As stated previously, the Reverend Mr. Cummings, Rector of Gethsemane Church, replaced the Reverend Dr. Knickerbacker when he left in 1883, but Mr. Cummings served only one year. A Mrs. Alice Pew was named Matron and Acting Superintendent in 1884. She served in this dual role until 1890. She was replaced as matron by a Mrs. A. K. Howey, who died only a year later. Board minutes indicate Mrs. Howey was succeeded on the day of her death in October 1891 by a Miss Lois Eastman. Like Mrs. Howey, Miss Eastman was called matron and there is no reference to a dual position for either of these people. The decade of the 1890s must have been a period of turmoil at the hospital, with frequent turnover in the position of matron. If there was no hospital director during those years, that might explain the frequent turnover of matrons who may have found it difficult riding a ship without a captain in charge. It is known there was an attempt to open a nursing school in the late 1880s or in 1890, but that failed.

Harriet S. Hartry was appointed Superintendent of Nurses on December 2, 1899, and on August 15, 1907, was promoted to Superintendent of the hospital. Miss Hartry was a trained nurse, a graduate of Brooklyn Hospital School of Nursing in New York. But the identity of the person in administrative charge of the hospital from 1890 to 1893 (when the hospital was closed for demolition and construction of the Martin building) and 1894-1907 is unknown. It appears that members of the board may have had more "hands-on" responsibilities for the day to day administration of the hospital than would be true in later years.

In 1931, Miss Hartry included a lengthy summary of the history of the hospital in her annual report for the year. She stated in that summary there were five matrons, beginning in 1884 with Mrs. Pew and ending with Miss Hartry's appointment as Superintendent of Nurses in 1899. The five she listed were: Mrs. Alice Pew, Mrs. Howey, who died in service, Miss L. V. Jones, Miss J. A. Purdy and Miss L. M. Staples. She does not include tenure dates for any of these, but since we know that Mrs. Howey died in 1891 and that the hospital was closed for more than a year in 1893 and 1894, it appears each of these ladies could have served only a year or two. Miss Hartry makes no mention of Miss Lois Eastman, who took Mrs. Howey's place (according to Minnesota Board of Nursing records.)

In an article they wrote for the *Bulletin Of The Hennepin County Medical Society*, April and May 1959, Robert Bachmeyer and Frederick Gibbs reviewed the early history of the nursing department at St. Barnabas. Their description of the sequence of directors indicates a Miss L. B. Jones was appointed matron in 1895 and that she organized the School of Nursing and served as its first head. The discrepancy in Miss Jones' middle initial (was it V. or was it B.) is minor, though it does indicate confusion in the records. That same article referred to five students in the first class, enrolled 1894, while further on they refer to fifteen students who applied for admission and seven who were accepted. The source records used by Bachmeyer and Gibbs are not indicated.

To confuse the issue even further, records at the Minnesota Board of Nursing state the first Superintendent of the nursing school was a Miss Eleanor Weston, who was a graduate of Indianapolis Hospital School of Nursing. There is no mention of Miss Weston in hospital board minutes or in annual reports. Since Board of Nursing records indicate she came to Minneapolis from Indianapolis, where the Reverend Dr. Knickerbacker was living and serving as Bishop of Indiana, one is led to wonder whether or not she knew the bishop and whether she may have been steered by him to Minneapolis. Perhaps we will never know exactly who did what during that tumultuous decade of the 1890s. After Miss Hartry arrived, Board of Nursing records indicate an unbroken line of nursing superintendents or directors on up to the time the school closed.

Mr. Black, president of the hospital board, comments in the 1903 Annual Report on many improvements being made with the building of the Corridor building. He makes reference to reports being submitted by various departments in the hospital such as nursing, housekeeping and dietary, so we know the organization of hospital administration was proceeding on modern lines. The report also includes a lengthy account of the planning and building of the Corridor building. Benefits to be derived from the new building included more private patient rooms, increased space for operating rooms, laundry and the kitchen as well as increased storage space. For the first time, mention is made of the establishment of a maternity ward. Apparently they changed plans regarding the first floor, substituting a maternity department there for some of the extra private rooms they originally wanted. He includes a lengthy account of the financial state of the institution indicating that financing the operation of the hospital was a continuing problem, though he was hopeful with the addition of the new building to attract more patients in the coming year. Overbuilding of hospital space was a problem in the city then as it would be again in the middle of the twentieth century.

The demand for more hospital facilities was increasing because members of the public were beginning to feel differently about being admitted to a hospital than they had in the past. The change in public attitude regarding admission to a hospital is highlighted in this quote from the President's address to the Sixth Triennial Congress of American Physicians and Surgeons, held in Washington DC on May 12, 1903:

> The old repugnance to entering a hospital when sick or when an operation is demanded is rapidly fading away. The immense advantages of a good hospital over the most luxurious home are now acknowledged on all hands. The poorest patient in a hospital is better cared for, his case more carefully investigated by bacteriological, chemical and clinical methods in a hospital than are the well to do in their own homes. Indeed, wise surgeons, in cases of emergency, now very properly refuse to do operations in homes instead of in hospitals. In many instances, lives that would be lost in homes are saved in hospitals, where the many and complex modern appliances for every surgical emergency are provided.

An X-ray machine for the hospital was on the horizon when Mr. Black wrote his report, though he makes no mention of the purchase. The machine was installed December 5, 1903, and so began the nucleus of a radiology department. It is obvious, also, from Mr. Black's report that a clinical laboratory was not far in the future. He extols the advantages of having a clinical laboratory on site in the hospital and makes reference to a committee which was looking into the matter. He said the board had already agreed to give up a room in the hospital for a laboratory.

After expressing great faith in the future growth of the hospital, he includes a recommendation at the end of his report which must have elicited considerable comment from the members of the board. He questions the wisdom of building any more buildings at the current location of the hospital on South Sixth Street. He cites the noise factor in that railroad yards and factories have been built in the area. And the streetcar which ran on Sixth Street also created a great deal of noise. He suggests the board look at new sites farther out into the country where noise is not a factor. While his concern about noise being a hindrance to recovery from illness might have had some validity, the fact that the board had a large building, well equipped and only ten years old, on site must have caused many board members to question moving and starting completely over in a new location, which could well become as noisy as the Sixth Street location as the growing city expanded. In any case, the more desirable sites further out in the country were being gobbled up at a great rate by other hospitals so nothing ever came of the recommendation to move the hospital.

Instead, beginning in December 1905, the board began to buy up all the lots in the block between Sixth and Seventh Streets and Ninth and Tenth Avenues. Did this mean the board rejected the premise of Mr. Black's report that the noise factor on Sixth Street was beginning to make that site undesirable for hospital usage, or was it apparent that the kind of distant site which Mr. Black envisioned was not going to be available and economically feasible. By this time, Swedish, Asbury, Northwestern, Abbott, Lutheran Deaconess, Fairview and St. Mary's had all opened their doors in neighborhoods south and east of St. Barnabas.

To demonstrate how much the services of the hospital increased from its beginning in 1871 when daily census averaged five to eight patients, no diagnostic services were available, nor were there surgical and maternity services, we add the following data from Miss Hartry's 1931 annual report. Similar data, published years after the new hospital was built in 1958, are included in the chapter on that era.

Number of patients admitted	3,224
Total number of patients cared for	2,399
Average number of patients per day	93
Number of X-rays	733
Number of pathological specimens	4,444
Basal Metabolisms	53
Cystoscopic examinations	23
Physiotherapy	92
Operations performed	1,610
Births	401
Deaths	132
Stillborns	1

Number of hospital days—wards	19,549
Number of hospital days—private rooms	11,420
Combined hospital days	30,969
Autopsies	23
Patients discharged	3,244
Death rate	0.04
Medical	584
Surgical	1,169
Orthopedic	53
Specialties	301
Obstetrical	412
Newborns	382
Children	343

Miss Hartry also wrote at the end of her 1931 annual report, "In common with other hospitals save those where patients may be cared for free of charge, the beds during the year were only a little more than fifty per cent filled."

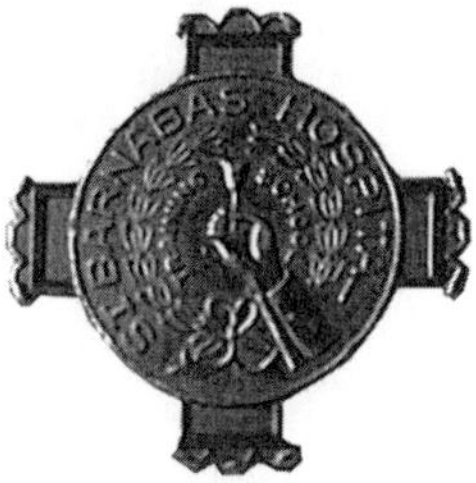

Chapter 4

Another St. Barnabas First: A Home for Nurses

Only four years after construction of the Corridor building, a new residence for nurses was built on the corner of Ninth Avenue South and Seventh Street. It stood several feet west and south of the Corridor building. The Women's Auxiliary had planned, beginning around the turn of the twentieth century, to build a nurses' residence for the hospital. They had accumulated nearly the sum required to finance the construction when funds were needed to finish the Corridor building in 1902. The women deferred their residence project and made a three-year loan of $5,000 to the Board of Trustees for construction of the Corridor building. By 1906, that money had been repaid, along with interest, and the building of the residence could go forward. The cornerstone for the new home was laid on June 11, 1906.

The motivating factor behind the residence project was the urging of Miss Catherine Welles that it be done. Both Miss

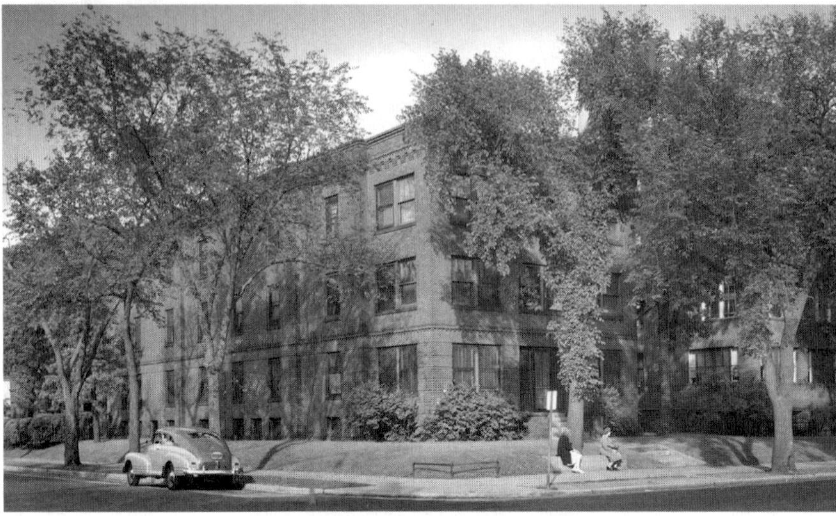

Wellesmere residence, late 1940s.

Welles and her mother were longtime members of the auxiliary and tireless workers for the hospital. Rewarding their efforts, the Women's Auxiliary named the new residence, "Wellesmere." The Welles part of the name was obvious; *mere* was the Welsh word for "home." Wellesmere was the first residence of its kind, built for the housing of nurses, to be constructed in Minneapolis. It was built to house both graduate and student nurses. Its capacity is unknown, but may have been as many as seventy women housed in 35 double rooms. A 1935 report at the Board of Nursing described it as "gloomy" and the board called for improvements. A year later, in 1936, the board record notes improvements had been made, but still rated it "inadequate."

Wellesmere continued to serve as a residence for all students until 1943. At that time, the school made its contribution to the war effort by participating in the Cadet Nurse Program and the size of classes admitted to the school was increased dramatically, so Wellesmere was no longer large enough to even nearly accommodate all students. Not long before that time, Asbury Hospital, which stood on the northwest corner of Ninth Avenue South and Sixth Street, had outgrown its facility and had been moved to another building a few blocks away, facing the south edge of Elliot Park. The old Asbury building was purchased by St. Barnabas and the Women's Auxiliary financed the remodeling and redecoration necessary to turn a hospital into a dormitory. It was named Knickerbacker Residence in honor of the good Bishop and founder of St. Barnabas.

The earliest reference to a housemother at Wellesmere was in 1942. Records indicate that Mrs. Gertrude Noyes was the housemother at that point. She may have been the first in that position. When there were substantial numbers of graduates living at Wellesmere, one of them may have been given charge of the building in case of emergency. Students worked much longer hours in the days preceding World War II than later in the 1950s and beyond, and their classes were scheduled at 4:00 P.M. and 7:15 P.M., leaving them very little of what latter day students knew as leisure time. So perhaps the need for someone like a housemother was not evident until 1942. When Knickerbacker opened its doors in 1943, Mrs. Noyes moved over there and Mrs. Grace Wittig was hired as housemother at Wellesmere. Mrs. Wittig retired in 1953, being replaced from 1953-1955 by Mrs. Helen Jahrow, who was in turn replaced in 1955 by Mrs. Daisy Lau. At Knickerbacker, when Mrs. Noyes retired in 1948, a St. Barnabas graduate, Mrs. Helen Cribbe Dick (class of 1917) was hired to be a combination student health director and housemother at Knicker. This combination did not work out as well as planned, so in 1952, Mrs. Dick vacated the housemother position and moved to a room set aside on 4 Martin as a Health Service for both employees and students. Mrs. Ruth Gallup was hired for Knickerbacker. When Whitney Residence was opened in 1959, both Mrs. Lau and Mrs. Gallup moved there, each with the new title of house director. Mrs. Gallup left in 1962 and thereafter there was just one house director who was assisted by residence receptionists, who were on duty twenty-four hours a day. When Mrs. Lau retired in 1965, she was replaced by Mrs. Helen Bachman.

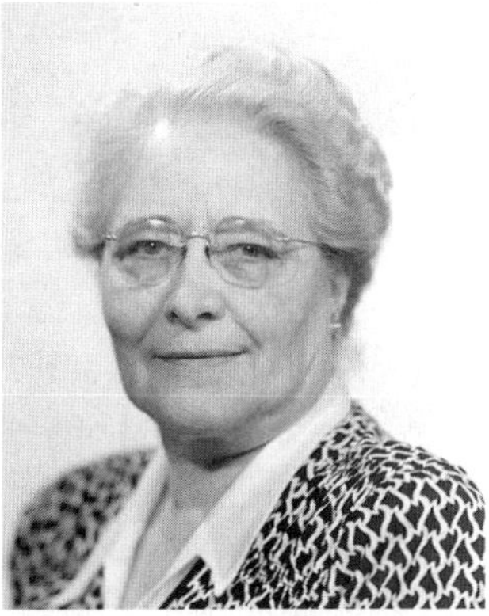
Gertrude Noyes, housemother at Wellesmere, then the first housemother at Knicker.

"Knicker," as Knickerbacker Residence was known to students, housed second and third year students, leaving Wellesmere for first year students and a handful of RNs and women house staff doctors who lived there. This arrangement continued for 17 years until the opening of Whitney Residence

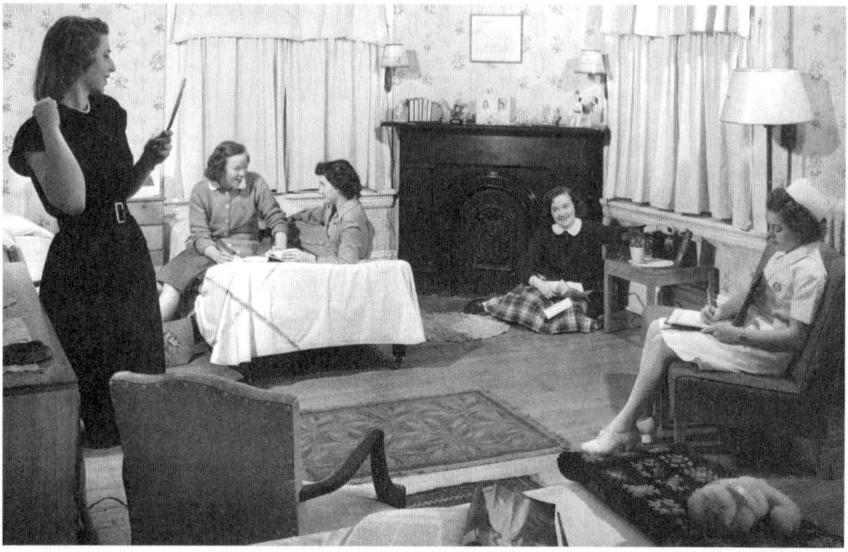

Student room at Knickerbacker, 1947.

on November 29, 1959. At Whitney, students were again housed all in one building.

The number of RNs and women interns housed at Wellesmere varied from time to time. In later years, the number of students admitted to the school determined the number of graduates who could be accommodated at Wellesmere. Students had priority in assignment of rooms in those years. In earlier years, it appears that graduates may have had priority. Minnesota Board of Nursing records indicate that in 1923 the school had fifty four students housed in one residence and twelve in another, possibly the large private home which sat in those days where the horseshoe drive in front of the Whitney building would be only fourteen years later.

All of the rooms at Wellesmere were double rooms except four private rooms that faced Seventh Street. Usually these four private rooms were occupied by RNs or women house staff. Depending on space available, some RNs might also have been assigned to double rooms, but usually they were given rooms at the front of the building so that all students were together and all staff members were also together.

Dr. Elizabeth Brumbaugh lived in one of the private rooms while she was serving her residency on Pediatrics, before her marriage to Dr. Bourne Jerome. A St. Barnabas graduate and University of Minnesota student in the late 1940s was Katherine Ness, who lived for some time at Wellesmere. She was a great friend to students then as well as later when she joined the faculty, first as a med-surg instructor and in the early 1950s as associate director of the school. By that time, she had vacated her room at Wellesmere.

There were two other RNs who lived at Wellesmere for several years. Both were long term employees at the hospital and were well known and well liked by students, Dorothy Eddy and Hazelle Lundell. Dorothy Eddy, a graduate of Kahler School of Nursing in Rochester, came to St. Barnabas in 1946. She worked on Maternity, primarily in the Newborn Nursery and later was head nurse in the Premie Nursery. She lived at Wellesmere until the early 1950s when she moved to an apartment at 1005 Portland Avenue South. The Portland Avenue apartment was her home until she died of cancer on July 21, 1963.

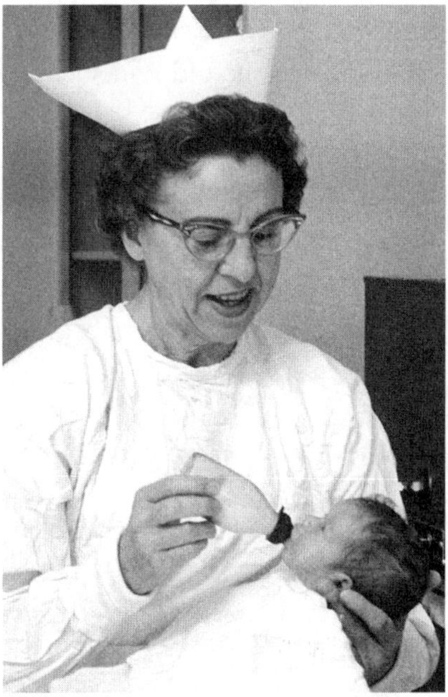

Dorothy Eddy in Premie Nursery

Hazelle Lundell, a graduate of St. John's Hospital School of Nursing in Red Wing, came to St. Barnabas, also in 1946. Though she was a graduate of St. John's she spent almost her entire professional career at St. Barnabas. She worked for several years as a staff nurse on 2 Pavilion, a medical service devoted to the care of patients who were treated with medication only, rather than surgery. After several years on 2 Pav, Hazelle moved to a faculty position, teaching Fundamentals of Nursing. She possessed particular skill in relating to young, possibly frightened, small town students (as she had been) new in the big city and new to health care. She was much beloved by students who showed their devotion to her in numerous ways. One example of their high regard for her was the dedication of the 1964 school yearbook, the *Sabarho*, to her. She was the first person ever to receive this honor. The description of her used in the yearbook said: "A friendly smile and generous attitude characterize the instructor to whom the *Sabarho* of 1964 is dedicated. In our freshman year, she introduced us to the fundamentals of nursing and aided in our adjustment to life in the dorm. Through our remaining years at St. B. we know there is a friend in Room 107 who will listen to any problem and suggest a solution. It is with sincere gratitude and affection that we, the students of St. Barnabas, dedicate our yearbook to you, Miss Hazelle Lundell."

Hazelle remained on the school faculty until the school closed its doors in 1973. Her father died in the late 1950s and Hazelle moved from her room at Wellesmere to an apartment in south Minneapolis where she made a home for her mother. The two had an exceptionally close relationship. Mrs. Lundell was a salt of the earth lady who didn't hesitate expressing her opinions, but she did it in such a pleasant way that it didn't interfere with her congenial relationship with her daughter.

On March 17, 1974, Hazelle married the Reverend Philip Featherstone. At the time of their marriage, Philip was serving a small Lutheran church in Colfax, Wisconsin. Later the couple moved to Pukwana, South Dakota, where Philip had two small churches as his pastorate. He also quickly became involved in community activities in Pukwana and was a popular figure

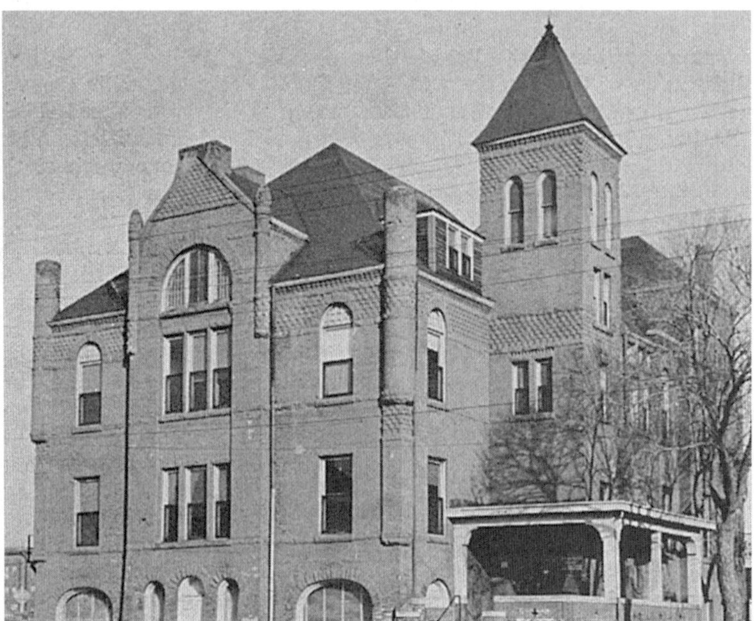

Knickerbacker residence, late 1940s.

in this little town. Philip retired from the ministry at Pukwana and the couple stayed on there in the comfortable little arts and crafts bungalow which they had purchased. When Hazelle and Philip were in their late seventies, they moved to Osceola, Wisconsin, in order to be nearer to their children and grandchildren. Philip had been married originally to Hazelle's sister, Delores, who died of cancer in 1972 or 1973. His son and four daughters were not only Hazelle's stepchildren, but were also her nephew and nieces, with whom she had shared a doting relationship from the day each was born.

Discussions in the faculty break room at St. Barnabas often included the latest on the activities of Sid, Linda, Martha, Patrice or Miriam. As of this writing, both Hazelle and Philip were living still in Osceola. Through the years, Hazelle, health permitting, and her compatriot from student days at St. John's, Norma Seebach, were regular attendees at annual banquets of the St. Barnabas Nurses Alumnae. Norma, like Hazelle, spent most of her professional career at St. Barnabas, though she was a graduate of St. John's. She worked originally as a staff nurse, later a head nurse on 4 Martin, a surgical unit. When the new hospital was built in 1958, she moved with the rest of the staff from 4 Martin to 5B in the new building and remained with St. Barnabas until she retired.

Knickerbacker was torn down in 1960 and for a time the land was used for parking for hospital staff. Later it was sold when the Hubert Humphrey domed stadium was built in the area. Wellesmere became a residence for interns and other house staff members. They had been housed at St. Andrew's Hospital in southeast Minneapolis, but that location was inconvenient, especially for the foreign doctors assigned as interns and residents at St. Barnabas. Wellesmere served as the home for these young doctors for a few years, but then it, too, fell to the wrecking ball in the 1960s. And so ended one era at St. Barnabas as a new era began.

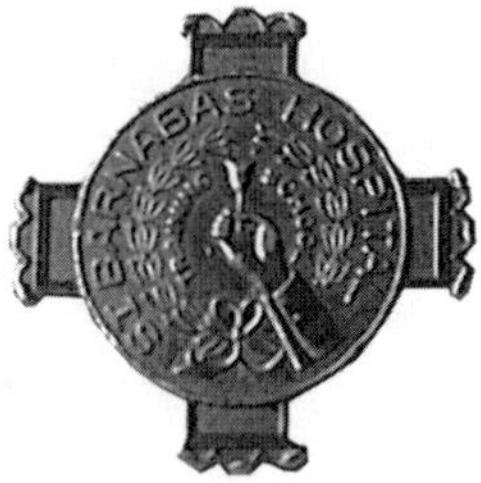

Chapter 5

Keeping Competitive in Hospital Circles, Circa 1910

The opening of the Corridor building met the space needs of the Hospital for only a few years. Being hospitalized for care when ill or injured had become the accepted thing to do and whereas at an earlier time all babies were born at home, by the end of the nineteenth century, doctors were recommending a hospital delivery for safer childbirth. They cited advantages for both infant and mother.

Early in the twentieth century competition entered the hospital scene in Minneapolis. The Cottage Hospital in 1871 was without competition, but only a few years later pressure was building for construction of hospitals all over town to meet the needs of several different constituencies in the city. Even the city fathers, so reluctant to become involved in establishing a hospital in 1871, opened Minneapolis General Hospital in 1887 on Sixth Street, only two blocks west of St. Barnabas. The Methodists built Asbury Hospital, a small hospital across Sixth

Street from St. Barnabas at the northwest corner of Ninth Avenue South and Sixth Street. In 1898 a new hospital was opened on Eighth Street between Ninth and Tenth Avenues South. It was built to meet the needs of Swedish immigrants who were pouring into the city of Minneapolis. A few decades into the twentieth century one of the most popular national magazines of the day would say there were more Swedes in Minneapolis than anywhere else in the world except Stockholm. And immigrants from the other Scandinavian countries had their own hospitals too, Fairview and Lutheran Deaconness, in south Minneapolis. In 1912, the German Lutherans opened their own hospital, St. Andrews, in Southeast Minneapolis. And over on the banks of the Mississippi, next to Fairview, the Roman Catholics built St. Mary's. Even with the burgeoning population at the time, it was inevitable that patient census would eventually suffer for all with this explosion in hospital construction. But that day was still in the future and in the early part of the twentieth century the word was "build"—build a hospital larger and better equipped than any other in town.

The Reverend Dr. Knickerbacker's dream that St. Barnabas would become a hospital resource for the University of Minnesota faded when the university opened its own hospital. Like Minneapolis General, the university hospital would serve some of the indigent people of the state and the city as well as patients who had complicated maladies that required the services of specialists who were on the faculty of the University Medical School.

In order to compete, or even to survive, St. Barnabas had to improve and expand its facilities. By December 1, 1908, the mortgage debt on the hospital had been paid off. On December 5, 1908, a new building was proposed to the board that then authorized purchase of more lots on the north side of Seventh Street, adjacent to Wellesmere Residence, then only two years old itself. The board secured a loan of $60,000 from the Minnesota Loan and Trust Company and construction of the Pavilion building was authorized.

The first contract for construction was let on May 14, 1910, for $45,864, but this turned out to be an insufficient amount to complete the project. So on June 11, 1910, the mortgage was increased to $65,000, allowing the construction to proceed at a rapid pace. The building was finished on February 11, 1911, and the first patient admitted entered the next day, February 12, 1911. Completion of the Pavilion building brought the bed capacity of the hospital to 172. To furnish the new building, the board turned again to the Women's Auxiliary which, along with 13 individual contributors, gave $4,788.20.

On March 7, 1909, the medical staff had contributed $3,750 "for hospital improvements."

Aesthetically, the Pavilion building was uninspiring. Basically, it was a five story rectangular box, one end of which was attached to the existing Corridor building. The Martin building had style, but adding this large rectangle, which projected like the upright portion of a T from the Martin building (which was the crosspiece of the T), made for an ungainly looking structure. The Corridor-Pavilion part of the T extended for the full block between Sixth and Seventh Streets. Those of us living today who remember the old St. Barnabas remember it with the Whitney building in place and that handsome building off to the east side of the Pavilion changed the appearance of the whole structure. But for the twenty-six years between the building of the Pavilion and Whitney buildings, it must have been an ugly sight to behold. In June of 1916, Mr. Edwin C. Whitney of Ottawa, Canada, visited Minneapolis and contacted the hospital regarding a possible future bequest he was considering for the hospital. He was taken to see the hospital complex then in existence. His comment was, "Your buildings do not impress me as having anything very attractive about their exteriors. I would not care to put up a building as ordinary looking as your new wing."

In March of 1911, the appearance was slightly improved with the addition to the grounds of a fountain, given by Clinton Morrison. It had stood originally at the mansion of his father, Dorilus Morrison, first mayor of Minneapolis. It was installed in the yard west of the Corridor building and north of Wellesmere. On the interior, the Pavilion building was set up with a majority of two- and four-bed ward rooms. The nurses' station sat at one end of the hall with patient rooms along both sides of the hall for the length of the building. A small diet kitchen, a medicine room, a service room, a conference room, a linen room and the elevator were all in the area of the nurses' station. This did consolidate noisy areas away from patient rooms. But the long hall made it difficult for the nursing staff to keep tabs on the patients in rooms near the sunporches which looked out on Seventh Street. There were many steps taken by staff many times a day to deliver diet trays, linens, medications, and needed supplies, and in performing

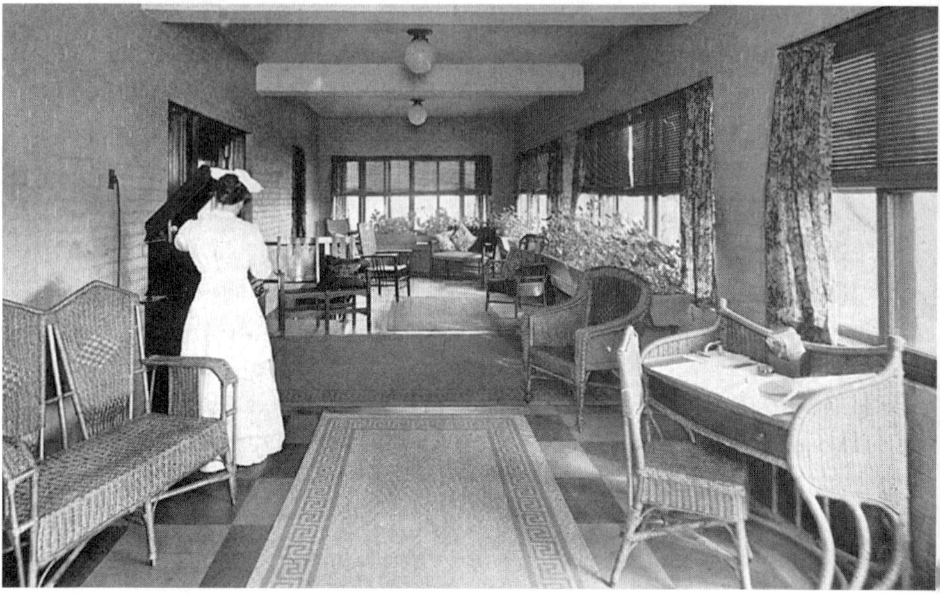

Sunporch, Pavilion building, 1925-1930.

general patient care. At a later time, nurses would become more involved in the planning of hospitals to utilize space in different ways, minimizing the miles nursing feet had to travel daily on the job and maximizing the ability of the staff to maintain close observation of patients, but in 1910 such a thing was unheard of. Architects were almost always men, as were construction crews, and they consulted with men on the board. Women in architecture and construction were rarities for the day. And, of course, the Board of Trustees included no women then. Interestingly, the superintendent of the hospital at the time was a woman, Harriett Hartry, but if she had any concerns about the length of the halls and the long distance between the nurses' station and rooms at the end of the hall, they were not reflected in the design of the building.

The second, fourth and fifth floors of the Pavilion building were laid out basically the same. Fifth floor was primarily for surgical patients, fourth for maternity and second was for medical patients. The original use of third floor isn't known, but later a pediatric unit was placed on third floor and it did vary in physical layout from the other floors, utilizing more glass walls and patient cubicles to facilitate observation of the sick children. And the nurses' station on pediatrics was centered among the patient rooms and cubicles, also facilitating continuous observation of the children. There was a playroom on pediatrics, a facility not necessary on the adult floors. Whether the playroom was part of the original design or a later addition is unknown.

The first floor of the building housed the kitchen and employee dining room as well as some office and maintenance areas. There was an entrance from that level which opened into a tunnel leading to the basement level of Wellesmere—a convenience as well as a safety measure for student nurses who could go directly to the hospital without going outdoors during late night or early morning hours.

In her 1931 annual report, Miss Hartry, the hospital superintendent, referred to a particular use of the hospital following World War I. She said: "St. Barnabas has twice cared for men returned from active service in the Army and Navy. After the great war and before Asbury was leased by the Government, 458 ex-service men were cared for in the wards and rooms of the hospital and the Annex fitted up for study, recreation and occupational therapy under the supervision of the Red Cross and other agencies."

Apparently the old Asbury Hospital on Sixth Street served for a time as a service and veterans' hospital. The Annex to which she makes reference is unknown. Perhaps at that time St. Barnabas had some little-utilized areas in buildings of the hospital which were known as "the Annex."

Farther on in her report, Miss Hartry refers to charity care that had been provided by the hospital. Remember, the hospital charter still specified that care should be made available to patients unable to pay. In that 1931 annual report Miss Hartry said: "During the past twenty-five years, more than $78,000 in excess of that received from the endowment fund has been spent in care of free patients."

It appears that even with Minneapolis General down the street from them, St. Barnabas was still making a contribution to the need which Bishop Knickerbacker had identified so many years before. Miss Hartry goes on to say, "Since March, 1871, 105,803 patients have been admitted. We know of at least one patient cared for so long ago in the little Cottage Hospital who 'returned to give thanks.'"

She was referring, of course, to Mrs. Whitney, whose husband had shown such great interest in donating money for construction of a new hospital. Mr. Whitney passed away in 1924 and in his will, left a substantial bequest to the hospital.

In spite of being an aesthetic failure, at least the Pavilion building was sturdily built. Many years later, after the 1958 hospital building was opened and patients were moved out of Martin, Corridor, Pavilion and Whitney rooms, the interior of the Pavilion was remodeled, as was the interior of the Whitney building. Together, the two buildings became the Whitney Residence, housing all three classes of nursing students as well as the school library, school and faculty offices and house director apartments. A new classroom wing was added on the east side where earlier there had been part of a parking lot for the hospital.

When the school was closed in 1973, the Whitney Residence facilities were leased to South Dakota State University to house their nursing program which had contracted for use of the clinical facilities of Metropolitan Medical Center. Later the Whitney Residence was utilized by St. Olaf College Department of Nursing which also had contract agreements for the use of Metropolitan Medical Center clinical facilities. Gustavus Adolphus College and the University of Minnesota also contracted for use of clinical facilities at Metropolitan Medical Center for their nursing programs. All three of these were baccalaureate programs, so the position taken at mid-century by the American Nurses Association that education of all professional nurses take place in institutions of higher education rather than the single purpose hospital school of the nineteenth and early twentieth centuries, was accomplished at St. Barnabas and its successor, Metropolitan Medical Center.

Chapter 6

Administering to Spiritual Needs

During his tenure at the Cottage Hospital, the Reverend Knickerbacker probably served not only as administrator, but also as chaplain in the hospital. The bed capacity of the hospital was very small then. Daily census varied from five to ten patients in the days before the move to the Sixth Street location. The record does not indicate how many beds the Garland House added to the hospital, but likely it didn't exceed a half dozen more in addition to those it replaced from the old building. The brick building put up next to Garland House added sixteen beds and the Welles Pavilion built to house surgical patients, added only six. It is probable that during the Reverend Knickerbacker's tenure, the maximum capacity of the hospital wasn't over forty, a number which he could easily have served himself with the help of his Gethsemane Brotherhood and of clergy from other churches in the area. It would have been advantageous to have clergy who could communicate with the non-English speaking patients in their own languages, understanding their cultural and religious traditions. As each new wave of immigration occurred, undoubtedly there were clergy among those arriving in the city and these men would shepherd little flocks of the newcomers into new churches established to serve their specific needs. With the Reverend Dr. Knickerbacker's talent for recruiting people to help with his hospital project, it is reasonable to assume he would have known these new pastors and would have had no hesitancy in asking them to help with patient visitation at the hospital.

The man who replaced the Reverend Dr. Knickerbacker at the hospital was also his replacement at Gethsemane, the Reverend Mr. Cummings. Since he served only one year with the hospital, it is likely he continued to follow the pattern, whatever that was, set by the Reverend. Dr. Knickerbacker.

It was during the tenure of Mrs. Alice Pew, 1884-1890, that a chaplain was added to the paid staff of the hospital. Mrs. Pew was employed originally to be the matron of the hospital, in charge of nursing, but soon she became acting superintendent as well after the departure of the Reverend Mr. Cummings. It would appear she had her hands full with these two jobs and since she was not a clergy person, she probably was the first to see the need of adding a chaplain to the staff. That first chaplain was a Reverend Mr. A. Alexander, who joined the hospital staff in 1886. Not much is known about him except that he was the first chaplain and we can assume the job organization that he developed was followed by those who succeeded him. We know that between 1886 and the appointment of the Reverend Mr. H. L. Russell in 1916, three other men in addition to the Reverend Mr. Alexander, served as chaplain. They were the Reverend Dr. Frederick Webb, the Reverend Mr. Irving P. Johnson and the Reverend Mr. C. E. Haupt. We know little about any of them except the Reverend Dr. Webb served a stint on the Board of Trustees so he must have been from one of the Minneapolis parishes. We also do not know tenure dates for these men. We just know that collectively, these four served a total of thirty years as chaplains for the hospital.

The Reverend Mr. H. L. Russell was appointed chaplain in 1916 and served for fifteen years until 1931, the longest tenure we can verify of any of the chaplains employed up to that time. We do not know with certainty how many men served as chaplain between the departure of the Reverend Mr.

Russell in 1931 and the employment of the Reverend Dr. Frederick D. Tyner in 1948. We know that a Reverend Mr. Joseph T. Walker apparently was the chaplain during the 1930s for he is listed as the chaplain on the program for the dedication of the Whitney building, April 17, 1937. It is possible he served the entire 17-year period between 1931 and 1948 since precedent had been set for that length of service by the Reverend Mr. Russell.

In 1948, the Reverend Dr. F. D. Tyner was appointed chaplain. Many St. Barnabas nurses living today will recognize his name. Those of us in the older generation remember him well because he taught an ethics course to all entering freshman students. One of the assignments for the course was to write an essay expressing what becoming a nurse meant to the student-author. Dr. Tyner read and evaluated each essay himself, then awarded a silver candle holder to the winning author at her Capping Service. Even graduates who came later and did not know Dr. Tyner personally would recognize his name, for on Easter Sunday, 1945, he penned the words of the St. Barnabas hymn, which was used for every capping and graduation ceremony after that time. At least one graduate, Shirley Land Fasth ('51) requested that this hymn be sung at her funeral service. The author of this book has left instructions that it also be sung at her Memorial Service when that day comes. In the program for each capping and graduation ceremony was this notation regarding the St. Barnabas hymn: "Written by the chaplain for all workers in St. Barnabas when he was a patient in the hospital and realized how every member of the hospital staff does everything possible to help a patient back to health and strength."

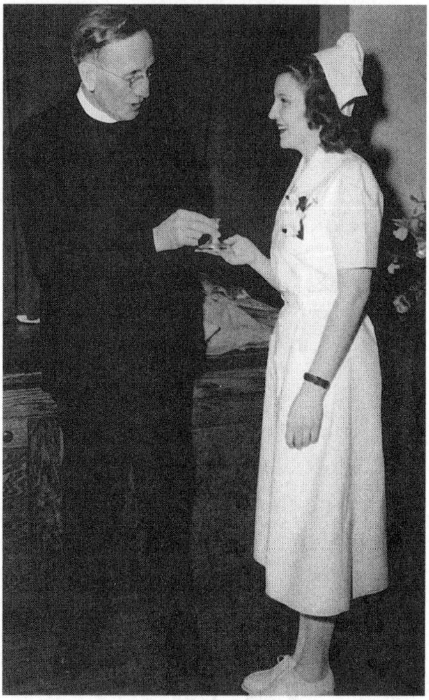
Dr. Frederick Tyner presenting silver candle holder award for the best essay on "Why I Want to Be a Nurse," Capping Ceremony 1948.

So the words were meant to apply to all hospital staff members, though it was the nursing school that perpetuated the hymn by using it in its official ceremonies twice each year. The words of the hymn are as follows:

Go heal the sick and suffering, it is our Lord's command
Be patient, firm but gentle, in look and word and hand.
The sick revert to childhood no matter what their age,
The rich, the poor, the cultured, the foolish and the sage.

When tempted to be angry, your patience sorely tried,
Let nothing blight your vision, He's always at your side,
To guide, direct and strengthen throughout the night and day,
He never fails the faithful who with Him watch and pray.

Oftimes you will grow weary, your task will lose its glow,
His strength will give you courage, His life through you will flow;
In times of tribulation, in times of doubt and fear,
In times when you are downcast be strong, for He is near.

Rejoice, then, in His power, be thankful for His grace,
We all are His co-workers and have our special place;
Think not of self or comfort, life's struggles never cease.
He fought the fight that we fight, in Him we all find peace."

The hymn was sung to the tune of "Go Forward, Christian Soldiers," #553 in the Episcopal hymnal of the time. Presbyterians use the same tune for "Lead On, O King Eternal."

The Reverend Dr. Tyner continued as chaplain until 1951, when ill health and the infirmities of old age forced his retirement. His interest in the hospital continued, however, and it was at St. Barnabas that he died in 1958.

Readers of the *Minneapolis Star and Tribune* during the 1940s would have known Dr. Tyner as the author of a regular feature on the sports page entitled, "What's Your Score?" In that column he combined comments on sports events with a religious message. One column included an athlete's prayer, which was clipped and posted in sports locker rooms all over the

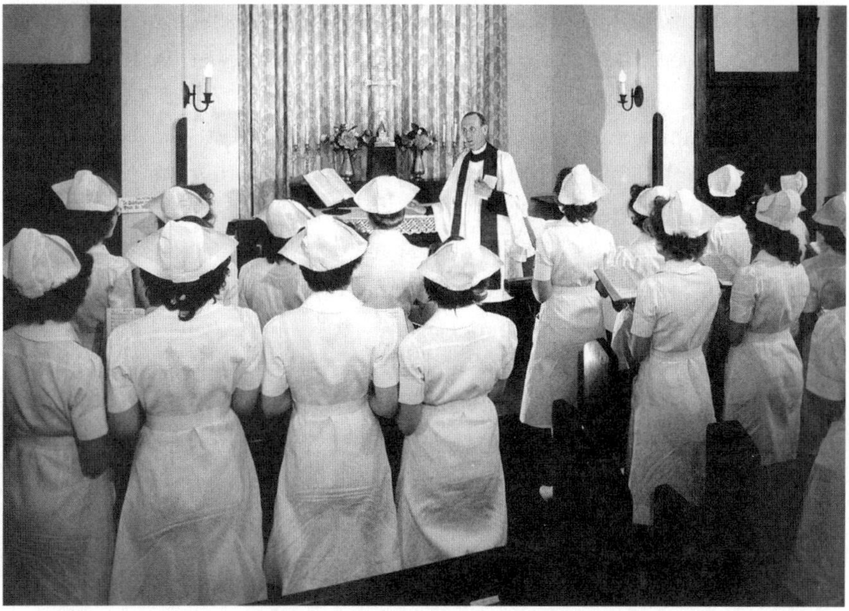

Chapel service with Chaplain Tyner, late 1940s.

state. Mr. Tyner's interest in sports stemmed from his father, who was active in team sports in ninteenth century Toronto, Canada, where Frederick Tyner was born and educated.

Mr. Tyner was ordained as a priest in 1903 in Toronto. He came to Minneapolis in 1915, first as an assistant at St. Mark's Cathedral. In 1917 he accepted appointment as the rector of St. Luke's Episcopal Church, then a congregation of only 40. When he retired from St. Luke's 31 years later in 1948, that small congregation of 40 had grown to 1,000.

In 1952, Dr. Tyner was replaced by the Reverend Mr. Perry M. Gilfillan, who served the remaining years of St. Barnabas and even on into the years of the Metropolitan Medical Center. This made him the chaplain who had the longest tenure in the histroy of the hospital, eighteen years with St. Barnabas plus the years he continued on at Metropolitan Medical Center.

Chaplain Gilfillan was a member of a distinguished St. Paul family. He graduated from Harvard University and from Seabury-Western Theological Seminary. He began his ministry in the Twin Cities in 1934. In addition to the Twin Cities parish, he also served churches later in Detroit, Michigan, and in Iowa before entering the chaplaincy at St. Barnabas. A mild-mannered, low-keyed, but very intelligent man, the Reverend Mr. Perry Gilfillan was a popular figure during his long tenure at St. Barnabas. He was the Right man in the right place at the right time. He was a part of the planning for the "new" St. Barnabas in the 1950s. After the move to that facility he had a chapel complex never available to previous chaplains. Because of his ability and tireless efforts, he developed many new programs.

In the old hospital, the chapel was in the Martin building and space was limited for it was a very small room. There were pews fastened to the floor and little space for wheelchairs, so if patients were to use that chapel, they had to be ambulatory. The chapel in the 1958 building was much larger. Instead of pews as in the Martin chapel, there were chairs which could be moved around, making space for patients in wheelchairs, or even in beds, to attend. It had been a longstanding tradition, possibly begun by the Reverend Dr. Knickerbacker himself, for nurses to attend a ten minute chapel service before going on duty at 7:00 A.M. Usually those assembled would sing a hymn and recite in unison the St. Barnabas prayer. Authorship of the prayer is not known, but it is thought to have been composed by the Reverend Dr. Knickerbacker. It went as follows: "O Almighty God, who callest Thy holy Apostle Barnabas to follow in the steps of Thy blessed

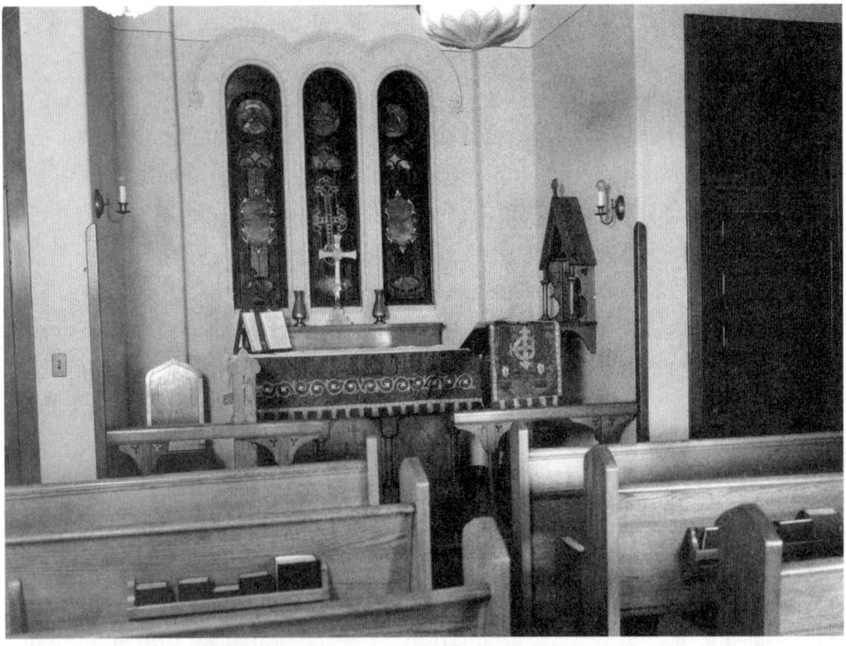

The chapel on the ground floor of the Martin Building in the old hospital.

Son in administering to the sick and suffering, grant to us the same spirit of consolation that by gentleness and love, through faithfulness and patience, we may serve Thy afflicted children. Support us in Thy work; endow us with wisdom and skill; give us sympathy for one another; deliver us from temptation and at last bring us to Thy rest and peace through Jesus Christ our Lord. Amen"

Until 1949 or 1950, attendance at these morning services was compulsory for all students assigned to duty that day. The services were held every morning. Later, attendance became optional and the services were held only on Sundays, Wednesdays and Fridays. The chaplain often was not in attendance at the early morning services, but every Monday at 6:00 P.M. he conducted a longer service in the chapel, including a short sermon at that time. With the greater amount of space available in the new chapel, the number of longer services was increased to serve more patients and visitors. There was an afternoon service, at 5:00 P.M. every Thursday and a Sunday morning service at 9:30 A.M. During Lent, Easter and Christmas, special services were held. There was Holy Communion, open to persons of all Christian faiths, on Ash Wednesday each year. On Maundy Thursday there was a service of Holy Communion at 5:00 P.M. An additional service was scheduled at 11:30 A.M. on Good Friday. Then again on Easter Sunday, there was another service of Holy Communion at 8:00 P.M. On Christmas Day, the customary early morning prayer service was lengthened to allow staff to have Communion before going on duty. After that service, the chaplain would take Communion to any patient desiring to have it.

Serving nursing staff on duty was always an "iffy" proposition, whether it was for class or for chapel service. Since it was necessary to have some staff always on the clinical units, times had to be planned when staff could expect to be less busy, and thus able to attend. Even with such planning, sometimes a nurse who planned to attend a service could not because of a patient emergency or a patient she just felt she could not leave for any length of time.

A program in which Chaplain Gilfillan was a participant involved a course offered for Lutheran seminary students by Northwestern Lutheran Seminary. It was a course on pastoral care in the hospital setting. Students taking the course were assigned to Twin Cities' hospitals, including St. Barnabas, for three months of practical experience in hospital pastoral care.

The chaplain for each hospital would serve as a preceptor for the students assigned to his service. St. Barnabas usually had three students assigned for three months in the spring of the year. As preceptor, Chaplain Gilfillan was their on site resource and guidance person.

In 1967, a similar program was developed as a joint project with Swedish Hospital. It was called the Clinical Pastoral Education Program of Swedish and St. Barnabas Hospitals. The program was conducted by Chaplain Mark Anderson of Swedish Hospital with the cooperation and assistance of Chaplain Gilfillan. It differed from the seminary course in that it was designed particularly for clergy serving Minneapolis churches. Participation was open to interested seminary students, but the focus was on the parish minister rather than the hospital chaplain. The purpose of the course was not to make hospital chaplains of the participants, but to help pastors become better prepared to serve the hospitalized members of their congregations. Each man taking the course spent approximately twenty hours per week for a twelve-week period on duty at either St. Barnabas or Swedish. The remaining twenty hours of each week were devoted to seminars, consultations and conduct of services in the Geriatric Building at Swedish, as well as other projects the man would develop in association with his classwork. So it really was a full-time commitment for a pastor to make for twelve weeks.

The Women's Auxiliary provided fresh flowers regularly for the chapel. They developed a program whereby they provided fresh flowers on the first Sunday of each month to memorialize any auxiliary member who had died during the previous month.

Youth members from two Minneapolis parishes, St. John's and St. George's, were enlisted to volunteer at the hospital transporting patients to chapel services every Sunday morning. The program began in the fall of 1961. The *Voice of St. Barnabas* reported in the May-June issue of 1962 the following relative to the chapel services for the Easter day: "The triumph of Easter was evident this special of Sundays, and the gifts of Easter lilies added the extra touch of spring. The attendance was the highest it has ever been and included patients and visitors. This could be attributed to our loyal teenage escorts who have faithfully performed the service of taking patients to and from the chapel every Sunday."

It appears the offer of escort to and from the chapel was enough of an incentive to encourage patients and visitors who may have hesitated going down to the service without the offer from the teenage volunteers. Whether the idea for this kind of volunteer service originated with the auxiliary volunteers or whether this was Chaplain Gilfillan's idea is not known. But obviously it was a productive idea.

That May-June 1962 issue of the *Voice of St. Barnabas* also includes an article about another way the chaplaincy of the hospital was reaching out to the community. It said, "Tuesday, May 1, twenty members of the Episcopal Social Workers Guild were present at a special Corporate Communion Service conducted by the Reverend Perry M. Gilfillan and the Reverend George F. LeMoine, Director of Christian Social Relations. Following the service, the group group breakfasted together in the cafeteria before going their separate ways."

In 1963, large print copies of the *New Testament And Psalms* were purchased for the chapel. They could be checked out from the chapel and used in their rooms by patients who had visual problems. Chaplain Gilfillan would deliver the copy in person to any patient whose nurse reported the need. In 1964, equipment was installed which made it possible to broadcast services from the hospital chapel to the bedsides of patients. The services could be tuned in through the pillow speakers each patient had for radio and television reception.

On May 26, 1965, the Reverend Mr. Gilfillan became the Reverend Dr. Gilfillan when he was awarded an honorary Doctor of Divinity degree by his alma mater, Seabury-Western Seminary. He received the degree during commencement exercises held at the seminary in Evanston, Illinois.

From time to time there were weddings in the chapel, usually involving hospital staff members or students. On May 29, 1965, another kind of wedding was held, one which involved a patient as one of the members of the wedding party. On that day, Beatrice Hass and James Rachner were married in the chapel by the Reverend Willis W. Velde, pastor of Hobart Methodist Church of Minneapolis. The bride's only sister, Mrs. Ralph Peterson, was a patient then in the hospital and having the wedding in the chapel made it possible for her to attend and serve as her sister's matron of honor as planned before the need for her hospitalization arose. Mr. Peterson served

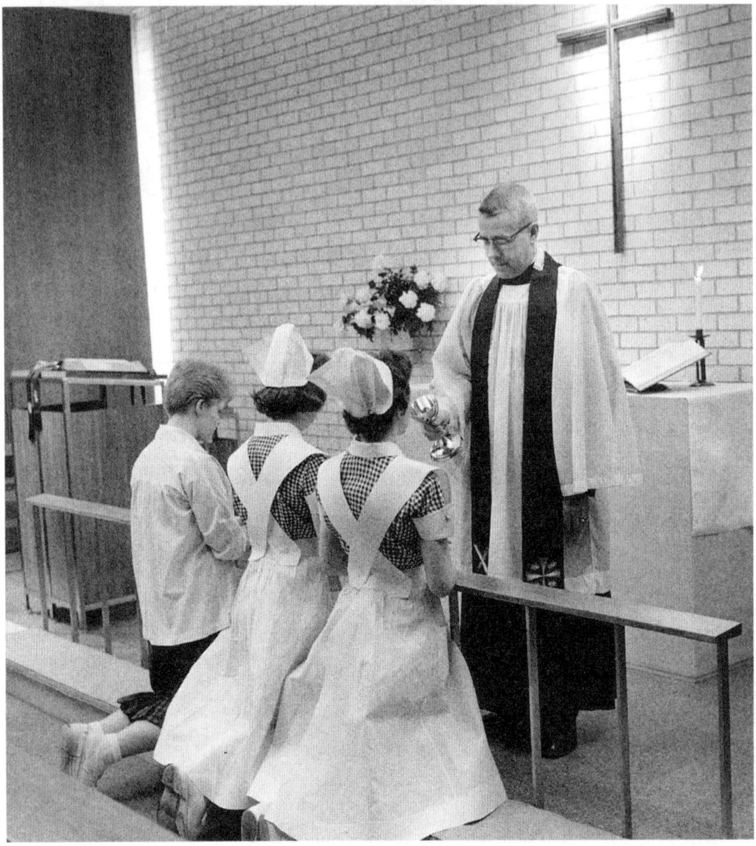

Chapel service in Leonora Christian Memorial Chapel, Chaplain Perry Gilfillan.

as best man. Following the service, those in attendance at the wedding had a reception in the small dining room, one floor below the chapel.

There were also baptisms from time to time. The first baptism to be held in the chapel was on January 19, 1964, a special one for many St. Barnabas staffers. On that day, infant Carlos P. Del Plaine was baptized during the regular Sunday service. He was special because his father was Dr. Carlos W. Del Plaine, longtime member of the medical staff of the hospital, and his mother was Marilyn Huntley Del Plaine, graduate of St. Barnabas School of Nursing, class of 1954. Marilyn was a supervisor in the Nursing Service Department when she and Dr. Del Plaine were married.

For ten years, the Reverend Dr.Gilfillan served as Chairman of the Health and Welfare Committee of the Diocesan Department of Christian

Social Relations. He was also founder and the first treasurer of the Minnesota Mental Hygiene Association, which later was renamed the Minnesota Association for Mental Health.

Chaplain Gilfillan was a regular contributor of articles to the *Voice of St. Barnabas*. Twice, in the issue of June-July 1955, and again in the April-May issue of 1958, he wrote articles answering the question, "Who was St. Barnabas?" The 1955 article was particularly informative. We quote it in its entirety as follows:

> "Who was St. Barnabas, anyway?"
>
> "You've got me."
>
> This dialogue actually took place outside Central Service one day, but perhaps you have repeated it somewhere else. At any rate, a number of people have asked about our 'patron' saint and so here is a brief story about him.
>
> The few references to Barnabas in the Book of Acts of the Apostles make us realize he was quite a man. Although he did not attain the stature of St. Paul, and he did not write immortal letters (however, some think he wrote the Epistle to the Hebrews) it was he who paved the way for his famous friend.
>
> Barnabas, we are told was a "good man, full of the Holy Spirit and of faith." Because of his additional qualities of tact and judgment, furthermore, he had been placed by the Apostles, with headquarters in Jerusalem, in charge of the Christian Church at Antioch.
>
> When he heard of the dramatic experience of Paul's conversion and realized what a powerhouse the latter would be, he invited the former persecutor of Christians to join him at Antioch. Evidently, "the great Apostle" made a fine impression there for subsequently that local church sent the two men on a missionary journey. During this trip they were stoned and driven from several towns, a real test of their courage and faith and they did not fail.

> The Church fathers at Jerusalem, however, were still fearful of Saul, the terror of Christian believers. When he tried to take counsel with them, they refused to have anything to do with him until Barnabas spoke up on his behalf.
>
> The word of our "patron" carried weight in Church councils, and when he vouched for the sincerity of the converted persecutor, Paul was finally recognized as a true and valuable co-worker.
>
> Two outstanding things may be said about Barnabas. He was a pioneer in the thinking (so strongly advocated by Paul, too) that said, "The Church must reach out to people not on the basis of creed but of need." This point of view certainly is appropriate in the "patron saint" of a hospital, which serves on the same basis. His nickname, a rough estimate of his reputation among his fellows also tells us much. He was called "Son of Encouragement" or "Son of Consolation," a truly prophetic name for one who was to have a hospital named for him!

Three other articles written by Chaplain Gilfillan for the *Voice of St. Barnabas* are included because they provide a glimpse of the character of the man who wrote them. The first one appeared in the December 1957 issue and was entitled, "Captured By Christmas."

> Have you ever been captured by Christmas? For Christmas is a mighty conqueror which has swept down the ages until our day. Many, indeed, have "fallen prey" to it during this time. There are those, however, who think they've been, only to discover, to their sorrow, that their conqueror was some lesser power. The glamour and the tinsel, charming and pleasant though they are, are not really Christmas. Yet is it not true that frequently these transient trimmings are thought to be the real thing? How sad it is , then, when they are gone to realize just how temporary is their influence, how ineffective they are. In the long run they actually "pack no punch."
>
> But Christmas itself—ah that's something else! Here we have a feast far older than the customs often either associated with it or practically replacing it. Here we have a celebration firmly grounded

in an historic event. And what an event it was! To be sure it apparently consisted only in the birth of a baby—one among millions. The captives of Christmas, however, have discovered that it was really far more and greater than it seemed. Grandeur, power, and love filled it, for herein (the truly captured know) God gave Himself uniquely and supremely. Because this is so, life has become different not just on December 25th, but every day. The captivity lasts and lasts! They find themselves caught up in the continuing need to express their gratitude for so amazing a gift and to reflect its glorious radiance in the mirrors, which are their lives.

Have you been captured by Christmas? If you have, you're "in"—not for one day, nor for 365, but for life. If you have, the generous spirit of the day will penetrate every corner of your life. With or without decorations and under all circumstances you, too, will radiate something of the grandeur, the power and the glory of the Creator of Christmas. Captured yourself, you will help Him to bring others into this same joyful bondage.

Have you been captured by Christmas? I hope so. If not, I sincerely trust you will find yourself this year among its newest victims!

The next one appeared in the February-March 1963 issue:
Since some may not be familiar with the ancient pious custom of praying for the departed, let me explain it. It rests on the belief that not even death can separate a believing (though imperfect) Christian from the fellowship of Christ and his disciples, the Church. Since, however, the usual desire to draw close to God is not automatic in the future life any more than now, people have always wanted to help both the departed and the living. Thus it has been as natural for believers to pray for the growth of those who have "gone on ahead" as for those still in their earthly pilgrimage.

Prayer is an expression of love in both instances, and throughout Christian history and even earlier, devout people have offered intercession for their loved ones in both stages of life.

And the last article, from the March 1965 issue of the *Voice*, discusses the meaning of Lent and Easter:

> Lent this year begins on March 3. Now there is an interesting parallel between this season of the Church year and the season of the calendar year which we call Spring. The world "Lent" itself, indeed, comes from the word "Spring." Each one of them, certainly, is a time of renewal. Just as the Spring of the year prepares us for the full blossoming of Summer, so Lent is intended to be a time of preparation for the great event of Easter. It is a time, therefore, of getting down to basic realities in order that one may more fully appreciate the significance of the triumph of Christ as we see him on the first Easter. Since our lives are always so full of many activities, this kind of concentrated preparation often is difficult to achieve. It has therefore been found necessary by people through the ages to take time from other activities in order that they may bear down upon a better understanding of Easter and the great events associated with it.
>
> Lent, therefore, has always been a time for study, a time for prayer, a time for meditation. Because of the necessity of taking extra time for these purposes, many people have found it necessary to go without other activities in order that they may concentrate upon the things which are important to them. Surely, those who have put in extra effort in this way have found a great reward in better appreciation of the whole significance of their faith and life as they see it hallowed by the Cross and Resurrection of Jesus, the Christ.
>
> We all recognize that as a rule we don't get out of anything more than we put in. Of course, in this particular instance, our labors do bring us a dividend far greater than anything we might expect. Nevertheless, it is essential that we give of ourselves if we are to receive; because the kind of giving we do makes us more aware of our own need and of the resources which are available to meet our needs. Unless we face these facts we cannot receive and we do not.

So, Lent is a time of self analysis, if you like, a time when people holding a mirror before their own lives contrast them with the great God whom they seek to serve. In this way they are enabled to go "from strength to strength in the life of perfect service." This, indeed, is what Lent is all about—an attempt to enable each one who observes it to be more perfectly the kind of person he is destined to be and (at his best) wants to be. May you, therefore, have an effective and happy Lent. In this way you will come to know the wonders of Easter in its richest significance.

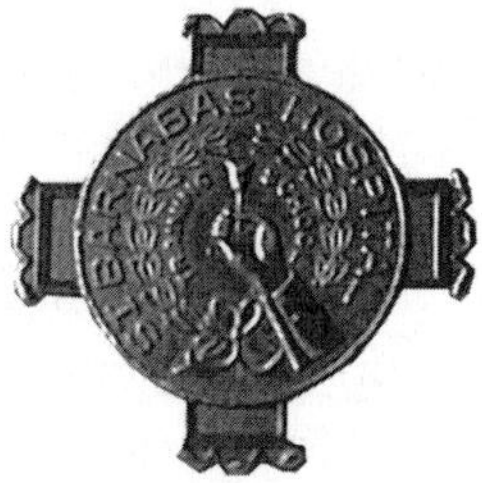

Chapter 7

Establishment of Diagnostic Services

A hospital in the nineteenth century was still looked upon as a last resort recovery and a place for those who had no home or no one at home to provide care for them. Antiseptic surgery was new in the 1890s. It came about largely due to the work of Joseph Lister in England. He was a professor of surgery at the University of Glasgow about 1860. At that time in history, almost everyone who had surgery developed a post-operative infection. The prevailing opinion then was that infections were caused by some force in the air or were a result of trauma to tissues associated with the surgery. Lister observed that patients who had simple fractures, with no breaks in the skin, tended not to develop infections. He reasoned, therefore, that trauma to the tissues was not the causative factor in development of infection. So he turned to study ways that bacteria might be introduced through breaks in the skin, using the work that Pasteur had done on the actions of bacteria. By keeping wounds clean, employing careful hand washing and cleaning of instruments, he was able to drastically reduce the incidence of postoperative infections among his patients.

In Minnesota, the pioneering work of the Mayo brothers, both surgeons in Rochester, led to the development of antiseptic procedures and therefore safer surgery in hospitals all over the state. The new Martin building boasted one of the finest operating rooms in the whole region. And gradually the hospital added to its staff surgeons who performed not only emergency surgeries, but more and more elective surgeries as time went on.

As the practice of surgery increased at St. Barnabas, so did the need for better diagnostic facilities increase. X-rays were still very new at the turn of the twentieth century. They were discovered in 1895 by a German physicist, Wilhelm Conrad Roentgen, working at the University of Wurzburg in the Franconia area of central Germany. He discovered, somewhat by accident while doing an unrelated experiment, that these mysterious rays could penetrate soft tissue and outline bones. He named the newly discovered rays "X-rays" because so little was known about them. The application of the new technology was made first in the treatment of bone fractures. For the first time a closed fracture could be visualized on X-ray and the bone could be set more precisely than possible previously. It wasn't long before it was also discovered that X-rays could be useful in locating metallic foreign items in the body. Examples of some of the early foreign bodies located by X-rays were: a broken needle in the tissues of a seamstress, a coin swallowed by a youngster, a metal bead accidentally aspirated into the bronchi and a bullet lodged in a wound.

At first the medical establishment was unimpressed with this new diagnostic tool. They viewed it more as some sort of hoax and urged caution and further study before putting the technology to work in the practice of medicine. In spite of skepticism, many physicians recognized the value of the new discovery and the advent of the use of X-rays as diagnostic tools had begun. For his discovery, Roentgen was awarded a Nobel Prize December 5, 1903, saw the installation of the first X-ray machine to be used at St. Barnabas. By 1911, the department was doing an average of slightly over one X-ray per day, a total of 380 for the year.

Not much is known about the X-ray department in those early years at St. Barnabas. It seems reasonable to assume there was a doctor in charge of the apparatus. Whether that was his fulltime occupation or not is not known and whether or not there were other employees in the department also is not known. Twenty years later, in 1922, Elmer J. (Jack) Leffingwell joined the X-ray staff and served as chief technician of the department for the next 36 years, until his retirement in 1958. Jack was a barber for several years prior to World War I. He served in the armed forces during that war and on his return, he elected not to go back to the barber trade, but rather to try his hand in the new field of X-ray technology. He took a training program at the Veterans' Hospital and shortly after that came to St. Barnabas. His wife was a St. Barnabas School of Nursing graduate, Gertrude Moses Leffingwell, class of 1921. In 1936, Jack was joined on the X-ray staff by a 1936 graduate of the nursing school, Helen Parker Hayden. During her time as a student nurse, Helen had worked part time in the X-ray department. Upon graduation from nursing, she worked for a while as a nurse until she had written and passed State Boards. Then she transferred to the X-ray department, working there for the rest of her professional career.

During the 1930s and 1940s, Dr. Russell Morse was the hospital radiologist. He served as chief radiologist until his death in 1951. In 1935, the department had expanded enough to warrant the hiring of an associate radiologist. Dr. Ames Naslund was appointed to that position and on the death of Dr. Morse in 1951, he became the chief radiologist, a position he held for many years. Dr. Naslund came to St. Barnabas with prior experience at the State University of Iowa Hospital and the Lewis Gregory Cole Hospital in New York. He spent four years during World War II in the United States Navy, Pacific theater. His hobbies were playing golf and hunting, activities which he shared with a number of members of the medical staff.

The X-ray department of the 1930s and before was housed in just one tiny room on the top floor of the Martin building. But with the opening of the new Whitney building in 1937, the department moved to a suite of rooms at the east end of the first floor hall. It was on the north side of the hall while the clinical laboratory was on the south side. When the new hospital was built in 1958, the X-ray department moved to much larger quarters in the new building than they had at Whitney and the volume of work done in the department increased. Dr. Naslund then had three associate radiologists, Dr. Philip Olson, Dr. Harley Calin and Dr. Frank Mork, Jr. Dr. John McDonald also served as an associate radiologist. He died in the 1950s of the scourge of radiologists, leukemia.

Close to the end of Dr. Morse's life, a radiologic technician program was established. From the beginning, Helen Hayden was a driving force in developing the program and she became its director as well as the instructor who supervised day-to-day activities and progress of the students. During the early years, the radiologic technician program was one year in length. Later it was expanded to become a two-year program. Early classes numbered five to six students per year.

Between 1950, when the first class graduated, and 1961, 56 students graduated from the program. Graduates took National Registry examinations to become Registered Radiologic Technicians. The record indicates that consistently all members of every class passed the examinations, indicating the high quality of instruction they had received. Most graduates returned for professional practice to the communities from which they had been recruited. Whether this was because of limited openings in Minneapolis hospitals or whether most just preferred to go back home after graduation is a question not answered. There were some who joined the armed services immediately after becoming registered. This was particularly true during the Korean War. It might be pointed out that St. Barnabas sent nurses and doctors, too, into the armed services during that war as they had done in the two World Wars.

When Jack retired in 1955, he was replaced by Walt Rasula, a former St. Andrews employee. Walt remained at St. Barnabas for ten years. After his resignation, he went back to college for more academic preparation, earning a BA in 1972 and an MA in Education in 1978. His replacement at St. Barnabas was Jerry Galde. Both Walt and Jerry worked closely with Helen in maintaining and improving the technician program. Jerry Galde had sixteen years of experience in radiology before he came to St. Barnabas. He was a graduate of the radiologic technician program at McKennan Hospital in Sioux Falls, South Dakota, and had worked at McKennan as well as St. Joseph's Hospital in Mankato prior to accepting the position at St. Barnabas. He had been active in his professional association in South Dakota and was also a member of the American Radiologic Society, so he came to St. Barnabas well prepared academically for the job to be done.

After the new hospital was built in 1958, it became possible, because of the greater space and increased volume of work in the department, to increase the class size annually to eight or nine. After that, more graduates stayed on to work at St. Barnabas following graduation. The radiologic technology program continued after St. Barnabas and Swedish merged to become Metropolitan Medical Center. In 1976, the program was rated among the top 25 of 750 programs nationwide. Helen Hayden retired in 1968, having been on the staff at St. Barnabas for more than 30 years, her entire professional career. The success of the program on which she had worked so hard must have been a source of great satisfaction to her. Though her identification during all those years was with the X-ray department, she never forgot her nursing sisters and was a regular attendee at nursing alumnae banquets. Helen was physically small and for years was known to many as "Peewee", an appellation she did not appreciate and she was not afraid to express her feelings about it. Looking back over her accomplishments, we can say the name did not fit the personality.

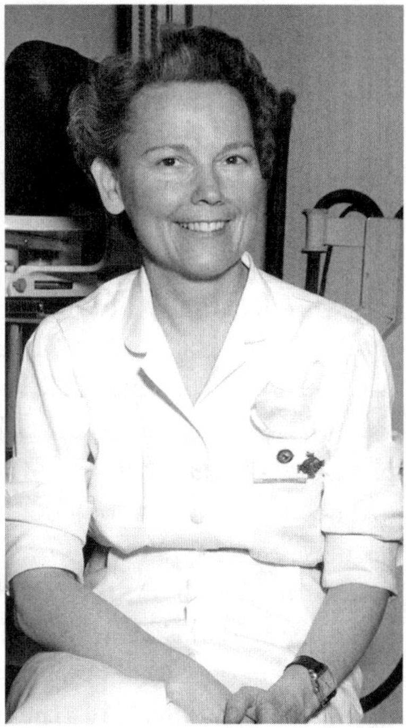
Helen Parker Hayden

During her many years at St. Barnabas, Helen regularly authored articles for the *Voice of St. Barnabas*. One such article, which Helen recalled in a 2002 letter to me, was a description of the demolition of Wellesmere. In her letter she recalls "the headache ball" which made short work of the old building.

In 1968, Helen published a book on The Vocabulary Of Roentgenographic Reports. She dedicated the book to Dr. Naslund, who had been her long-time colleague in the X-ray department.

No dormitory space was available to the X-ray students. Rather, they were responsible for making their own housing arrangements. This may have contributed to their desire to return home after graduation since the majority came from small communities where living tended to be more relaxed than in the city. Local need for their newly acquired skills may also have been a factor pulling them back to hometown hospitals.

As new equipment came on the market to improve the services the hospital could offer, purchases were made to allow the hospital to provide the best care and diagnostic service possible. One piece of equipment added to the X-ray department in 1965 was a magnascanner. A patient for whom this machine would be used was given a radioactive isotope, then the machine was used to scan the area of the body in which the isotope would concentrate, making it possible to visualize soft tissues more effectively. The machine picked up the distribution and concentration of the radioactive material, then recorded the data on both graph and photographic formats. Some of the most useful applications of this technology were in diagnosis of tumors or abnormalities in the thyroid gland, brain, kidney and liver.

After St. Barnabas and Swedish became Metropolitan Medical Center, a CT (computerized tomography) scanner was added to the radiology department, adding another way to better diagnose and treat patients, particularly those who had tumors. The scanner, costing $1,000,000, allowed physicians to view internal body parts with non-invasive techniques and provided them more diagnostic information than available before, short of opening the patient to view the part directly. The savings in pain and recuperation time for patients was enormous. The use of the CT scanner was shared with Hennepin County Medical Center. At the time it was installed, it was anticipated it would be used in diagnosing more than 4,000 patients annually.

A later generation of this kind of miracle diagnostic tool was the MRI, Magnetic Resonance Imager or NMR, Nuclear Magnetic Resonance. In place of radiation, as in X-rays, NMR uses magnetic forces. It is capable of "looking through" more dense body tissues (such as bone) making it possible to pick up abnormalities which could not be visualized using earlier technologies. In 1952, Felix Bloch and Edward Purcell shared a Nobel Prize for their work with NMR. Forty years later nearly every major medical center had both CT and MRI equipment available to serve the diagnostic needs of physicians and patients.

In his 1902 Annual Report, John I. Black, President of the Board of Trustees referred to the need for a clinical laboratory at St. Barnabas. He indicated the Board of Trustees had voted to give one room at the hospital to be utilized as a clinical laboratory. The report doesn't indicate whether he was speaking of an independently contracted laboratory to be housed in this room or whether, perhaps, members of the medical staff were willing to pay to get the laboratory started. But soon after that, the hospital did have a clinical laboratory on premises.

As with the X-ray department, little is known about the early days of the laboratory. It is likely there was a physician in charge, but whether or not he was a fulltime employee is not known. It is known that it operated from one small room in the Martin building. Also unknown is how many staff members were in the early department, but it is likely it was a one-man operation at first. Use of the laboratory grew quickly. By 1911, approximately six patients each day had lab procedures ordered for them, a total of 2,222 for the entire year 1911. Just five years later, that number had almost doubled for a total of 4,242 patients for the year 1916. It is not clear whether that number, labeled "patients" was the same as the number of procedures done, or whether the procedures done might have been greater since there were undoubtedly some patients who had more than one procedure done on any given day.

A long-term member of the St. Barnabas laboratory staff was Dr. Nathaniel H. Lufkin, a much-loved figure in the history of St. Barnabas. He arrived at the hospital in 1939 with an undergraduate degree from Carlton College and an MD from the University of Minnesota plus ten years experience as the chief pathologist at Minneapolis General Hospital. At the time of his appointment to the St. Barnabas post, he was also an associate professor at the University of Minnesota. His talents as a teacher were soon recognized at St. Barnabas and it wasn't long before he became a member of the School of Nursing faculty.

Many St. Barnabas nursing graduates of the '40s and '50s remember taking a course in Pathology from Dr. Lufkin. Through the course he came to know the nursing students well and always went out of his way to provide learning experiences for them Several could recall receiving a call at the dormitory announcing that an autopsy would be performed at a given hour and that nursing students were invited to be present. The author attended a number of autopsies announced in this way. Otto Jahnke, house orderly (years later administrator of Ancker Hospital in St. Paul), assisted with the procedure, which was done with the utmost decorum to protect the dignity of the deceased Dr. Lufkin provided a running commentary on his findings, stopping at times to quiz the student or students in attendance and praising them for correct responses. His friendship with students and his interest in them continued beyond graduation. He was always pleased to learn of the professional accomplishments of those students to whom he had taught pathology.

Dr. Lufkin retired in 1965. He had been associated then with St. Barnabas for twenty-six years. Only twenty of those years found him on site. He served for six years in the Navy in the South Pacific during World War II. An article in the *Voice of St. Barnabas* announcing Dr. Lufkin's retirement said he had been one of the first fulltime private hospital pathologists in Minneapolis. The article continued, "Dr. Lufkin has helped the lab grow from a staff of two or three in one small room to the present lab with its staff of thirty eight clerical and technical personnel. The medical staff and lab personnel will miss his broad shoulders and sympathetic ear. He has never been too busy to listen to the troubles of others and offer moral support."

The author of that article isn't listed, but it was likely either Mary Conroy or Pat Taylor. Both served as reporters from the lab for the *Voice of St. Barnabas*. Both were, like Dr. Lufkin, longtime staff members. Mary, head medical technologist, came to St. Barnabas in 1945 and was still on the laboratory staff twenty six years later, perhaps even longer, but the records available indicate she was there at least that long. When Mary joined the staff in 1945, there were only five technicians. Ten years later, that number had doubled and with the move to the more spacious laboratory in the new hospital in 1958, it continued to increase. Mary had a baccalaureate degree in chemistry from the College of St. Catherine. She learned medical technology while enrolled during the late 1930s in a training program at Minneapolis General Hospital.

Pat came in 1948 and was still on the laboratory staff in 1964, the last year about which we have data on her. She was a contemporary of Mary Conroy in terms of age and education. Her baccalaureate degree was earned at the University of Minnesota in the late 1930s, after which she took the same training program Mary did at Minneapolis General Hospital. Both ladies were involved in war-related jobs during World War II, Mary in Washington, DC, and Pat at Wright-Patterson Airfield in Dayton, Ohio.

Pat's area of specialty was cytology, for which she had special training in 1955 at the Mayo Clinic She was in charge of the tissue laboratory at St. Barnabas. Both ladies were great travelers and the *Voice of St. Barnabas* frequently included tales of their most recent trips.

When Dr. Lufkin retired in 1965, the post of chief pathologist went to Dr. Wayne Chadbourn. Dr. Chadbourn had been on staff for some time as the associate pathologist, so he was well prepared to progress to the chief position. Other associate pathologists who came on board during the '50s and '60s included Dr. Gerald K. Palmer, who joined the staff in 1958, Dr. Thomas Semba, who came in 1960 and combined the position at St. Barnabas with a like one at the new North Memorial Hospital, Dr. John Poppowich, who came in 1963 and Dr. Richard L. Reece in 1965.

The 1980 Annual Report for Metropolitan Medical Center states the center had received a $100,000 grant from the Surdna Foundation of New York. That grant was used to provide computer hardware for the laboratory. It was not the first grant provided by the Surdna Foundation, for, beginning in 1958, the St. Barnabas Hospital had received a total of $250,000 in smaller grants from the same foundation.

Some time in the years between 1958 and 1980, the name of the St. Barnabas lab was changed to the Andrus Laboratory in memory of John Emory Andrus, a long-term benefactor of the hospital. By 1980, it had become the largest hospital laboratory in the Twin Cities.

A doctor member of the staff who was not an MD was Dr. Emil Schleicher, chief of the hematology section. Beginning in 1950, Dr. Schleicher (a PhD rather than MD) was associated with St. Barnabas while working on research projects sponsored by the Parke-Davis Company. He became an official part of the St. Barnabas family in January 1958 when he was appointed director of the hematology and tissue laboratory. He was recognized as an authority on bone marrow, developing and refining techniques for harvesting bone marrow from live donors and transferring it to patients in need of its healing qualities. Most of the bone marrow procedures were developed at St. Barnabas during his years of association with Parke-Davis and the hospital. He was the first to recognize miliary tuberculosis could be detected by examination of an individual's bone marrow. This was an extremely important finding for at the time, bovine born miliary tuberculosis was rampant in post-war Europe. Tuberculin testing of cattle had not become a reality in Europe in those days and many who drank the milk from infected cows became tuberculosis victims themselves.

Another of Dr. Schleicher's pioneering projects was a study of vitamin C paralleling some of the work done by Dr. Linus Pauling, who received a Nobel Prize for his work. Dr. Schleicher's emphasis was upon the utilization of vitamin C by pregnant women and the relationship between a lack of the vitamin and habitual miscarriage. He postulated that cigarette smoking tended to destroy vitamin C in the body and was one of the early advocates of nonsmoking for pregnant women. Working in association with St. Barnabas obstetricians, Dr. Schleicher advised prescribing mega doses of vitamin C for women who had previously miscarried. Several women so treated were able to carry babies to term under the regimen. One such successful outcome was achieved by a St. Barnabas nurse who was visited by the good Dr. soon after the birth. His greeting, overheard by other nurses on the station was, "Where is our baby? I am anxious to see her." Since it was well known that Dr. Schleicher was a bachelor, this news provided amusement for all and perhaps fodder for gossip for some!

Like Dr. Lufkin, Dr. Schleicher enjoyed teaching and never missed an opportunity to share his knowledge with nursing staff and nursing students. He endowed an award which was given annually to the junior nursing student rated as the best bedside nurse in her class. One edition of the nursing school yearbook, *Sabarho*, was dedicated to Dr.Schleicher.

A devoted patron of the arts, he often also provided symphony tickets to interested students. He possessed considerable artistic talent and many a St. Barnabas staffer, the author among them, was the proud recipient of a watercolor painting done by Dr. Schleicher. Like Mary and Pat he was a great traveler. He was German-born and made a number of trips back to his homeland. Many of the watercolors he did were of beach scenes on the North Sea. He particularly enjoyed painting beach scenes. Several of his paintings were done in Hawaii and others on Pacific beaches in California. The painting possessed by this author is a beach scene from one of his California vacations. In 1959 he donated one of his paintings, entitled "Indian Summer," to decorate the doctors' lounge in the new hospital.

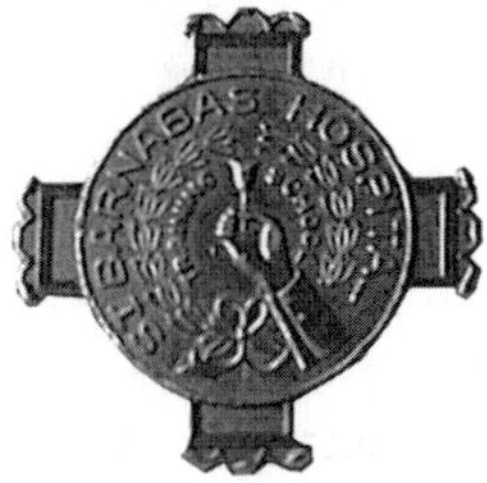

Chapter 8

St. Andrew's Division Is Added

In 1953, there was a joint announcement made from Robert W. Bachmeyer, director St. Barnabas Hospital and Telmer O. Peterson, director of St. Andrew's Hospital. St. Barnabas was adding to its corporation a new division, St. Andrew's Hospital, an 80-bed facility in southeast Minneapolis. St. Andrew's had been in existence since March 24, 1912, but it had fallen on hard times by 1953 and it was about to close its doors when an agreement was reached with the board and administration of St. Barnabas for purchase of St. Andrew's. Under terms of the purchase, St. Andrew's would become a division of St. Barnabas and would continue to operate with basically the same staff as before.

The acquisition of St. Andrew's on February 1, 1953, served both hospitals well. It preserved the jobs for St. Andrew's employees and satisfied the need for a local hospital in Southeast Minneapolis. There were also economic incentives since as a part of the larger corporation, supplies of everything from napkins for the cafeteria to sutures for surgery could be purchased in amounts which allowed quantity discounts. For St. Barnabas, it added eighty beds to their capacity at a time when hospital space was at a premium in town and long lists of patients were waiting for admission to St. Barnabas for elective procedures or diagnostic workups.

St. Andrew's had opened a school of nursing soon after the hospital opened. It operated the school for thirty-six years, but five years prior to the St. Barnabas purchase, the school had closed its doors. Senior students completed their studies at St. Andrew's, but underclass students transferred to other schools. Some of them elected to transfer to St. Barnabas where they graduated as St. Barnabas nurses in 1950 and 1951. When they wrote their State Board Examinations for licensure, they found that the executive director of the board presiding over the examinations was their former school director at St. Andrews, Leonora Collatz. Lee served in her position at the board for approximately twenty years after that. St. Andrew's, in its thirty-six year history, graduated three hundred thirteen nurses.

Looking back on the founding of St. Andrews in 1911, we learn that Charles Gluek, a prominent businessman in Minneapolis and a dedicated Lutheran layman, purchased the L. S. Gillette home, which stood at 712 Fifth Street Southeast. He donated the property, including the house, a large stable and most of a whole city block of land, to the German Lutheran Church. After remodeling and renovation, the home was converted to a hospital which could serve thirty five adult patients plus a small number of children. The building covered three floors plus the basement of the old house. The kitchen, employee dining room, a classroom, a laboratory and a drug room were in the basement. The street floor included offices, admitting space and a waiting room plus the children's ward and five rooms for adult male patients. The obstetrical ward and nursery were on the second floor along with rooms for adult women and an operating suite. Student nurses, the hospital superintendent and maids lived on the third floor. There was a medical intern on staff who had a cot in the drug room in the basement. There was also a house orderly who had a room in the stable which had been occupied previously by the Gillette family coachman.

Rev. Henry Hartig, one of the original founders of the hospital, served as its first president as well as superintendent. He remained in the position of superintendent for twelve years. Several doctors were on the original medical staff—a far cry from the beginnings of St. Barnabas forty one years earlier. St. Barnabas was served originally by one volunteer physician who was joined later by two others. The organization of a medical staff was years into the future after the founding of St. Barnabas. Members of the original medical staff at St. Andrew's along with their medical specialties were: Dr. William Chowning, chief of staff; Dr. W. Sheldon, medical; Dr. F. Schultz, pediatrics; Dr. F. Adair, obstetrics; Dr. Charles N. Spratt, eye, ear, nose and throat. Drs. Hartig, MacDonald, E. L. Baker, H.A. H. Bouman, I. A. Preine and G. Dezeil also served, though their areas of practice are not known. From this list one can deduce the care offered to the first St. Andrew's patients was a whole world beyond that available to the first patients at St. Barnabas. There was even an intern at St. Andrew's from the beginning, the first being Dr. Ed Hayes. When St. Andrew's became a division of St. Barnabas, there were several doctors who already enjoyed staff privileges at both hospitals, so the transition for the medical staff was relatively easy.

St. Andrew's, at its founding, was meant to serve the needs particularly of the German Lutherans who supported it. Many Germans at that time were immigrants or first generation people who were most comfortable among those who spoke their language and understood their culture and customs. Apparently there were a good many such people in Southeast Minneapolis at that time for by 1917, it was apparent that more space was needed than the old Gillette house afforded and though it was wartime, discussions began about building a new hospital. For various reasons, it was another ten years before the new building became a reality. The cornerstone was laid in 1927 and on February 8, 1927, the hospital was formally opened and dedicated. It continued to be operated under the auspices of the German Lutheran Church until 1938. By that time, the German immigrant population was well integrated and a special hospital to meet their needs was no longer required. Besides, with possible war with Germany looming again on the horizon in 1938, many German born and first generation German-Americans were anxious to identify as Americans, not Germans. When the relationship of the hospital was severed from the German Lutheran Church, a private corporation, the St. Andrew's Hospital Association, was formed to manage the hospital. Rev. Alfred Wilke served as the President of the new association. The hospital at that time was a 100-bed facility with bassinets for 18 newborns.

When the new St. Andrew's was opened in 1927, all patient services in the old residence were discontinued. Classrooms and residence rooms for student nurses were maintained there. In addition, that building provided quarters for interns, employee lounges and conference and office space for hospital administration. By 1919, the space allotted to student nurse rooms was insufficient, so a house in the same block was rented for student housing. Ultimately in 1930 the house standing at the corner of Fourth Street and Seventh Avenue Southeast was purchased to provide more housing for students. The old Gillette residence continued in service for the hospital until it was demolished in January of 1963. It had stood as witness to the entire history of St. Andrew's as a separate entity as well as a division of St. Barnabas.

Soon after St. Andrew's joined the St. Barnabas corporation, extensive remodeling and redecorating was done on the 1927 building. An article which appeared in the January-February 1954 issue of the *Voice of St. Barnabas* described the work which was done. That article, written by Mary Jane Suithoff, is quoted as follows:

> Would you like a glimpse of the St. Andrew's of the Future? The renovation has not been completed as evidence by what seems to be ceaseless hammering, the smell of paint and the presence of plumbers, plasterers, lathers, carpenters and the like interrupting the usual reposeful atmosphere. We are bearing up quite well, however; so, if you don't mind the inconvenience, come along. We'll start from the bottom and on up the ladder.
>
> The Pharmacy
>
> First things first, down in the basement where we find the pharmacy —a study in grey, with a combination of slate and summer smoke walls interrupted by a natural birch service window flanked by glass and transit panels. The new Dillon-Lilly tabletop refrigerator for storing biologicals is a source of great pride to our pharmacist, as well as the Schwatz-type unit of shelving. I don't hesitate to say that the pharmacy is the pride and joy of the whole hospital, for

what used to be an empty hallway materialized into what is now one of the finest of pharmacies.

We'll leave the basement now for the plumbers are busy in the dietary department and the falling plaster and noise are more than you would want to contend with at the moment.

Business Office

Taking the elevator to the first floor we find the business office which will in the future have a new "face" so we will describe that at a later date. Instead, let's go to the nursing section where we behold a veritable rainbow of color. The rooms are decorated in cameo, copper, aqua, grayed white and summer smoke with burgundy doors. The furniture is new, of course, the latest Simmons has to offer in Dusty Rose and Shell, Dove Green and Gray, Terra Cotta and Light Gray with new varihite beds. The nursing station, too, has the "new look" with a blonde wood desk; and, with centralization its motif, it is a great convenience to the nursing personnel. Last, but not least before we leave, notice the aeroflush bedpan washer and sterilizer. The utensils are placed directly inside and a complete flushing and sterilization process is carried out by merely applying pressure on the foot and hand pedal. This is progress!!!!!

Second Floor, Laboratory

Now to the second floor where we find the laboratory. It is so new that one is dazzled by the brightness of it, with its gray steel cabinets and tables and the refrigerator and centrifuge to complete the detail. As we look more closely, we notice the disposal unit for destroying old tissues and specimens, the water bath for serology and the dry heat oven for drying glass. Yes, this is advancement. Believe it or not the site of the laboratory was formerly a waiting room and hallway.

Surgery Modernized

The second, third and fourth floors are similar to the first floor in regard to the nursing section; let's get off the elevator at fifth and "see" what's happening in surgery. There have been changes here, too. An all-important Castle light over a new surgical table certainly adds to the appearance. The numerous new surgical instruments along with the electricosurgical unit were more than welcomed. There has been a rumor to the effect that the doctors rather like the new scrub sinks, too. The former obstetrical room on fifth has now been converted into an emergency room where minor surgery and cast work are done, thus allowing expansion for the surgical department—minor, yes, but none the less expansion.

X-Ray

Speaking of expansion, we might take a "peek" in the X-ray department. At the moment it is in a state of transition, what with holes in the wall and again the sound of the hammer and drill. The X-ray personnel are a patient group, however, for they have visions of a super-deluxe department. They feel that when the job is completed and they return to normal routine once again, the inconvenience will have been well worthwhile.

New Oil Burner

Although we didn't visit the engine room, I understand that many changes are taking place there, too, which will eventually make the boiler room fully automatic. A new oil burner was installed and another project now underway is the rebricking of the boiler units.

After St. Andrew's became a Division of St. Barnabas, the *Voice of St. Barnabas* devoted a column in every issue to "St. Andrew's Highlights." In 1955, the description of a wedding appeared in that column. Dr. Alfred Jerofke, intern, married Marion Stavenow, radiologic technician. The wedding took place on Tuesday, September 15, 1955, at Trinity First Lutheran Church. Marion graduated from the radiologic technician program at St. Barnabas. She was working at St. Andrew's when she met Dr. Jerofke. Dr. Jerofke was from East Germany. He served an internship at St. Andrew's before beginning his residency at St. Barnabas.

St. Andrew's employees were also included regularly in the "Familiar Faces" column of the *Voice*. Two people honored as "Familiar Faces" in the same issue as the article about the remodeling of the hospital were Marjorie Person and Arthur Manske, both key people in their departments and both long-term employees of the hospital. Both also moved to the staff at St. Barnabas after St. Andrew's closed in 1963.

Art Manske was the chief engineer at St. Andrew's, but over the many years he served the hospital, he actually was often a "jack-of-all-trades." When he first arrived at St. Andrew's, more than twenty years before the article was written, he really did not intend to stay in Minneapolis. He had come from Chicago to accept what he understood to be a temporary position. The interviewer summed it up by saying, "Fortunately, he remained and now we would venture to say is almost indispensable."

Marjorie Person, RN, was the director of nurses at St. Andrew's. She transferred to St. Barnabas as a supervisor in nursing service. Her biographical sketch, taken partially from this article in the *Voice*, appears in the chapter entitled, "At the Center of It All."

On April 22, 1964, the following press release came from both St. Barnabas Hospital and the Minneapolis Presbytery of the United Presbyterian Church:

> St. Andrew's division of St. Barnabas Hospital has been purchased by the Minneapolis Presbytery of the United Presbyterian Church. The Board of Trustees of St. Barnabas and the Presbytery made the announcement today.
>
> St. Andrew's will be remodeled by the Presbytery to be used as a church-sponsored residence for single young working people and students. It will be known as 'Andrew House', and will be opened by September 1.
>
> Approximately a half block of property between Seventh and Eighth Avenues Southeast and Fourth and Fifth Streets is involved in the purchase. There are three buildings in addition to the hospital proper. Andrew Presbyterian Church is located on the opposite corner of the block.

St. Andrew's stood near the University of Minnesota campus and housing for students in that area of town was always at a premium. In its days as a hospital, many University students, the author of this book among them, were employed at the hospital while living in that area. The new use of the facility by the Presbytery meant the building continued to meet a need for people in Southeast Minneapolis. The circle which was started with Richard Chute and his mill at the Falls of St. Anthony one hundred years earlier and the relationship of that and other mills surrounding the falls to the founding of St. Barnabas, was completed. The summer 1963 issue of the *Voice of St. Barnabas* was devoted almost entirely to the closing of St. Andrew's. Included in that issue, along with the official statement of the closing of the division was this step-by-step accounting, kept by Marjorie Person, director of nurses, of the activities of the staff during the last days:

> Closing a hospital, even a small one, is a tremendous operation. Immediately following the announcement, plans for the big operation began to be formed. With patients to be cared for by every department until discharge or transfer, much of the work had to remain in the planning stage. However, orders already in to replenish present supplies could be cancelled or modified.
>
> The nursing service office had work that could be started at once. Final evaluations were written on all employees, and personnel records were completed and transferred to the Mother Hospital. Miss Schmidt and Mrs. Devereaux, nursing administration at St. Barnabas, arranged time for interviews with nursing staff members who were interested in transferring to the St. Barnabas staff.
>
> Arrangements were made by Mr. Manthey, Personnel, for representatives from other Minneapolis hospitals to hold interviews also. Reference requests from various hospitals began to arrive and these were taken care of at once.
>
> The student records of St. Andrew's School of Nursing had to be cared for. They were transferred to the St. Barnabas School of

Nursing and the Minnesota Board of Nursing was notified of their new location.

Former patient records had to be preserved and moved to St. Barnabas. A microfilming crew was soon at work, and the process of reducing vast piles of forms to compact rolls of film was begun... When completed, the entire file of film was moved to the medical records department at St. Barnabas.

After June 15, when no more patients were to be admitted, the real physical labor began. The operating room staff could safely begin closing their department. They retained only enough staff to provide operating room call coverage for emergencies of the patients already in the hospital. They began counting, packing and labeling their instruments and supplies. After the long inventory was completed the operating room staff bid their farewells and were the first to leave St. Andrew's.

As the patient census began to dwindle, the patients were consolidated...first on two floors and then on one. As each floor closed, inventories were made of supplies and station equipment—then packed, labeled and stored.

It seemed necessary that the X-ray and laboratory be kept in operation as long as we had patients to care for. When the last patient was discharged those departments were inventoried and transferred records and some of their equipment.

The last patient at St. Andrew's was transferred at 2:45 P.M., Tuesday, June 25, 1963.

Dietary began closing before the discharge of the last patient though meals continued to be served to personnel until noon, June 26. Delivery services were stopped after first estimating how much of each perishable item would be needed.

Then...inventory! Every pot, pan, piece of silverware, dish and gadget had to be counted, packed and labeled. Few of us realize what an enormous amount of equipment is used nor the quantity and

> variety of foods needed to provide balanced and varied diets for a hospital of patients and personnel. Even with the planning, there was some perishable food to be taken out for immediate use when meals were terminated. Pharmacy counted pills, vials and tubes, packed them with care and moved them to St. Barnabas. Narcotics and alcohol had to be checked out with the government officials before they could be transferred. Central supply inventoried all equipment and supplies and packed box after box. The business office packed and transferred all their accounts and records. Housekeeping had a tremendous task throughout the whole period.
>
> Finally, all departments were closed and inventories were completed. The vending and servicing companies had been notified. It seemed just about everything was completed. But…we had supplies and equipment on every service and every floor. Most of these supplies were returned to the storeroom at St. Barnabas. Some equipment in every department could be put to use at St. B; so inventories were re-checked and those items which were to be transferred were listed and removed from the inventories, then carried by van to their destination.
>
> The remaining equipment was finally moved to one storage location to await the future.
>
> Everyone has gone now except for the chief engineer and his assistant, and the work has been completed…? Even today I wonder, 'Did we forget to do anything?'"

The remainder of the page in that summer 1963 issue of the *Voice* was devoted to the plans of St. Andrew's staff members for their futures after the hospital was closed. That section is also quoted in its entirety:

> We have tried to find out what plans the staff members at St. Andrew's have made. Some will be found in the 'Spotlight' column, and here are some of the others…

Several RN's have joined the staff at St. Barnabas: Olga Aspers, Amy Backlin, Mayme Baldwin, Vera Johnson, Lillian Meyers, Rose Peterson, Florence Simonson and Rose Mary Tschida. Sharlot Ahlgren has joined the staff at Gillette; Sharon Bergstad has taken time off to have a baby; Freda Carmichael has gone to Sister Kenny; JoAnn Culligan to Eitel; Sandra Fisher to Montana with her husband; Lavilla Hering to Swedish; Margaret Janes to Mt. Sinai. Aileen Tottori will vacation in Hawaii and then to Texas with her army husband; Marlene Wasson to Shriners. Betty Aspenson and Lillian Blechert are retiring. The rest of the RNs will relax for the summer and some may join the St. Barnabas staff in the fall.

Several of the LPNs and PNs will take it easy for the summer also. Ruby Butz is going to Swedish and Janice Griswold will go to Eitel. Others who have joined the St. Barnabas staff are JoAnne Bendel, Anne Marie Collier, Renee Compton, Anna Salovich and Gladys Thompson.

Aides Maria Buryes, Sharon Espeland, Katharine Frydrych, Ida Kleven, Ellen Moore have gone to St. Barnabas. Edna Castleman will retire.

Orderly David Allan Lee has gone to Fairview, and Bennie Mathison and Ronald Wilson have gone to St. Barnabas.

Head dietitian Betty Griffen has gone with the Minnesota Public Health Department. Eva Beihoffer, Anna Holovka, Karen Helland, Martha Howe and Anna St. Cyr have retired.

In Housekeeping, Alton Anondson and Joseph Kaufman stayed at St. Andrew's temporarily and then went to St. Barnabas. Amelia Cochran, Gladys Peters and Genevieve Templeton have gone to Fairview.

Chief engineer Art Manske and Martin Sorenson are on duty at St. Andrew's with Pinkerton's taking over at night. Michael Siegmund, business manager, is at St. Barnabas as is Carol Wolff. Muriel Mc-

> Intire, cashier, has gone to Mt. Sinai and Jessie Wood, admitting, is relaxing for the summer.
>
> Irene Butters, PN on switchboard, has been ill at St. Barnabas. Ann Lohse has gone to Fairview. Operating room technician Helen McCarthy has come to St. Barnabas. Mary Salonen, medical records, is working for Dr. Bofencamp. Carol Geier, laboratory, has taken time off for a baby, and Janice Reynen has gone to St. Ansgar's in Moorhead.

This, in microcosm, is the procedure which had to be followed years later when Metropolitan Medical Ceneter-Mount Sinai closed its doors. Knowing how many details were involved in closing this small hospital, it is mind-boggling to think of all which had to be considered in closing a large medical center which had originally included two nursing schools and thousands of their graduates.

Chapter 9

Another First: The First Air-Conditioned Hospital

According to a short historical sketch included on the program for the dedication of the Whitney building April 17, 1937, a laundry building "fully equipped and furnished with machinery" was constructed in 1909 with funds provided by Miss Kate J. Welles. The short historical sketch also includes notation of the building in 1929 of an engine room, boiler plant, laundry and ice plant building. The funds for this construction were provided by Edwin C. Whitney and Sarah Whitney. That sketch indicates the cost to have been $162,000. Another report indicates the sum was $143,005. Whatever the cost, it constituted a substantial gift from the Whitneys. The cost of the 1909 laundry facility is not known, but taken with previous gifts from Mrs. and Miss Welles, including a substantial amount they contributed in 1916 toward debt liquidation, certainly put them in the category of unusual friends of the hospital. No wonder there were buildings named for both the Whitneys and the Welles.

Apparently the 1909 laundry building became obsolete and was replaced twenty years later with the facility financed by the Whitneys. The record doesn't so indicate, but it appears the 1929 building was constructed nearly in the middle of the block between Sixth and Seventh Streets and Ninth and Tenth Avenues. Many will remember it as the building which stood between the parking lot which faced Sixth Street and the approach to the ambulance entrance to the Whitney building.

The negotiations which resulted in the bequest with which the Whitney building was constructed, were carried out over a period of more than twenty years, during which Mr. Whitney died, so he never saw the building he worked so hard to finance. In 1916, Mr. Whitney, then a resident of Ottawa, Canada, visited Minneapolis and initiated the discussions that finally culminated in his providing for the construction of a new hospital wing. His outspoken, negative opinion of the Pavilion building is included in a previous chapter of this book. During the nineteenth century, the Whitneys were living in Minneapolis, and, at one point Mrs. Whitney became very ill and was treated at the Cottage Hospital. They were indigents then, but during the almost fifty years which had elapsed since that illness, Mr. Whitney achieved what he described as "moderate success" in the lumber industry. Knowing what we know today of his bequests to the hospital, we probably would be more inclined to describe him as highly successful. At any rate, by 1916, his mortality was on his mind as he was advancing in years and he was considering ways he might be able to reward the hospital for the kindness shown them and for the saving of his wife's life so many years before.

During those intervening years, he had become friends with James J. Hill and through correspondence with Mr. Hill he had kept tabs on the growth and fortunes of the hospital after he left Minneapolis. It appears he had not returned to Minneapolis in all that time. By 1916, Mr. Hill could no longer provide information to him for he had passed on, so the Whitneys returned for a visit to the city of their early years. Mr. Whitney made arrangements to meet with James E. Freeman, then president of the hospital board, and inquired of him how much debt the hospital was carrying at the time. When he learned it was $95,000, he admonished Mr. Freeman by telling him the hospital should not have a debt. He advised steps be taken to liquidate that debt, since paying interest reduces the amount of income available for operating expense

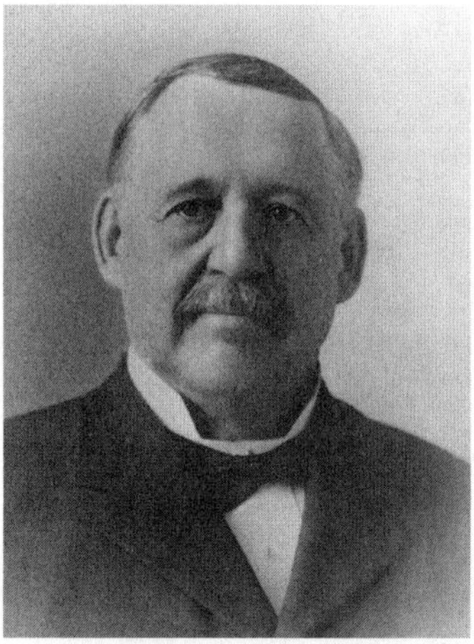
Edwin C. Whitney

He went on with Mr. Freeman, proposing that if the board would liquidate the debt, he would more than match that amount by presenting the hospital with $100,000. He also learned from Mr. Freeman that in addition to the outstanding $95,000, the board had either recently borrowed another $7,500 or was about to borrow $7,500. This amount was to be used to buy two small homes which, apparently in addition to Wellesmere, would house nurses near the hospital. Mr. Whitney offered to give an additional $7,500 to liquidate that debt, this amount being in addition to the $100,000 already offered. In offering the additional $7,500, Mr. Whitney made clear the fact that he wanted to give money in recognition for the care given Mrs. Whitney, but he wanted the board to be prudent in handling its funds. He proposed giving a reasonable amount of time for liquidation of the $95,000 debt, but cautioned that it should not take too long for he was concerned about his health and wanted everything in order before he died.

Like Richard Martin had done years before, he was throwing a challenge to the board and stating the conditions which had to be met in order for them to receive the prize of his moneys. In 1916, there were still lots on the east end of the block between Sixth and Seventh Streets and Ninth and Tenth Avenues, which were not owned by the hospital. Mr. Whitney asked how much it would cost to purchase those properties, making possible future expansion of the hospital complex. He was given an estimate of $50,000 to purchase the remainder of the block. They discussed the possibility of erecting a well-equipped pathological laboratory on the property to serve the hospitals of the region and to engage in research work. Although the idea was discussed, it never came to fruition.

Following the meeting with Mr. Whitney, Mr. Freeman met with the board and they agreed to mount a campaign to liquidate the debt of $95,000

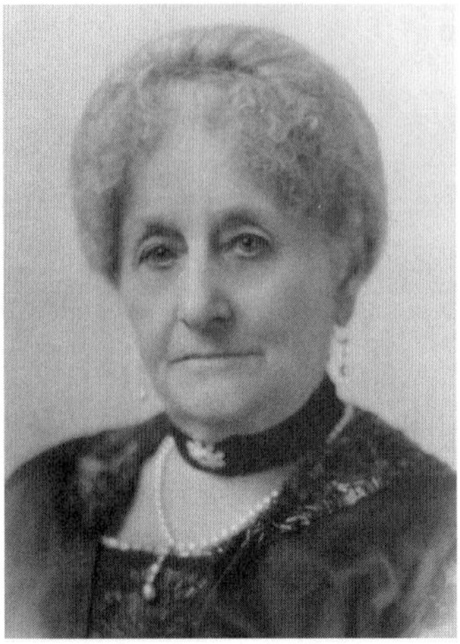

Mrs. Edwin Whitney

by January 1, 1917. Mr. F. M. Prince, chairman of the board of the First Security National Bank and member of the hospital board, agreed to lead the campaign. Ultimately the campaign for the liquidation of debt was successful. It appears that among the donors who contributed heavily to the campaign were Mrs. Thomas Welles and her daughter, Catherine (Kate). The board voted to send a letter to Mrs. and Miss Welles thanking them for their generous contributions of both time and money to the hospital over the years.

On January 22, 1917, Mrs. Sarah Whitney sent a check for $7,500 to pay for the properties purchased earlier to house nurses. She was in receipt of certification that the hospital debt had been liquidated by the campaign of 1916, so on the same date she also enclosed a check for $100,000 as promised by the Whitneys during their visit with Mr. Freeman in 1916.

In the letter of thanks to the Whitneys for their generous contributions, the board secretary, L. R. Robertson, wrote, "The Board of Trustees of St. Barnabas Hospital acknowledges with profound gratitude the gift by Sarah C. Whitney, wife of Edwin C. Whitney…of One Hundred Seven Thousand Five Hundred Dollars for the purposes of the hospital. Realizing that words are inadequate at such a time to express our real appreciation of such kindly and helpful generosity, this board can but assure the donors of this magnificent gift that for themselves and those who may succeed them, they pledge their utmost endeavors to the end that the Christian service of this institution shall ever be kept to the high standard that such interest and helpfulness as (yours) demands."

Letters were also sent to parties who had contributed funds to the debt liquidation campaign as well as a special letter to Mr. F. M. Prince for his outstanding leadership of that campaign. The board treasurer was instructed to deposit the Whitney check for $100,000 on a certificate of deposit drawn with the First and Security National Bank or the Minneapolis Trust Company. A building committee of three persons was appointed to develop plans for a new building in accord with the wishes expressed by Mr. Whitney at the time the proposal for the bequest in reward for debt liquidation was made.

From 1917 on through 1918 and all the years to 1934, the board did not act on the building project which Mr. Whitney had suggested and hoped to see come to pass. They were notified that Mr. Whitney died on February 18, 1924. In March of 1925, the board was notified the hospital had received a bequest in accordance with Mr. Whitney's will. It included eight shares of stock in the Mississippi Land Company plus one-fourth of Mr. Whitney's estate.

Finally in 1934, at the prodding of board member Mr. J. Fred Quest, the construction of the Whitney building was authorized. It had been fourteen years since Mr. Whitney's death.

In defense of the board over those fourteen years they had studied various ways the money should be spent. For example, in 1925 they made an agreement with Magney and Tusler, Minneapolis architects, to draw up plans for a power plant and laundry and to make a survey to recommend future construction for the hospital. As for the survey, no further reference is made to it in board minutes. An architect's sketch and block plan are on file at the Metropolitan Medical Center Historical Library, which may be the plan referred to above from Magney and Tusler, although the sketch has a signature which says "Hewitt & Brown, Architects-Engineers." The plan is not dated. It could be the plan from 1925, or it may date back to 1917 when there was a building committee looking at the possibility of adding a new wing to the hospital. Whether this plan was ever used by the board in planning further construction is unknown. The one known fact about it is that it predated the Whitney building, for the proposed building was on the site later occupied by the Whitney building.

The architect's plan showed an H-shaped building facing Seventh Street with a long arm on the west looking much like the Pavilion building already on that site and an identical arm on Tenth Avenue extending the full length of the block between Sixth and Seventh Streets. The crosspiece of the H would have been approximately where the Whitney building was built. The block plan labeled that cross piece "Administration" and showed a chapel attached to the north side of that part of the building.

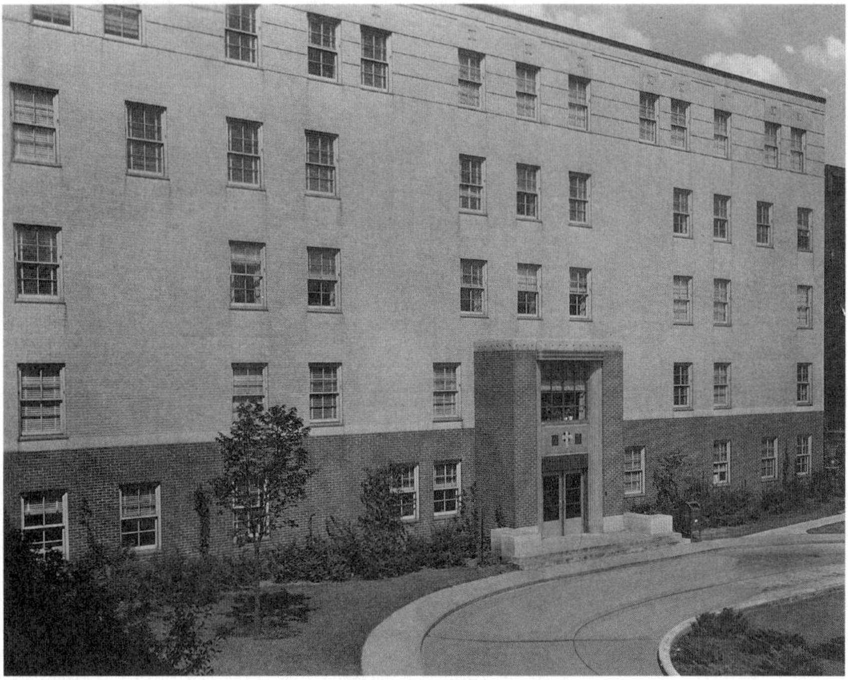

Whitney Building, 1940s and 1950s.

In March of 1930 the board had voted to build a new hospital and had engaged an architect, but the project was cancelled when the value of the stock from the Whitney bequest declined dramatically. It could be that the plans described in the previous paragraphs were those for the building that was to be constructed at that time. Board minutes for 1931 indicate the value of the Whiney bequest at that time was $300,000.

Finally, on January 22, 1936, the board authorized the construction of the building and the project went forward. Notes included on the program for the dedication of the Whitney building in 1937, the completed cost of the building was $275,000, almost twice the amount ($150,000) authorized, but still within the amount left of the Whitney bequest.

The program from the dedication service also notes, "From the very first, St. Barnabas Hospital has been known as a Church hospital, and is under the care of the diocese of Minnesota. The chaplain at the present time is the Rev. Joseph Walker, who is always ready to respond to a call from any patient, whether a member of the Episcopal Church or not. The diocese of Minnesota is justly proud of the standing and reputation of St. Barnabas

Hospital, and diocesan authorities are keen to cooperate in all that belongs to the spiritual and material welfare of the hospital."

Listed in the program as features of the new building were these descriptions:

> Fire proof five story building with a new entrance at 920 South Seventh Street; Year around air conditioning with three separate systems, one each for operating rooms, nursery and general floors, whereby temperatures and humidity can be controlled in any room.
>
> Accoustically treated throughout; One floor devoted to maternity patients, with delivery rooms, nursery and a father's room; Two general patient floors; One floor for administrative offices; X-Ray department, newly equipped for radiographic work, and 200,000 and 400,000 volt deep therapy X-Ray equipment; Pathological laboratories; Central Supply room; Pharmacy; Doctors Lounge.

Not included on the list, but included in the new building were a telephone switchboard and an ambulance entrance with an emergency room.

The Whitney wing was the first air-conditioned hospital built in the United States, so in that respect it was a model for all hospital construction after that. It is likely that for a period of years after it opened, other hospitals were watching to determine what the reaction of patients, families and visitors would be. Even today with a large number of private residences being built with central air, there are skeptical people who would rather live without it. One thing learned early on was that one thermostat setting would not please everyone. The patient in 231 might find the temperature exactly right, while the one down the hall in 237 was complaining that it was too cold and across the hall in 240 the patient was asking if anything could be done to "cool it off in here." Different strokes for different folks, as the old saying goes.

The new entrance to the hospital opened on a horseshoe drive off of Seventh Street, which made it easy for a patient to go directly to a private vehicle from the front entrance without blocking traffic on the busy Seventh Street. East and north of the new wing were parking lots for visitors and staff.

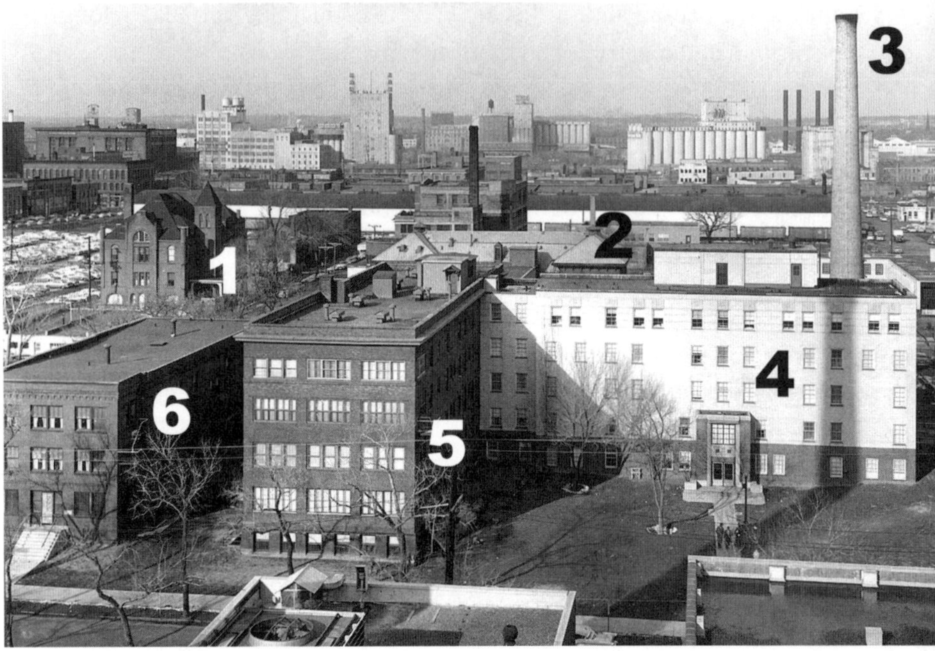

St. Barnabas Hospital, 1940s and 1950s. 1) Knickerbacker Residence; 2) Roof of Martin Building facing Sixth Street; 3) Smokestack adjacent to laundry building; 4) Whitney building; 5) Pavilion building; and 6) Wellesmere Residence on the corner of Seventh Street and Ninth Avenue South.

The new building was built of a cream colored brick with reddish brown brick trim. It provided a nice contrast with the red brick of the Pavilion building and Wellesmere and the red brick trim helped to tie the design of the buildings all together. The horseshoe drive and the color difference in the Whitney building decidedly improved the whole appearance of the St. Barnabas Hospital complex.

With the addition of the Whitney building and the conversion of some of the Corridor rooms to purposes other than patient rooms, the bed capacity of the hospital was listed as 195 patients plus 42 bassinets and space for 10 premature infants.

Chapter 10

The Phoenix Rises: 1958

In the February-March 1957 issue of the *Voice of St. Barnabas*, Helen Hayden wrote of the demolition of Smith House, the last vestige of a bygone era during which the area around Sixth, Seventh and Eighth Streets South was a grand residential neighborhood. Elsewhere in the same issue of the *Voice* was a picture of the dilapidated old apartment houses on Chicago Avenue between Seventh and Eighth Streets South as they, too, fell to the wrecking ball. The Griddle, that old diner on the corner of Eighth Street and Ninth Avenue South, earlier had gone the way the apartments and Smith House went in 1957. Students of the 1940s and 1950s had long enjoyed the convenience of the Griddle when a hamburger seemed more appealing to them than the fare in the hospital cafeteria. Helen ended her article about Smith House with these words: "We hope soon to see a new St. Barnabas arising like a Phoenix bird from the ashes of the old buildings of a bygone era."

Following World War II, the whole scene in health care changed markedly. The worth of sulfa and antibiotic drugs in treating infections was proven by their extensive use in treating wounded and sick servicemen during the war. Once the war ended, these miracle drugs became available for the civilian population. The great volume of surgeries that were performed in treating battlefield injuries brought improvements in that specialty to civilian patients at war's end. Weddings postponed because of the war were conducted when the men returned home in the late 1940s. And soon after, a baby boom was the natural result. A comparison of hospital statistics from 1931, 1941 and 1951 at St. Barnabas demonstrates the dramatic changes that had taken place. The 3,224 patients admitted to the hospital in 1931 had nearly doubled (to 6,189) in 1941 and quadrupled (12,434) by 1951. The same could be said for the number of babies born—401 in 1931, 1,051 in 1941 and 2,081 in 1951. And operations—1,610 in 1931, 2,658 in 1941 and 4,638 in 1951. Even more dramatic were the increases in X-ray and lab procedures done. In 1931, 733 X-rays were taken, averaging about 2 per day, while by 1941, the number had increased to nearly 10 per day (3,340) and by 1951, that number had increased again by more than three fold to

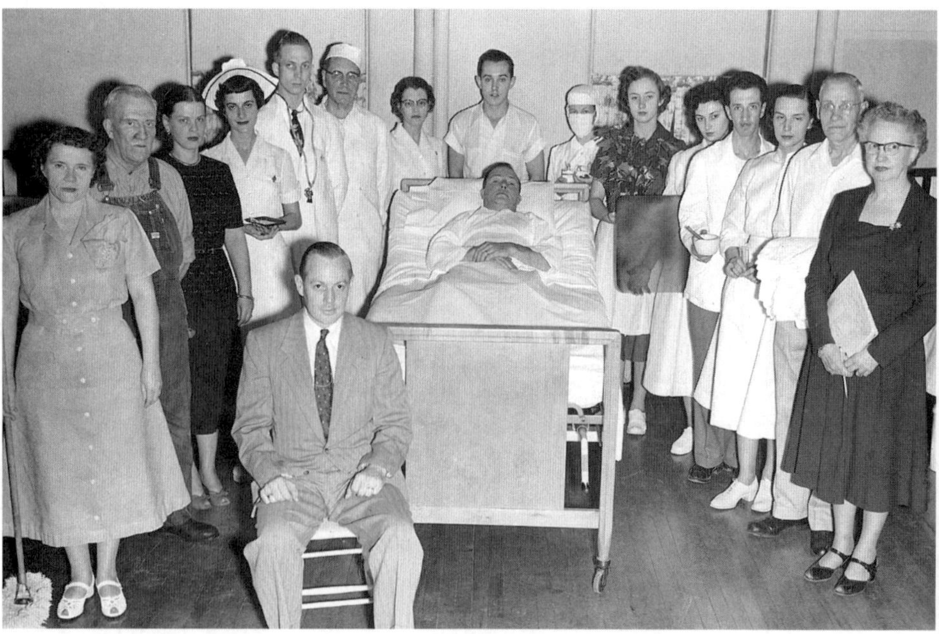

Sixteen of more than thirty categories of personnel involved in patient care, early 1950s

11,363. Lab procedures totaled 4,444 in 1931, more than five times more in 1941 (25,930) and about twenty-four times as many in 1951 (102,733). The hospital board, looking at these dramatic changes in hospital utilization, came to the realization that the time was again approaching when the physical plant that was St. Barnabas Hospital would be inadequate to meet the needs of the population, especially in services like X-ray, the laboratory and pharmacy.

Charles Bolles Rogers was elected president of the board in June of 1937, only two months after dedication of the Whitney building. With the new building, state of the art in hospital construction of that day, and the high quality of leadership provided by Mr. Rogers, St. Barnabas entered the modern era. Then came the war—both doctors and nurses left civilian life to serve the military during the national emergency. Even Mr. Rogers left civilian life to offer his services with the Red Cross overseas. When he returned to Minneapolis at war's end, he was again elected president of the board. And discussions were held regarding the need for new hospital facilities.

A bequest of $200,000 came to the hospital from the George H. Christian estate. The money was to be used to build a new wing at St. Barnabas. Mr. Christian, a pioneer flour miller and member of the first Board of Trustees of St. Barnabas (1883), had served as first treasurer of the hospital. He knew well the financial problems the hospital had faced in the last two decades of the nineteenth century and resolved a portion of his estate would go to the hospital upon his death for the purpose of expanding its facilities. There was a question of space for a new wing, however. A potential site existed on the east side of the Whitney building, but it would have eliminated parking spaces which were already at a premium for the hospital. And just adding a new wing probably wouldn't have solved the problems, for at that point the once glorious Martin building had passed its prime and really needed replacement more than updating or repair. The same could be said for the Corridor building. Magney, Tusler and Setter, Architects, were engaged to draw up plans for a new wing. Mr. Rogers threw himself not behind the new wing proposal, but behind one to build a large downtown medical center in the area today covered by Hennepin County General Medical Center. It would have been a joint project of Minneapolis General and several of the nearby private hospitals, St. Barnabas among them. That idea went nowhere, however. There was insufficient support from any of the hospitals involved and so the proposal died.

As the decade of the 1950s wore on, it became more apparent to the board that an entirely new hospital would be more cost effective than adding a new wing to the existing hospital complex. In 1955, Mr. Newell P. Weed Jr., chaired a building committee of the board. About that time, the United Hospital Fund of Minneapolis and Hennepin County had been formed and funds they provided allowed the board to proceed with plans for an entirely new facility. The first step was to purchase the rest of the block between Seventh and Eighth Streets and Chicago and Ninth Avenue South. The hospital already owned the property on which Smith House stood, at the corner of Seventh Street and Ninth Avenue South. But there were several old apartment buildings along Chicago Avenue which had to be purchased, then demolished, to make room for the new hospital. During the following two years, all the necessary purchases were made and all the old structures in the block were leveled in preparation for the construction of the new building.

Ground breaking for the new St. Barnabas took place on April 17, 1957. Mr. Newell Weed was the keynote speaker for the ceremony. He opened his remarks saying, "Many of the Trustees of the Hospital are here today and certainly every member of the board shares with me the thrill and satisfaction in seeing this long-awaited project officially commence."

Then he went on to pay tribute to the vision of St. Barnabas leaders of the past and to past building projects. He said, "The buildings which were built in these past years and the building on which we are to start construction today are not in themselves the answer that we seek. They are only a vehicle that we are trying to provide so that the skills of our medical and nursing staffs have the best physical facilities surround them and so that this community will have the best medical service that it is possible for us to provide within the scope of our vision and abilities."

The cornerstone of the new building was laid on June 11, 1958. Participating in the ceremony that day were the Right Reverend Hamilton H. Kellogg, Bishop of Minnesota, the Reverend Perry M. Gilfillan, hospital chaplain, and Mr. Valentine Wuertele, president of the Board of Trustees. The student nurse choir under the direction of Mr. Howard Englund, sang two hymns. The program opened with a welcome by Mr. Wuertele, followed

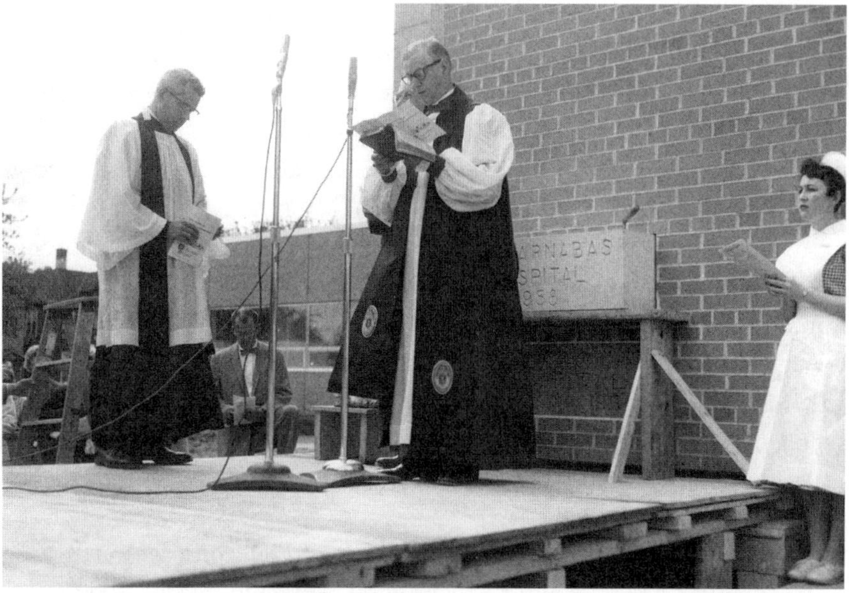

Laying of cornerstone, 1958 building. The Rev. Perry Gilfillan and the Right Reverend Hamilton Kellogg, 11 June 1958.

by the choir singing "Faith of Our Fathers." Next came responsive readings from Psalms led by Chaplain Gilfillan. Bishop Kellogg gave brief remarks in which he said, "Brethren, we are assembled to lay the cornerstone of a house which is set apart to the healing of the sick in body and soul and to the service of Almighty God in the name of Christ our Lord. Hearken therefore, and consider how our Saviour commends this work to us."

He then quoted the words of Jesus from St. Luke 9:1-2, 6, following it with prayer. The cornerstone was put in place with a responsive reading led by the Bishop and Mr. Wuertele and the saying of the St. Barnabas Prayer. Prayers by the Bishop followed and finally the people assembled repeated the Lord's Prayer. An appropriate closing to the ceremony was the singing by the student nurse choir of the St. Barnabas Hymn, followed by the benediction given by Bishop Kellogg.

Of interest are the documents which were placed in the box within the cornerstone on that day. They included a copy of the hospital annual report from 1888-89, the Articles of Incorporation from 1893, a copy of the 1893 Prayer Book, A short history of the hospital up to 1893, The Annual Report of the Bishop and Council of 1957, the hospital annual report of

1957, Articles of Incorporation and corporation bylaws for 1956, the bylaws of the Research Foundation, 1956, the bylaws and list of current Medical Staff, 1955, the Constitution and Bylaws of the Women's Auxiliary, 1958, a copy of the Diocesan Journal of 1957, a history of the new hospital and the United Hospital Fund, prepared by Mr. Newell Weed, 1957-58, a copy of the Star Tribune, June 11, 1958, a copy of Minnesota Missionary, 1957-58, Minnesota Statehood Stamps, Issued May 11, 1958, a patient admitting folder, the Personnel Handbook and Directory of 1958, pictures of the St. Barnabas buildings as of 1958, a copy of the program of the cornerstone laying, June 11, 1958, a copy of the program of the ground breaking, April 17, 1957, a School of Nursing catalog and a school brochure of 1958, a sketch of history, 1893-1958 by J. Fred Quest, Sr. and a copy of the *Voice of St. Barnabas*, 1957-58. Several of these documents have been used in writing this story of the hospital.

Also listed on the program were the names of all the officers and trustees of the hospital. This list will be found in the appendix of this book along with lists of all the known officers and trustees through the years from the beginning of the hospital. The *Voice of St. Barnabas* for December 1958-January 1959, gave this account of the dedication of the new building on November 19, 1958: "Formal dedication services took place Wednesday, November 19, when the Right Reverend Hamilton Kellogg, Bishop of the Episcopal Diocese of Minnesota, snipped a ribbon of gauze strung across the lobby with a pair of surgical scissors. Then a solemn procession of student nurses, clergy and trustees wound its way down the corridor to the chapel for further ceremonies.

Actively participating were Mr. Valentine Wuertele, president of the Board of Trustees; the Right Reverend Philip McNairy, Suffragan Bishop of Minnesota; the Reverend Perry Gilfillan, chaplain of the hospital and Mr. Stanley Hawks, president of the United Hospital Fund. An open house was held for hospital personnel and their friends and families for two days, November 22 and 23, 1958. Members of the auxiliary hosted the 5,000 people who attended on the two days and conducted them on guided tours of the building. One of those in attendance at the Dedication Ceremony was Mr. Charles Bolles Rogers whose leadership in the 1940s and early 1950s began the process which culminated in the building of the new hospital.

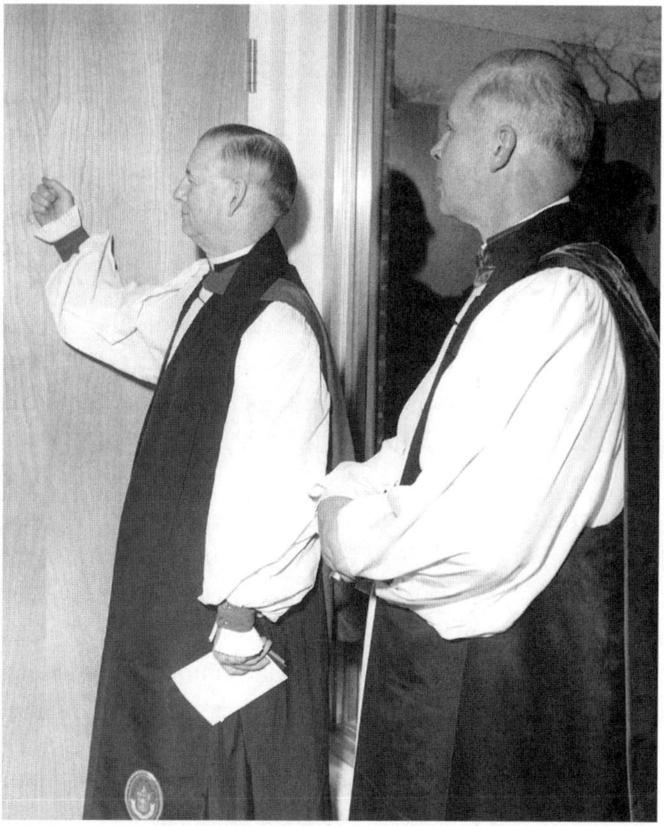

The Rev. Henry Hancock and the Rt. Rev. Philip McNairy knocking on the door of Whitney Residence, dedication service, fall of 1959.

The hospital was the first to be built with moneys from the United Hospital Fund.

The 1958 hospital was a five and one half million-dollar building. It had a capacity of three hundred eight adult beds, including eighty-eight private rooms, fifty-two double rooms and twenty-seven four-bed rooms. In addition, there were twenty-one rooms for pediatric patients and sixty-six cribs and bassinets on the maternity floors. The accommodations were changed over time, but never to larger than four-bed rooms and the great number of private rooms as compared to multiple bedrooms continued.

A twenty-four hour shift required the services of one hundred ninety RNs and LPNs assisted by one hundred twenty two ancillary nursing staff. Staff for all other departments in addition to nursing are not included in those figures, so there was a sizeable group of employees working every day just to keep the services to patients going. In addition, there were many members of the Women's Auxiliary on duty every day carrying out all the activities which have been described for them in an another chapter of this book. Long gone were the days when students were the only nurses on duty in the hospital. The nursing school in 1958 was taking about fifty students per year, but the service they provided in patient care days was incidental to their courses in nursing. Every station had at least one instructor assigned to pick and choose patients to whom their students would be assigned, based on what they were learning in the classroom at the time. There were two hundred twenty five MDs on staff covering all the usual areas of practice plus most of the medical specialties of the day. The ground floor and tunnel levels of the new hospital were shaped like a large square. The floors from two-five were arranged on the top of the square in an offset cross pattern. The core or center where the arms of the cross intersected was the service area of every floor. There were dumb waiters to the tunnel level and a tube system which allowed quick transfer of messages and small items to and from services located in the tunnel level, (for example Central Supply, Pharmacy and Dietary.) Carts of meal trays were set up in Dietary and brought to the stations by Dietary employees who helped with distribution of trays and came back to pick up the used trays at the end of a meal. A nurse-saver communication system allowed every patient to speak to someone at the nursing station when they needed assistance or had questions. Every effort was made to relieve the nurse of non-nursing duties so that maximum effort could be geared to meeting nursing needs of patients.

On the main floor of the hospital, a large lobby occupied the southeast corner of the square. The main entrance faced Ninth Avenue South on the east side of the building. Directly ahead of the front entrance was the Information Desk. In addition to consulting personnel on duty at the desk, visitors and others could follow colored stripes on the floor that led to X-ray, Laboratory, Physical Medicine and the elevators in the core of the building. Nowadays, those colored stripes are in widespread usage in hospitals, but at the time they were considered an innovation.

Behind the Information Desk and to the left (facing south) was the administration corridor. Hospital administration personnel and community relations were on the east side of the hall with a board conference room at the end of the hall. On the west side of the hall were nursing administration offices with their own nursing conference room. Returning from the administration wing to the center of the hospital one came to the Christian Memorial Chapel. A bronze plaque outside the chapel carried the inscription, "This chapel is given by the Citizens' Aid Society in grateful remembrance and loving memory of Leonora Hall Christian, 1845-1916, wife of George Henry Christian." One of the stipulations made in the bequest from George Henry Christian's estate was that a portion of the money be used to build a new chapel in memory of his wife, so the new chapel fulfilled that obligation, incurred years earlier when the Christian bequest was accepted by the board. Mr. and Mrs. Val Wuertele donated a new electronic organ that was installed in a small room at the front of the chapel. The organ in the chapel of the old hospital was a reed pump organ. Having the new, easier to play electronic organ facilitated securing volunteer organists for chapel services.

Also in the core area of the ground floor were elevators which had buttons and lights for an eight story building, though there were only five stories in the building at the time of construction. The extra buttons and lights were meant to be activated should the building be extended three floors higher at some future time. The foundations were constructed to be able to handle such expansion when and if it were needed.

Beyond the elevators was a corridor leading west and another leading north. Looking west in that corridor, on the left was the operating suite and the emergency room. At the end of the hall was the ambulance entrance. There were nine operating rooms in the new suite, double the number in the old Whitney building. Gone were the days when anesthetic agents were so explosive that operating rooms were placed on the top floor of the hospital to minimize damage to patient areas should an anesthetic explode. Having the operating suite adjacent to the emergency room enabled staff to move critically injured patients or critically ill patients requiring emergency surgery quickly from the emergency room to surgery.

Across the hall from the emergency room was the hospital laboratory with space dramatically larger than they had occupied in the Whitney building, enabling the laboratory to provide more services to patients.

Going back to the center of the building, on the left was another corridor, leading north. Facing north, on the left side of the hall was Physical Medicine. Like the laboratory, the physical medicine department had much more space in the new building than they had in the old St. Barnabas. Across the hall from Physical Medicine was X-ray, and they, too, had much more space than the small area they had on first floor of the Whitney building. They were able to increase the size of their X-ray technology program after the move to the new building.

The layout of the rooms for inpatient care was similar on each of the floors from the second through the fifth floor. There was the core area service room convenient to two nursing stations. The nursing desk for each station was just outside the service room and patient rooms were in two wings radiating out from the nursing desk. On the A side of the building, the wings radiated to the north and west. On the B side of the building the wings radiated to the south and the east. No matter which direction the wing faced, the room arrangement was all private rooms on one side of the hall and multiple bedrooms, almost all doubles, were on the other side of the hall. This facilitated moving staff from one station to another since they always knew the floor plan whether the station wasmedical, surgical or maternity. Maternity was on the second floor. Third floor was Pediatrics and one surgical station, primarily orthopedic and urologic surgical patients.

Florence Buck, who had been the head nurse on 5P in the old hospital, moved with her staff to 3B when the new hospital was opened. This was consistent with the plans carried out throughout the new facility. Insofar as possible, the staff of a unit in the old building was carried over intact to a station in the new building. Because there were more beds in the new building, each staff was augmented with some new people, but otherwise, unless a staff member requested transfer, they were moved together and continued to work together in the new building. There were two stations for medical patients on the fourth floor. The staff headed by Clara Johnson on

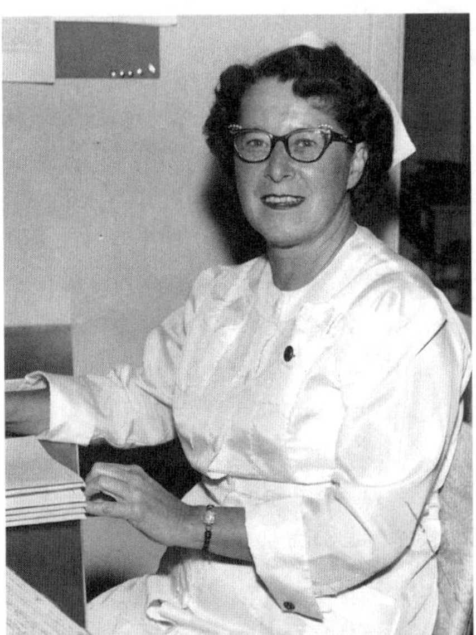

Clara O. Johnson.

2W moved to 4A in the new building. The staff from 2P, headed by Irene Nelson, moved to 4B. On fifth floor were two surgical units. 5A staff came from 3W in the old building. Helen Krieg had been the head nurse on 3W for years, but she moved to head of Central Supply in the new building, so the head nurse on 5A was Irene Peper, who had been Helen's assistant head nurse during the Whitney days. On 5B was the staff from the old 4 Martin, under the direction of Norma Seebach, who had been head nurse on 4M for several years.

There were several ways the new building itself led to improvements in patient care. Among the advantages were as follows: 1) Having the core area service and supply room meant more supplies were kept on the station so there was less running and less time lost in waiting for supplies to come from another area of the hospital; 2) The pneumatic tube allowed requests for Pharmacy, Dietary and/or Central Supply to be filled much faster than previously when an unexpected need for something meant a staff member had to run to the department in question to obtain the needed item or items; 3) In the new hospital, there was a chart nurse trained and assigned to every unit. They reviewed patient charts after doctors had been on the unit and began implementation of any orders left by the doctor, preparing requisitions which would be needed to implement doctors' orders. They also were trained to chart routine things, leaving the RN or LPN free to concentrate on charting professional observations and treatments; 4) The meal carts which brought meal trays to the nursing units had both a heated and a refrigerated side. Foods were loaded in the appropriate side of the cart, then trays were assembled on site at the station so that hot foods were hotter and cold foods were colder. When Dietary supplied staff to help deliver and pick up trays, nursing staff were freed to concentrate more on tasks only they could do; 5) The direct connection between the emergency room and the operating suite saved time in getting critically injured patients into surgery as quickly as possible. That also decreased emotional trauma for families since emergency patients could be taken directly to the treatment modality they needed without waiting for elevators and traveling through public hallways; 6) Oxygen piped into one hundred four medical and surgical rooms and all twenty one rooms on pediatrics meant the oxygen was always there, readily available when a need was identified. In the old hospital, an orderly had to go to the supply room, select a tank and the needed gauges and transport all of that to the station after the need for oxygen was identified and the order obtained; 7) The "Nurse-saver" communication system was reassuring to patients and families, for the patient could speak directly to someone about a need. Nursing staff were also better served by the system for they could take the needed supplies with them on one trip to the patient's room rather than answering a light, getting the needed information, then running back to the service or medication room to get what they needed to serve the patient.

When it was time to transport patients from the old hospital to the new, extra staff and volunteers were on hand to help with the process. The whole business was facilitated by the presence of a tunnel which had been constructed under Seventh Street connecting the old buildings and the new. The tunnel was a necessity for the regular operation of the new hospital because all of the laundry facilities and some of the maintenance facilities were kept in their buildings on the north side of Seventh Street. There was a motorized vehicle which was used to pull carts of soiled linens to the laundry and to pull carts of clean linens from the laundry to the new building. On moving day, priority was given to patients in wheelchairs, on Gurneys or in beds over the laundry train with its carts. The move went off smoothly in spite of cold weather outside and traffic on Seventh Street since all of that was bypassed in the tunnel. The tunnel also served students well, for after the new hospital was built, the Whitney and Pavilion buildings were converted to student housing and school offices. Students could go through the tunnel from their rooms to a duty station without exposure to the elements on the street above.

In an appeal for employees to adopt a demeanor in keeping with the physical environment surrounding them in the new hospital, Helen Hayden wrote the following article for the February-March 1959 issue of the *Voice of St. Barnabas*. The article is quoted in its entirety:

> Let us look to ourselves and consider the intangible responsibility that must be ours in helping to create the personality of the New St. Barnabas Hospital—the personality that will clothe the stern and unyielding walls of brick and mortar with a warmth and softness that only the hospital personnel can impart—creating an outgoing personality as patients leave with a memory of a single

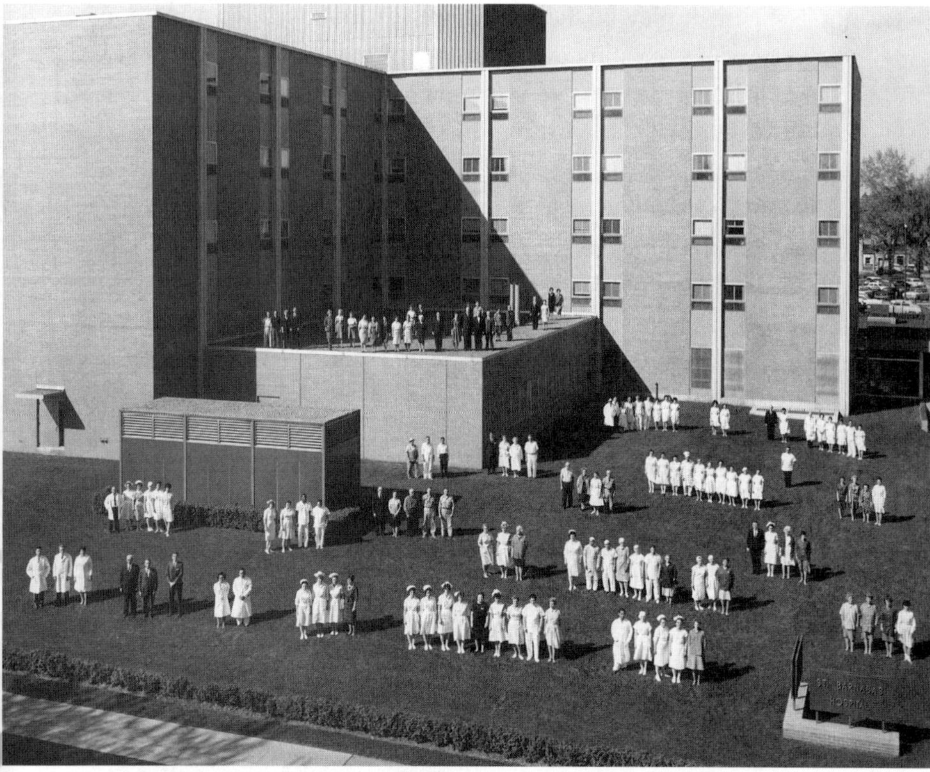

Each person in this photo represents one job category required to operate St. Barnabas Hospital. Hospital Week, 1962.

outstanding act of kindness and understanding or the patina of a general solicitude.

Evaluation of the technical skill and exactitude of nursing procedures is assumed as 'value received' but the special bit of kindness is an extra dividend and it is this that is remembered. When two or more friends get together and their 'main event' is under discussion–the 'rare and unusual' surgery or the equally 'unusual' sequence leading to the birth of a child–it is then that these extra dividends color the stories and are the memory fragments of their hospital stay. It may be the understanding given by the admitting clerk as the patient sits panic stricken trying to remember his telephone number for the records; it may be the courtesy shown by the floor nurse who puts them at ease as they stumble numbly off the elevator; it may be the student nurse who takes the trouble to explain away a question in the patient's mind—a question that has lost its importance by its very familiarity and routineness; it could be the orderly who was so inordinately gentle in his handling of a patient in his helplessness; or the quiet concern and help given by the business office personnel as the patient checked out. These could, any or all, be bits of memory in the minds of patients—bits that endure through the months and years and become a lasting part of the intangible personality that will enhance the New St. Barnabas Hospital.

When all was said and done, the people of Minneapolis and the board and staff of the hospital got their money's worth from the five and one half million dollars it cost to build the new hospital. It would serve all well for another generation until the next phase of the hospital began. Several features which were innovations to staff at the time the building was constructed became standard in hospital buildings after that. Like the air conditioning in the Whitney building, what was new at the time became run of the mill in later times. But in Minneapolis St. Barnabas did it first!

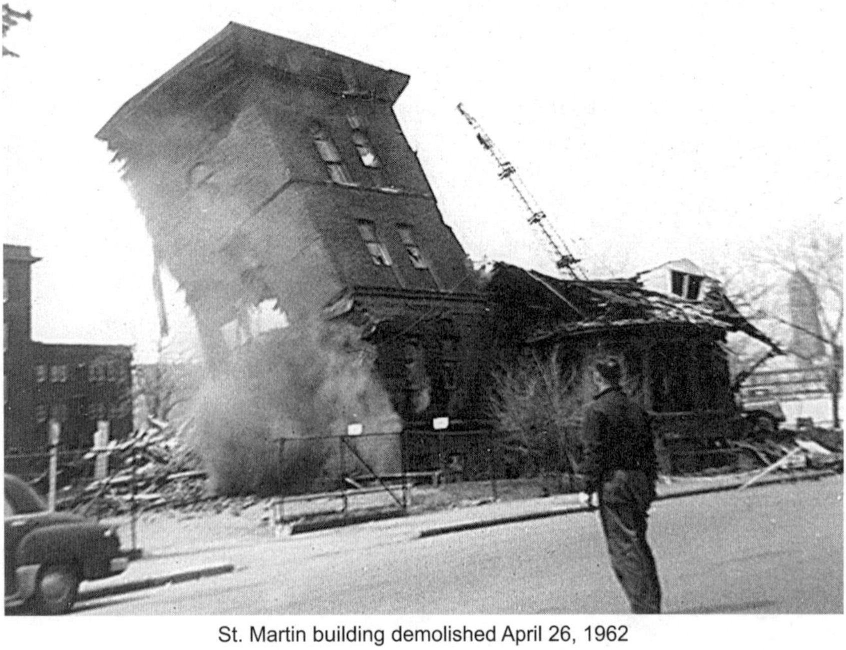

St. Martin building demolished April 26, 1962

Chapter 11

A Medical Staff Is Organized

A booklet describing St. Barnabas Hospital in detail was published in 1916. In it was a short history of the hospital that included the names of the first physicians to be associated with the hospital. Listed were Doctors A. E. Ames, J. J. Linn and Edwin Phillips. We have little information about these three. One, Dr. Ames, was a member of the good rector's Gethsemane Brotherhood. He was Surgeon-General of the state militia in 1859. Reports of the time also indicated he was held in high esteem among the poor of the city. Nothing is known about Doctors Linn and Phillips other than their names and nothing is known about the preparation of any of the three to practice medicine. It is understood all three gave their services without charge to either the patient or the hospital.

The quality of medical education and resultant quality of medicine practiced in the large cities of the eastern states was fairly good for the times, but the best doctors there were likely to stay in those eastern cities to practice rather than to venture out to the frontier, which Minnesota was in the mid nineteenth century. The Mayo brothers, practicing during the last part of the century in Rochester were among the first doctors in Minnesota to insist on university preparation for the practice of medicine. Even their father, William Worrell Mayo, good doctor that he was, came up through the ranks of apprenticeship as his preparation for medical practice.

Medical practice in those early days in Minnesota was limited not only by the preparation of the doctor for practice, or lack thereof, but also by the diagnostic tools at his disposal. And if he were able to correctly diagnose the patient's problem, the treatment modalities available to him were limited.

In Minnesota, most physicians of the time were men, though there was an occasional woman, with a strong will to learn and practice medicine, who was willing to face such obstacles as an attitude that the place of the woman was in the home, but if she were inclined to work in the medical field, then she should do it as a nurse rather than a doctor. Nurses were viewed by most doctors as their handmaidens. Even as late as the middle of the twentieth century, there were still Minnesota hospitals in which the nurse was expected to stop whatever she was doing and stand when a doctor came on the scene.

With doctors in short supply on the frontier, many people, especially in the rural areas, learned to treat their own illnesses with a variety of methodologies learned from family, friends, and sometimes from the Indians who lived around them. Some of the treatments could stand the test of modern scientific inquiry, while others seem bizarre by today's standards.

Some examples of treatments known to have been used in the nineteenth century were:

- Asthma: Cut a piece of bark from a red oak tree, get close and breathe deep into it, then put the bark back on the tree. (?)
- Bee sting: Apply freshly cut onion or wet tobacco.
- Burns and bruises—three different treatments: 1) Apply a poultice of crushed onions; (2) Apply strong tea to the area; (3) Apply Vaseline or lard which had salt added to it.
- Cancer of the skin: Apply leeches or maggots and allow them to eat away the bad tissue, then remove them and apply salve.
- To hasten childbirth, give whiskey. (!)

- Consumption (tuberculosis): Inhale fumes of boiling apple vinegar. An alternative was to take a concoction three times a day which was made from boiling together cherry bark, pine buds, sweet gum leaves, mullen leaves, honey and whiskey.
- Dropsy (Edema): Wear an eelskin around the neck and waist.
- Flu (LaGrippe): Wear an asafetida bag around the neck containing asafetida, onions and turpentine; sprinkle same on underwear. (!)
- Heart burn: Chew mustard seed mixed with chimney soot.
- Internal bleeding: Drink strong salt water.
- Nausea: Drink tea made from boiling the lining of a chicken gizzard. (!)
- Nightmares: Put a pan of cold water under the bed. (?)
- Restless babies: Give them catnip tea.
- Rickets: Eat and apply poultices of raw onions.
- Typhoid: Split a fat hen and while it is still warm, put entrails against the soles of the feet, or put fresh cut onions on the soles of the feet to draw out fever. (?)
- Warts: Rub with an old bone found in the yard, then put the bone back where you found it. (?)

Apparently raw onions were seen as the miracle drugs of the era. Today one can only imagine the problems faced by a doctor who was consulted only after these home remedies had failed to work.

From the beginning, St. Barnabas was an "open hospital" meaning any doctor practicing in the city was welcome to admit patients to the hospital for care. After the hospital was incorporated in 1883, attention was directed toward organization of a medical staff. In 1884, thirteen doctors were organized as the first medical staff of St. Barnabas. The list included four surgeons, four identified as "medical" and five specialists. Their first chief of staff was Dr. Thomas S. Roberts. Presumably by that time at least some of their number had attended medical school somewhere although the quality of the schools at the time was variable. As stated earlier, the best schools tended to be those in the large eastern cities. The 1916 booklet describing the hospital's first medical staff, stated, "This body of men gave of their best to St. Barnabas Hospital, caring for the poor and spending much valuable time in the Free Dispensary, lecturing to nurses and conducting medical clinics for students as we recall with pride that St. Barnabas was for a period of years the first and only center for the practical instruction of medical students."

During the late 1880s, two private medical schools operated in Minneapolis, the Minnesota Hospital College and the Minneapolis College of Surgeons. The University of Minnesota had not at that time opened its Medical School. In 1885, the hospital offered the opportunity to these two private institutions to participate in clinics at the hospital. Staff physicians were allowed to take a maximum of four students with them on rounds to observe dressing changes. This, in rudimentary form, was a kind of medical education offered at the hospital. The first intern to be assigned to the hospital was a Dr. F. E. Wright, appointed in 1894. The record doesn't indicate from where he got his formal medical education, but this internship marked the beginning of medical education as we would recognize it today.

A free dispensary was opened in the basement of the hospital on October 29, 1894. The objective of the dispensary was "to treat, free of charge, any person too poor to pay for medical or surgical attention", continuing the charitable philosophy upon which the hospital had been established. Funding to carry on the work of the dispensary (presumably for supplies since the physicians gave the time they devoted to the clinic) came from the Ladies Auxiliary to the Medical Staff. In June of 1899 the suggestion came from a member of the medical staff to close the free dispensary since the University of Minnesota hospitals were available for the care of indigent patients. Ultimately the suggestion was accepted and the dispensary was closed permanently on September 1, 1899.

Another of the charity services offered by the hospital was a program for medical inspection of children in the public schools. The program was organized in 1909 under the direction of a St. Barnabas nurse, Miss Helen Stevens, class of 1906. She began first at nearby Washington School where she examined every student in the school and referred those in need of medical and/or surgical care to one of five volunteer physicians: Dr. Margaret Nickerson, Dr. Jane Kennedy, Dr. Robert Campbell, Dr. Homer Annis and Dr. A. E. Benjamin. A second school, Jackson School, was added in 1911. In June of 1912, the Board of Education established its own program to examine students and refer them for treatment, but St. Barnabas had been the first to get the ball rolling for an ongoing program of medical surveillance of students in the Minneapolis public schools.

After the Board of Education established its own program, the St. Barnabas Social Service Nurse was used to render similar service to children who came before them who were identified in need of medical, surgical or dental care were treated at the hospital, free of charge if they were unable to pay for the needed services. Miss Helen Stevens, the nurse who began the program at Washington School, went on to a distinguished career in public health nursing in Pennsylvania and New York before returning years later to the Visiting Nurse Association in Minneapolis. In 1960, she was recognized with an award from the Public Health Nursing Service of the Pennsylvania Public Health Association for the twenty-three years of distinguished service she gave in Pittsburgh and Allegheny Counties.

An article, written in 1959 for the *Bulletin Of The Hennepin County Medical Society* by Robert W. Bachmeyer and Frederick W. Gibbs ("Minneapolis Hospitals, St. Barnabas and St. Andrew's Division," April and May 1959), notes a tug of war between the Board of Trustees and the medical staff over control of use of the hospital during the early twentieth century. The article states, "By 1911, the number of the staff had reached the proportions of a town meeting and its efficiency increased adversely in proportion to its size…a series of disagreements and counter proposals between the Board of Trustees and the medical staff. The medical staff held out for greater control over the hospital and being turned down, resigned and refused reappointment. So ten years passed without an organized medical staff."

The article goes on to say the issue was not resolved until it became apparent that without an organized medical staff, accreditation of the hospital was in jeopardy. Finally in April of 1922, a new medical staff was organized and the hospital was put on the accredited list of the American College of Surgeons.

An earlier portent of the coming conflict between the board and medical staff appeared in an 1893 report prepared by the board president, John I. Black. He reported that early in 1892 the board found members of the medical staff were taking their patients to some of the newer hospitals in town which had better facilities than those at St. Barnabas. Concern over this issue of declining census led to the closing of the hospital and construction of the Martin building the next year.

As the hospital grew, so did the number of doctors who chose to practice there. By 1970, there were two hundred eighty five men and women on the

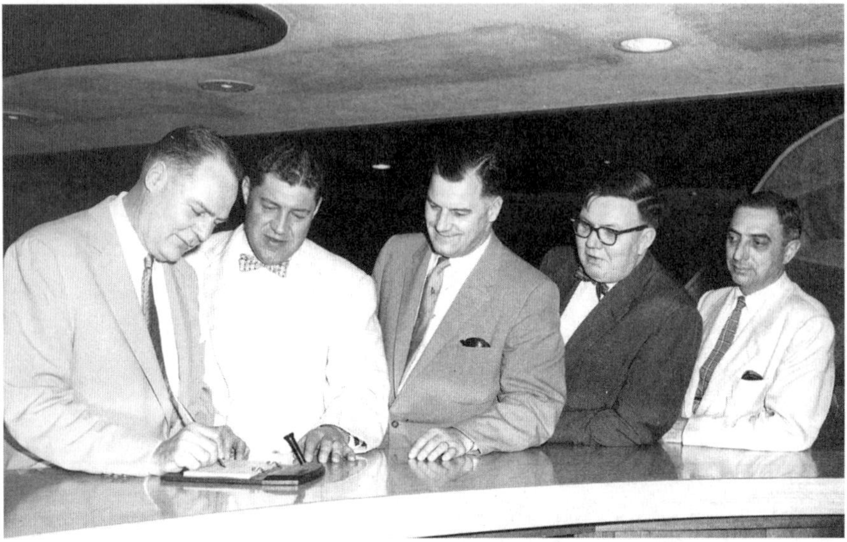

Five long-time members of the Medical Staff, late 1950s. Left to right are Owen F. Robbins, Robert Tenner, Harold Hall, O.L.N. Nelson and Harold Buckstein.

medical staff, representing all areas of medical practice. Eighty-four of this number had served twenty or more years at St. Barnabas, twenty one had served more than thirty years and one, Dr. Frank Kucera, had served on the medical staff for forty nine years.

Communicable disease was a constant problem for doctors of the nineteenth and early twentieth centuries. Since there were no drugs available to cure these diseases, prevention was the primary method the doctor had for dealing with them and isolation was the usual preventive method employed. Children were particularly susceptible to a number of the communicable diseases—whooping cough (pertussis), mumps, measles, chicken pox and scarlet fever made the rounds of most schools every year. Scarlet fever, for which a family would be quarantined, or isolated, for a period of six weeks or more, was seen as the most dangerous among them, with whooping cough and diphtheria close seconds. It was almost expected every child would get measles, mumps and chicken pox at some time and these were viewed by many as more of a nuisance than a danger to children though there were children who died from even these diseases.

Typhoid fever from contaminated water and hepatitis and botulism from mishandling of food were common. Meningitis was also common, though usually it was not the epidemic form of the disease which affected most children, but rather it tended to be a complication from ear and mastoid infections. After World War II, the advent of the sulfa drugs and antibiotics changed the outcome on most of these diseases.

Immunizations were developed for diphtheria, pertussis, measles, mumps and finally chicken pox to prevent the diseases from happening at all. An antibiotic could quickly knock out meningitis or scarlet fever, so in a period of only fifty years or so, these once common maladies were nearly a thing of the past.

Influenza epidemics were periodic in the United States beginning as early as 1647. The years 1889, 1890 and 1893 had particularly severe influenza outbreaks. And of course, well known is the 1917-1918 epidemic of Spanish Influenza. An article in the *St. Paul Dispatch* in December of 1918 stated that in only two months time, October and November 1918, there were 350,000 deaths from Spanish flu. By comparison, loss of life from the war (WWI) totaled only 60,000. In other words, nearly six times as many people died during two months of that influenza epidemic as died in all the battles of the first World War.

Tuberculosis was another common communicable disease for which isolation was the most frequent control measure utilized. State sanitaria for TB patients were established and did a booming business for years. The first graduate of the St. Barnabas Nursing School, Minnie Paterson, had a hand in the opening of the Glen Lake Sanitarium, the facility to which Minneapolitans were sent for treatment of tuberculosis, many achieving successful outcomes from the treatment they received there.

During the 1930s and 1940s, epidemics of infantile paralysis (poliomyelitis) occurred almost every summer and scores of young people especially, were left with permanent paralysis as a result. The disease thrived in the warm summer weather, often curtailing summer water sports and gatherings of people. Before Sister Kenny brought her revolutionary treatment of the disease to Minneapolis and founded the Kenny Institute, numbers of polio patients were treated at St. Barnabas. As with the childhood diseases, polio can now be prevented by immunization, and the paralysis and epidemics once so common have been relegated to history.

By 1959 a program of medical education had been developed between St. Barnabas and Swedish Hospitals. Though internships had for years been required for every doctor immediately following medical school, often these programs resembled apprenticeships more than educational programs. The joint program with Swedish was based on more formal education principles. Dr. Lyle J. Hay was appointed to direct the program and to serve as the surgical co-ordinator for both hospitals. Two physicians, one from each hospital were appointed as co-ordinators for medicine. They were Dr. Frank E. Martin from St. Barnabas and Dr. Wayne L. Hoseth from Swedish.

Three purposes guided the joint program: 1) to provide good training for the participants, giving them an opportunity to put into practice under the direction of experienced doctors the knowledge they had acquired in medical school; 2) to increase the competence of physicians on staff who improved their own practices by working with the young doctors in the program; 3) to recruit future members for the medical staffs of both hospitals.

Provision was made in the program for junior and senior medical students who could work as externs in both hospitals, their experiences limited by the levels and courses they had already completed in medical school.

Teaching rounds and ward rounds with experienced physicians in the lead were scheduled regularly. Service in outpatient clinics and participation in planned conferences were also included in the program.

By 1963, thirty interns had completed the program. Ten of those had joined the St. Barnabas medical staff and four had gone on to residencies following internship. The bane of the existence of some doctors on the staff was the ever- present pressure to keep medical records up to date, particularly discharge records. At some point the medical record department, with the cooperation of administration and the medical staff itself, passed a regulation suspending the admitting privileges of doctors who did not have their records up to date. This was a powerful stimulus to insure the record was complete. After all, who wanted to explain to a patient in need of hospitalization that he or she could not admit patients to St. Barnabas because of a situation that could have been prevented in the first place? Everything possible was done to make the job easier, including installation in the 1958 hospital of dictation equipment tied into medical records from little booths on each station. Medical transcriptionists in the records department transcribed the doctor's dictation directly into patient charts and the doctor was relieved of going to the medical records department to make his notes on the charts.

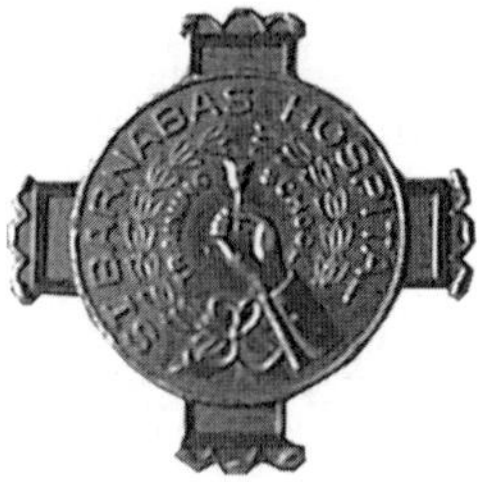

Chapter 12

Medical Staff Biographical Sketches

During the years of its existence, St. Barnabas Hospital was blessed with medical staff members whose standards of practice were equal to the best available in the area. Almost every issue of the *Voice of St. Barnabas* carried a biographical sketch of a member of the medical staff. Helen Hayden wrote most of those columns. She knew many of the doctors well, having been a part of the St. Barnabas scene herself for thirty years or more when the articles were written. Her articles and a few written by other people served as the resource material for this chapter. Where appropriate, quotations have been included from the original articles.

Hundreds of doctors served on the St. Barnabas medical staff over the years. The biographical sketches included here are representative of all those doctors. Even if information were available on every doctor, space limitations would preclude writing about all of them. The doctors are listed in alphabetical rather than chronological order of their times of service.

Dr. Charles Aling

Born in 1905 to a physician father who had served on the medical staff at St. Barnabas, Charles Aling was familiar with St. Barnabas years before he became a doctor himself. As a child, he often accompanied his father when he made rounds to all his patients. He graduated from the University of Minnesota Medical School in 1929, then served his internship at Minneapolis General Hospital. He was fortunate in securing an assistantship to Dr. A. A. Zierold, then Professor of Surgery at the University of Minnesota. He served with Dr. Zierold for five years, at the same time taking postgraduate courses, particularly in anatomy and pathology. During those years, he was married. When World War II came along, he served for four years, 1942-1946, with the United States Army, earning the Bronze Star among other awards. At war's end he returned to Minneapolis and went into private practice. He was a devoutly religious man who gave generously of his efforts to his church. His hobbies included photography and playing chess with his young son.

Dr. Silas Anderson

Dr. Anderson entered the practice of medicine in Minneapolis in 1924, though he did not join the St. Barnabas medical staff until 1948, only five years before his untimely death from a fall in 1953. Always active in community affairs, Dr. Anderson had served on the board of the Hennepin County Medical Society and the Judicial Council of the Minnesota State Medical Association. He was also a board member of Dana College in Blair, Nebraska. His father had founded Dana College many years earlier, so in serving on their board, he was carrying on the family business.

Dr. Stuart Lane Arey

Dr. Arey graduated from the University of Minnesota Medical School in 1931 and the next year served his internship at Minneapolis General Hospital. For a pediatric residency he chose Children's Memorial Hospital in Chicago. He frequently authored articles for professional journals and served as clinical assistant professor in pediatrics at the University of Minnesota. In addition to St. Barnabas, he had staff privileges at Minneapolis General where he was an attending physician in contagion and pediatrics. Along with his practice in pediatrics, he also studied allergic diseases in all ages.

Dr. Stuart Arhelger

Dr. Arhelger came from our neighboring state of Wisconsin. Born in Lancaster, Wisconsin, he attended the University of Wisconsin, in 1945 earning his MD degree there. He served his internship at St. Luke's Hospital in Duluth, Minnesota, and his residency in surgery at the University of Minnesota. He earned two postgraduate degrees in surgery, an MS and a PhD. During the Korean conflict, he served as a Captain in the United States Army Medical Corps (1951-1953). He returned from army service to a fulltime teaching position at the University of Minnesota where he was assistant professor of surgery and director of the tumor clinic. In 1958 he went into private practice, but continued as a consultant with the tumor service at University of Minnesota Hospitals. He was a diplomat of the American Board of Surgery. In 1953 he became an editor for *Minnesota Medicine*, a post he held for a number of years. Not only did he edit professional literature, but he authored several articles himself. He was married and had two children.

Dr. Clarence E. Arlander

Clarence Arlander, son of a Nebraska minister, was born in Valley, Nebraska, on June 22, 1905. When he was three years old, the family moved to Big Springs, South Dakota, where the youngster spent the boyhood he remembered. It included an introduction to the life of a farmer, as he worked as a farmhand during his teens. At age nine he was introduced to the sport of hunting pheasants, which were in large supply in the fields of South Dakota. Hunting became a lifelong hobby, though he knew from his earliest recollections that one day he would become a doctor. He attended the University of Minnesota, earning a BS degree in 1926, a BM degree in 1929 and his MD in 1930. Since his family was short on funds through all those years, he worked to put himself through college and medical school. He served his internship at Minneapolis General Hospital and a residency at Midway Hospital in St. Paul. During World War II (1942-1946) he served in the United States Navy, rising to the rank of commander during his forty months of service. On his return to civilian life, he went back into private practice. He had joined the medical staff at St. Barnabas in 1938, prior to his military service. He was married and had two sons. Mrs. Arlander (Ruth) was an RN, a graduate of the University of Minnesota nursing program. The couple had two sons. Tom, the eldest, followed his father in graduating from the University of Minnesota Medical School and joining the United States Navy. Like his friend Dr. Aling, Dr. Arlander was a deeply religious man, faithfully involved with the Baptist church. Reflecting his early years working on South Dakota farms, Dr. Arlander chose rural acreage on which to raise his sons. He loved caring for the woods which surrounded their home. Golf was another leisure time activity, a hobby he shared with many others on the medical staff. For many years Dr. Arlander was in practice with Dr. Carl Olson.

Dr. Paul J. Bilka

Dr. Bilka was born in New York City. He took his premedical college courses in Hartford, Connecticut, then went on to Columbia University for medical school, receiving his MD in 1943. He served both an internship and a residency at Hartford Hospital in Connecticut before going on to a three-year fellowship at the Mayo Clinic where he received special training in the field of rheumatology. Between his internship and his residency, he served a stint as a captain in the United States Army Medical Corps. In 1950 he joined the faculty of the University of Minnesota Medical School where he held the position of clinical associate professor. He also served as a consultant on rheumatology at the Veterans Hospital in Minneapolis and published numerous papers on rheumatology. In 1966, he was a guest lecturer at a meeting of the Peruvian Rheumatology Society in Lima, Peru. At the meeting, attended by five hundred Peruvian physicians, he was made an honorary member of the Peruvian Rheumatology Society. Dr. Bilka was engaged in clinical research on rheumatoid arthritis that led to the production of two different teaching films on the disease, one of which was translated into Spanish for use in Central and South American countries. Other areas of study in which he played a central role were disorders of the shoulder joint (this interest led to production of another clinical film) and evaluation of anti-rheumatic drugs as well as a study of the functions of the adrenal gland and the cortico-steroids produced by the adrenals.

Dr. Benjamin Bofenkamp

Dr. Bokenhamp, an otorhinolaryngologist, joined the medical staff in 1949. He remained on the staff for the rest of the years of St. Barnabas's existence as a separate institution. In the mid 1950s he designed an operation that enabled patients who had developed throat paralysis as a result of polio to swallow normally again. The operation, an extremely delicate procedure, involved severing the muscle constricting the esophagus so it would open normally again during the swallowing motion. In 1957, Dr. Bofenkamp had successfully performed this surgery on five patients, but estimated there were probably at least two hundred more people throughout the country who could benefit from it. Widowed while still a young man and the father of small children, Dr. Bofenkamp married St. Barnabas graduate Kathleen Griffin, class of 1953.

Dr. Donald G. Bohn

Donald Bohn was born on January 30, 1921, in Great Bend, North Dakota. He lived in Great Bend until the age of seven, during which time he attended a one-room school for his first two years of elementary school. The family moved to Minneapolis in 1928 and Don spent the rest of his boyhood and teen years learning to appreciate the joys of swimming and fishing in Lake Harriet, Lake Calhoun and Lake of the Isles. He attended the University of Minnesota and during his last years in the medical school he served as a junior intern (or extern) at St. Barnabas. After he received his MD in 1945, he served both his internship and a residency at Minneapolis General Hospital. During the Korean conflict, in 1953, he served in the United States Army, stationed at Fort Riley, Kansas. When he returned to civilian life in 1955, he picked up his private medical practice. Throughout his years in private practice, he enjoyed teaching and was involved in teaching internal medicine both at Minneapolis General Hospital and at the University of Minnesota where he held the rank of clinical associate professor. In 1957 he became a member of the American Board of Internal Medicine. He left private practice in 1964 and became medical director for North American Life and Casualty. He continued a relationship with St.

Barnabas as a coordinator in medicine of the St. Barnabas Joint Medical Education Program. Hunting, fishing and gardening were special interests during spring, summer and fall. Winter found him still involved with gardening for he had a "warm greenhouse" in which he grew orchids all winter long. Another winter pastime he enjoyed was playing bridge. His wife (Yvonne or Vonnie) shared his interest in bridge. She was also an active and conscientious member and worker in the hospital auxiliary. The Bohns had two children, daughter Merry Ann and son Bobby.

Dr. Wesley Howard Burnham

A native Minneapolitan, Dr. Burnham received his premedical education at Wheaton College in Wheaton, Illinois, and then attended the University of Minnesota Medical School from which he received his MD in 1939. He served an internship at Minneapolis General Hospital and then four different residencies at Minneapolis General, at the University of Minnesota hospitals, at Gillette State Hospital and at Veterans Hospital in Minneapolis. During the years of World War II, he served in the United States Army where he was Chief of Orthopedic Surgery, first at Fort Leonard Wood, Missouri, then in New Guinea. He held the rank of Lt. Colonel when he left the army in 1946 to resume civilian life. He enjoyed sharing his knowledge of orthopedics and was a frequent lecturer for nursing classes at St. Barnabas. He was also a clinical instructor in orthopedic surgery at the University of Minnesota Medical School for several years, during which time he also published a number of papers in professional journals. He was certified by the Specialty Board of Orthopedic Surgery.

Hunting was a favorite off duty activity and he enjoyed sharing his adventures with anyone who would listen when he returned from safari or from hunting big horn sheep or whatever. He also enjoyed music and had a nice tenor voice, so was often asked to sing for functions at the hospital. A thoroughly decent and nice man, he always found time in his busy schedule to talk to students or to nursing staff about their interests in his patients or in his chosen field of practice. The family home for Dr. Burnham, his wife Ester and their three children was on Willow Creek Road in Hopkins.

Dr. Orwood J. Campbell

Dr. Campbell joined the medical staff at St. Barnabas in 1945 after completing requirements for his MD at Rush Medical College in Chicago, plus internship at Presbyterian Hospital, Chicago. Following internship he took graduate programs in surgery at the Mayo Clinic and at the University of Minnesota. Earlier in his life, in 1927, he earned a PhD degree at the University of Minnesota. He had a large and successful surgical practice in Minneapolis and earned the respect of his medical colleagues not only by the example he set in his practice, but also by the contributions he made during years of active participation and leadership in the county and state medical associations as well as the American Medical Association. In 1966, he became the twelfth doctor to receive the St. Barnabas Bowl Award. At that time it was said of him (*Voice of St. Barnabas*, Spring 1966), "His recognition of current problems, his anticipation of future events and political trends, combined with a keen analysis of all their ramifications, have generated wholesome respect among his colleagues."

Dr. Lyman Clay

Lyman Birney Clay was born on November 21, 1911, at Winona, Minnesota. He attended the University of Minnesota Medical School, earning his MB in 1936 and his MD in 1937. At that point, he already had professional ties to St. Barnabas, having served as a junior intern during medical school days. He stayed on at St. Barnabas for his internship in 1937 and after completing that, joined the medical staff when he went into general practice in 1938. Later he went for graduate work in surgery at the University of Minnesota and at Cook County Hospital in Chicago. During World War II, he served in the United States Navy for forty-two months, having achieved the rank of Lt. Commander at war's end. He continued his naval career as a member of the reserves when he returned to Minneapolis and to the practice of surgery with Dr. Verne Cabot. He stayed with Dr. Cabot for twelve years before going into practice on his own.

His wife, Valleen, was a graduate of Kahler School of Nursing in Rochester. The couple had two children, son John Lyman and daughter Janet Lee. He and his family were avid bird watchers, keeping records of the various species visiting their back yard bird feeders. Another special interest was wild flower gardening. The family had a summer home at Lutsen,

Minnesota, and plants which sprouted from seeds at Lutsen often found their way down to the Twin City home. The north country home provided many opportunities for two other hobbies, fishing and rock hunting on the north shore of Lake Superior. During the winter months, they would cut and polish their finds of Thomsonite (Lake Superior agates), malachite, and thunder eggs.

In the June-July 1967 issue of the *Voice of St. Barnabas*, Helen Hayden recounts a childhood experience Dr. Clay had which he never forgot, but had no wish to live over. "At age 16, he and his brother were aboard the steamer Americana when she ran aground, sinking in about twenty minutes. The sinking occurred in early morning just off Isle Royale (in Lake Superior) at a time when there was no radio communication with the mainland. Lifeboats saved the boys, but they lost all their possessions—and their dog!"

Dr. Albert Corniea

One of the older members of the medical staff at St. Barnabas was Dr. Albert Corniea. He was born in 1888 in Glencoe, Minnesota. After graduation from the Glencoe schools, he went to the University of Minnesota for premedical and medical studies. He received his MD in 1913, then served an internship at Northwestern Hospital in Minneapolis and a residency at Mounds Park Hospital in St. Paul. He joined the medical staff at St. Barnabas in 1923 and continued his practice for nearly fifty years after that. He was a quiet man whose patient lists included the same people for forty years and more plus their children and grandchildren as well. That he spent so many years in medical practice could be attributed to the fact that he just couldn't see himself spending time on anything else.

Dr. James Sharpley Cole

Dr. Cole joined the staff of St. Barnabas in 1954. Born on July 24, 1924, in Winona, Minnesota, he spent most of his boyhood in Indiana and when he elected medicine as his future vocation, he attended Indiana University at Bloomington, Indiana, from which he received his MD degree in 1947. He served his internship at Memorial Hospital in South Bend, Indiana, and went on to residencies in internal medicine at Methodist Hospital in Des Moines, Iowa, and at Ancker Hospital in St. Paul. From 1952-1954, he was Captain Cole of the United States Army Medical Corps, serving both stateside and in Korea. He was board certified in internal medicine and active in the American Medical Association and the Minneapolis Society of Internal Medicine.

Dr. Cole, his wife, Helen, and their four adopted children lived with an assortment of pets acquired by the children at different times through the years. His home and his children were his prime interest in life in addition to his medical practice. He said that repairing broken toys was one of his specialties. And picking watercress growing in the creek that cut through the back of his property. The author who wrote about him in the March 1965 issue of the *Voice of St. Barnabas* stated, "He keeps trim by cutting wood from his own wooded grounds and he'll vouch that using a Swede saw calls for physical fitness."

Dr. Carlos W. Del Plaine

Dr. Del Plaine spent his boyhood years in Mexico where his American father was employed. He developed a love for that country that lasted for his entire life. In 1954 he wrote his memoirs of childhood in Mexico. Entitled *Son Of Orizaba*, it became popular reading among Minneapolitans of the time. It was through the efforts of Dr. Del Plaine that interns who had graduated from medical schools in Mexico were enticed to come to St. Barnabas in the early 1950s.

Widowed after a long, happy marriage, Dr. Del Plaine in the later years of his life married Marilyn Huntley, St. Barnabas graduate of the class of 1954. The joy of the couple was boundless when in 1963 a baby son was born to them. The doctor had no children from his first marriage, making this son, born in his father's twilight years, a special blessing. The child, Carlos P. Del Plaine, was baptized during a Sunday morning worship service in the hospital chapel on January 19, 1964. His was the first baptism to be held in the new chapel. Dr. Del Plaine was a general practitioner in Minneapolis.

Dr. Richard Frey

Dr. Frey joined the medical staff at St. Barnabas in 1954. A 1946 graduate of the University of Minnesota Medical School, he interned at Minneapolis General Hospital from 1949-1951. He served a residency in internal medicine at the University of Minnesota hospitals, following which he was a fulltime faculty member of the University of Minnesota Medical School for two years. Between graduation from medical school and beginning his internship, he served two years as a captain in the United States Army Medical Corps (1947-1949).

Dr. Frey and his wife, Evelyn, had seven children. He was a member of the American Board of Internal Medicine and the American College of Physicians.

Dr. Marian Grimes

Over the years, the vast majority of those on the medical staff at St. Barnabas were men. Not over one half dozen were women at any time until the very last years of the hospital. One of the half dozen women was Marian Grimes, who joined the staff in 1930. Her father, George Sutherland Grimes, served on the Board of Trustees of the hospital for more than fifty years in the early part of the twentieth century. The medical library, maintained for use of the medical staff, was named for him. Marian's family pedigree extended all the way back to colonial times and John Alden.

Dr. Grimes graduated from West High School in Minneapolis in the early 1920s. She attended Sweet Briar College in Vermont, then returned to Minneapolis where she enrolled for premedical and medical training at the University of Minnesota. She got her MD in 1926 and took her internship at Minneapolis General Hospital. Postgraduate work included study in New York and Vienna as well as the University of Minnesota. The highlight of her graduate study was a fellowship at Chicago Lying-In Hospital and study under world famous obstetrician, Dr. Joseph B. DeLee.

On completion of her experience at Chicago Lying-In, she returned to Minneapolis to go into the private practice of obstetrics. She also was married at that time to Dr. Francis Collins, a friend of longstanding from both high school and her church. Dr. Collins had become a dentist in the years Marian was preparing to become an obstetrician. They were married for twenty-eight years until his death from pneumonia in 1958.

Searching for wild mushrooms or the Minnesota state flower, the showy lady slipper, were hobbies along with gardening. During the years of her marriage, she and her husband loved also to hunt, fish and swim in the area around their summer home at St. Croix Falls, Wisconsin. She was an active committee worker on the medical staff, but the appointment she cherished most was being chairman of the medical library committee, overseeing operation of the library named for her father.

Drs. Bourne and Elizabeth Jerome

A husband and wife team who both served on the St. Barnabas medical staff were Dr. Bourne Jerome, an ophthalmologist, and Dr. Elizabeth Jerome, a pediatrician. Dr. Bourne was already serving on the staff when Dr. Elizabeth Brumbaugh came to St. Barnabas as a pediatric resident. After she finished her residency in the late 1940s, the couple were married. Motherhood came, but Dr. Elizabeth continued in her chosen profession. She was at first in practice with Dr. Joseph Spano and Dr. Maxine Nelson. Later, she opened an office and a practice of her own. Always a colorful person, she was perennially popular with nursing students. Many who observed her practice during their student days, married and stayed in Minneapolis brought their children to be cared for by Dr. Jerome. She was one of the handful of doctors and RNs who lived at Wellesmere for a time and she had a special gift of being able to relate to students. Dr. Bourne, an excellent practitioner in his own field, tended to be quiet, almost shy, but his love for his irrepressible wife was undeniable.

Dr. Arthur C. Kerkhof

Another physician who was perennially popular with nursing students, staff in all departments and fellow physicians was Dr. Arthur Kerkhof. He was a member of the St. Barnabas medical staff for twenty-seven years, 1940 until his sudden death in 1967. His wife, Florence, was an active member of the auxiliary. She also died an untimely death, a few years before the doctor.

Nursing students at St. Barnabas capitalized on Dr. Kerkhof's gregarious nature by asking him to serve as Santa Claus at the Christmas party they held each year for students from Washington School. He was pleased to be able to contribute a bit of holiday joy to the youngsters, most of whom would have little in the way of Christmas cheer in their homes. It was hard to judge who had more fun at these Christmas parties, the children or Santa Kerkhof.

Dr. Kerkhof was born in February 1904 in Minneapolis. He attended the University of Minnesota for premedical and then medical school. He received his MD in 1928, then continued on at the University of Minnesota, earning a master of science in medicine in 1931 and a PhD in medicine in 1935. As with so many others, he chose Minneapolis General Hospital for his internship and stayed on there for residency as well. He had great teaching talents and from 1932 to 1939 he was a fulltime teacher at Minneapolis General Hospital. He was also an instructor in medicine at the University of Minnesota at the same time. He continued teaching at the University, progressing from instructor to clinical assistant professor to clinical associate professor and in 1962 to clinical professor. During his years on the St. Barnabas staff he was also called upon frequently to teach nursing students, an invitation he never refused.

For years Dr. Kerkhof was actively involved with the Minnesota Heart Association and was named director of the Work Evaluation Unit of the Minnesota Heart Association. He was president and director of Mediclinics, a non-profit corporation, which annually offered instruction in cardiovascular medicine seminars.

Following the death of his wife, the Mediclinic Corporation set up a Florence A. Kerkhof Mediclinic Foundation that made interest-free loans to medical students. He was the driving force behind the St. Barnabas Coronary Care Unit in the 1958 hospital building. There was a red phone in that unit which was activated without dialing. It rang immediately in Dr. Kerkhof's home. EKG readings were transmitted through this phone line and by this means he could advise the nurse on duty regarding a patient any hour of the night.

He was a prolific writer of papers for professional journals and a popular speaker as well. He had worldwide recognition as an authority on heart disease and was called to be a speaker at several foreign meetings. He and Mrs. Kerkhof enjoyed traveling, making four leisure-time trips to Europe alone. After his wife's death, their two children continued to live with their father in their suburban Minneapolis home. Gretchen, the elder, was a French teacher at Northrup Collegiate School. His son, Arthur, also lived at home.

Dr. Kerkhof was a medical consultant at the Star Tribune and medical director at Federal Cartridge in New Brighton. He made daily visits to the Star Tribune before coming to St. Barnabas for patient rounds. He saw patients in his busy practice from his office in the Medical Arts Building in downtown Minneapolis.

Not only was Dr. Kerkhof a hard worker, but he also threw himself wholeheartedly into social activities as well, enjoying good food, and good conversation along with beverages for making merry. He died on May 3, 1967, only sixty-three years old and still in the harness of the career he enjoyed so much.

Dr. Frank Kucera

Dr. Kucera was a member of the medical staff at St. Barnabas for forty-nine years, beginning in 1921. He medical education was received at the University of Minnesota Medical School from which he graduated in 1921. Practicing a lifetime in Hopkins, he was active in the Czechoslovakian community there, which honored him as "Czech of the Year" in 1970. He was a member of "Sokol," a Czech athletic association, for fifty years. He also served on the school board in Hopkins for twenty-seven years. Dr. Kucera was a general practitioner.

Dr. Otto A. Lenz

South Dakota was the birthplace of Dr. Lenz. He was born in 1899 in Conde, South Dakota. In 1948, his mother was named South Dakota State Mother of the Year—quite an honor for a lady who arrived half a century earlier in a covered wagon. Her son had his early education in South Dakota, then turned to the University of Minnesota when it was time for college. He enrolled as a premed student, but changed his major a number of times from pharmacy to engineering and finally to science and business administration. When he graduated in 1923 his degree was in physics with a minor in business administration. Two years later he was back at the University, once again a student. This time he reverted to his original choice of medicine and in 1929 he received his MD degree.

He joined the medical staff at St. Barnabas in 1939. In 1947 he was a part of a group of doctors who organized and incorporated the General Practitioners in the United States, a forerunner of the American College of Physicians and Surgeons. He was also active in his Roman Catholic faith, being responsible in 1925 for writing the Articles of Incorporation for the Neuman group at the University of Minnesota. His education in business administration was bearing fruit. His interest in pharmacy he applied to cooking skills, enjoying preparing a good meal or baking a delicious pie—use only lard, never hydrogenated shortening in pie crust was his rule.

He was also an inventor of sorts, putting his education in physics to practical use. He loved to tinker with a mechanical device and make it better. His did acquire patents for some of his ideas. Probably his most notable invention was a rotary snowplow for sidewalks and driveways—a most useful item for a man living in snow country as Minnesota is every winter. Like many Minnesotans, however, his idea of a good way to spend the winter was on a warm southern beach.

Dr. Lenz was married and had four children. The three Lenz daughters chose to stay in the Minneapolis area when they became adults while their only brother looked to far away places. For example, in 1967 he was living with his family in Baghdad, Iraq, where he was administrator for a 1000 bed hospital.

Dr. Russell Cyrus Lindgren

Dr. Lindgren was a member of the St. Barnabas medical staff beginning in 1937. Born and raised in Stillwater, Minnesota, he attended the University of Minnesota Medical School from which he received his MD in 1932. He served both an internship and a residency in internal medicine at Minneapolis General Hospital. During World War II he served in the United States Army Medical Corps, earning the rank of lieutenant colonel. Returning to civilian life, he was appointed instructor in medicine and cardiology at Minneapolis General Hospital. He also served for twenty years in the University of Minnesota Outpatient Cardiac Clinic.

He was married and had two daughters and a son. The family lived in Edina.

Dr. John Blackmore Maunder

A native Minneapolitan, Dr. Maunder received his MD from the University of Minnesota in 1945. He served his internship at Detroit Receiving Hospital in Detroit, Michigan. Residencies in obstetrics and gynecology followed at Herman Kiefer Hospital and Florence Crittenton Hospital, both in Detroit. The years 1953-1955 found him in the United States Air Force, Captain Maunder then.

Dr. Maunder was the third doctor to join Dr. Owen Robbins in practice, the two preceding him being Dr. John Moehn and Dr. Mancel Mitchell. Dr. Maunder was married and the couple had four children.

Dr. Mancel T. Mitchell

Dr. Mancel T. Mitchell joined the medical staff of St. Barnabas in 1947, about the time that he and his colleague, Dr. John Moehn, joined the practice of Dr. Owen Robbins. Dr. Mitchell was a graduate of the University of Minnesota Medical School. He interned at Philadelphia General Hospital in Philadelphia, Pennsylvania. He was a teaching fellow at the University of Minnesota Hospitals from 1937-1940. Concomitant with his private practice he was also chief of obstetrical and gynecological services at Minneapolis General Hospital. He was a member of the American College of Obstetricians and Gynecologists and a fellow of the American College of Surgeons. In 1963, he volunteered to serve a tour of duty on the United States Ship Hope. The Hope was a twenty-year-old vessel on loan from the government for use as a mercy ship in various parts of the world. For example, in 1960 the ship was in Indonesia and Viet Nam; northern Peru was another destination (1962). The target for the tour on which Dr. Mitchell served was Ecuador.

A tour of duty on the good ship Hope was two months in length. In 1963, they were anchored off the coast of Guayaquil, Ecuador. Patients chosen on the mainland were ferried out to the ship for surgical treatment. The ship was fitted up with complete operating room facilities as well as postoperative beds for recovery.

In addition to the services provided aboard the ship, the doctors also set up clinics on the mainland, in the case of this tour it was an obstetric clinic in a suburban area outside of Guayaquil. It was a most interesting experience for the American-trained doctors for the mothers who came to the clinic brought their children with them. Only about half of Ecuadoran children at that time went to schooling. The rest spent all their time with their mothers.

Also a different experience for the American doctors was observing the maternity hospitals in Ecuador. The hospital in Guayaquil, where most of the mothers they saw at the clinic went to give birth, averaged 1,500 deliveries per month. In this very large, busy hospital, there was only one registered nurse on duty from 8:00 A.M. to 4:00 P.M. She was assisted by a staff of lesser-trained people. That hospital was supported by the sale of lottery tickets, a novel idea new to the American doctors.

Another maternity hospital in Quito was about half the size of the one in Guayaquil, only 800 deliveries per month on average. It had been built in 1930 with American funds During the time Dr. Mitchell was observing and working at the hospital in Quito, they were without running water, though there were 600 patients to be cared for.

The doctors learned that in all of Ecuador there were only two nursing schools with the result that nurses were in drastically short supply.

In spite of the heavy work load for the doctors assigned to the ship, there were relaxation times for them on the weekends when they visited various places tourists would go, such as a banana plantation or a ranch for race horses. One feature that tourists missed was being hosted by the United States Ambassador to Ecuador.

Dr. John T. Moehn

Dr. John T. Moehn joined the medical staff at St. Barnabas in 1947. A prewar graduate of Creighton University Medical School in Nebraska, he served an internship at Ancker Hospital in St. Paul, then entered the Army Medical Corps, serving 1942-1945 in the European theater of operations. In 1945, he returned to civilian life and to a general residency at St. Barnabas. He served in the general residency spot until April of 1946 when he became a resident in obstetrics and gynecology. Upon finishing his residency in 1947, he joined the practice of Dr. Owen Robbins. Dr. and Mrs. Moehn lived in Minneapolis in a home overlooking the south shore of Lake Harriet.

Drs. Harold, Frank Sr. and Frank Mork Jr.

Three members of one family were members of the medical staff in the 1950s and 1960s. Dr. Harold Mork joined the staff in 1949 after graduation from the medical school at Creighton University in Nebraska. He served a junior internship at Mercy Hospital in Council Bluffs, Iowa, and his senior internship at Ancker Hospital in St. Paul. He and his wife, Ruth, raised a family of five children, three boys and two girls in Anoka, Minnesota. They also raised a foster child, Kathleen Ann.

Dr. Mork's brother, Frank, also from Anoka, like his brother, joined the medical staff at St. Barnabas in 1949. At that time, there were no large hospitals closer to Anoka than the downtown hospitals of Minneapolis. In 1963, Frank Mork Jr. followed his father and his uncle to the staff at St. Barnabas when he was appointed as a radiologist.

Dr. O. L. Norman Nelson

Though he was born in Moorhead, Minnesota, Dr. Nelson spent most of his life in Minneapolis. His father was a dentist in Moorhead. Norman was only four years old when his father died and just seven years old when his mother also died. At that point, Norman and his brother were taken by their uncle and raised by him.

Obviously a bright youngster, Norman entered the University of Minnesota in 1924 when he was only fifteen years old. He had an eye on a career in medicine. Not only was his father a dentist, but the uncle who raised him was a pharmacist, so healing arts were very much a part of the Nelson family. He took his premed courses at the University of Minnesota, then went on to the University of Minnesota Medical School from which he received his MD in 1932. He was elected to Phi Beta Kappa in 1928 and in 1932 became a member of AOA, an honor society. Finishing medical school, he served both an internship and a residency in internal medicine at Minneapolis General Hospital. While at Minneapolis General he met a nurse, Helen Collard, who was to become his wife. The couple had two sons, Tom and John.

A member of the United States Naval Reserve, Dr. Nelson was on active duty from 1942-1946 as a lieutenant commander. While serving in the Bougainville and Peleliu areas of the South Pacific, he was attached to the marines.

The medical profession accorded Dr. Nelson many honors. He was president of the Hennepin County Medical Society in 1958 and served on various boards of the society. He also served on state committees and representing the Sixth District of the Minnesota Medical Association, he served as councilor. In 1958, he was general arrangements chairman for the clinical sessions of the American Medical Association convention, held in Minneapolis. He was certified by the Board of Internal Medicine in 1946. In 1932, fresh from medical school, he was appointed an instructor in internal medicine at the University of Minnesota. Later he would advance to clinical associate professor and finally to clinical associate preceptor at the medical school. He was a talented extemporaneous speaker and regarded as a good teacher by those who knew him.

Dr. Nelson was the sixth recipient of the Shotwell Award in 1976. This was an award established by Metropolitan Medical Center in 1971 in honor of the late Mr. and Mrs. James D. Shotwell, who left a gift of $670,000 to endow the award. Its purpose was to support research in medicine and in nursing. Unlike the St. Barnabas Bowl Award, the Shotwell Award could be and was given to a variety of health professionals, not just to physicians. In accepting the award, Dr. Nelson said, "It is especially heartwarming for me to receive this award because it came from a hospital that I've been identified with all my professional life. I care about MMC and it was an honor just to be considered."

He went on to reminisce about the old days at St. Barnabas and his partner in practice for a number of years, Dr. Arthur Kerkhof. He recounted the days when insulin was a new treatment for diabetes and when there were no antibiotics. He remembered prescribing cubes of liver for patients who had pernicious anemia. And he told of the long hospital stays for most patients. For example, a patient who had a hernia repair would remain in the hospital for two weeks as compared to today when the same kind of patient is sent home the next day, or possibly even the same day. In recognizing the revolutions in modern health care, Dr. Nelson expressed the opinion that something was lost along the way. He said, "Unfortunately, hospitals have gone from an intimate atmosphere to large, impersonal institutions. I also think it was more fun seeing patients during the Depression years because people were so grateful—today everything is 'my right.' Back then, you never thought twice about malpractice, which is a social cancer as far as the health care system is concerned."

Dr. Carl John Olson

Born in Gladstone, Michigan, Dr. Olson entered Gustavus Adolphus College for his premedical education. He enlisted in the United States Army in 1941, serving in the infantry until 1945. In 1946, he enrolled at Northwestern University in Illinois and received his MD from that school in 1949. He interned at Minneapolis General Hospital and took postgraduate courses at the University of Minnesota. He joined the practice of Dr. Clarence Arlander and became a member of the St. Barnabas medical staff in 1950. He lived with his wife, Marie, and their three children in St. Paul.

Dr. Eugene Ott

Born in Milwaukee, Wisconsin, August 23, 1929, Dr. Eugene Ott spent most of his life in Minneapolis. The family moved to Minneapolis when he was just one year old. He had all of his schooling in Minnesota, first in Minneapolis schools, then premedical courses at the College of St. Thomas in St. Paul. For medical studies he chose the University of Minnesota Medical School from which he graduated in 1954. He did leave Minnesota for internship, choosing Detroit Receiving Hospital for that phase of his medical education. He returned to Minneapolis in 1956 and entered private practice there.

Dr. Ott was a longtime advocate of physical fitness, choosing golf in summer and snow skiing in winter to maintain his own state of fitness. He enjoyed gourmet cooking, but with an eye to keeping the waistline trim. He and his wife shared enthusiasm for playing bridge. The couple lived in Minneapolis with their six sons.

Dr. Charles R. Peluso

A native St. Paulite, Charles R. Peluso was born May 19, 1922. Eighteen years later he enrolled at the University of Minnesota from which he earned his MD degree. He served internships at St. Mary's Hospital in Detroit and St. Mary's Hospital in Duluth. Following internships, in 1948, he joined in practice with Dr. Joseph Spano. In 1953, during the Korean conflict, he left Minneapolis to serve in the Army Medical Corps. When he returned to Minneapolis in 1956, he went into practice for himself. In 1958 he was elected vice chief of staff and in 1959, chief of staff at St. Barnabas.

Dr. Peluso had a marvelous tenor voice. While an undergraduate student at the University of Minnesota, he faced the choice of a career in music or in medicine. He had been appearing as a popular guest soloist at St. Paul Pop concerts. Many people thought he was a professional musician. Interestingly enough, he had never had a voice lesson in his life. He was able to use his musical talent to financial advantage during his years at University of Minnesota Medical School by directing the St. Thomas College Choir, serving as a paid soloist at St. Stephens Church and singing in clubs and at various special events in the Twin Cities. During the lean years of his internship he also supplemented the family income by singing engagements throughout the Twin Cities. He often loaned his vocal talents to St. Barnabas events after he joined the staff at the hospital.

During his junior year in medical school, he married his high school sweetheart. They had a family of eight children. At their northeast Minneapolis home, they raised German shepherd dogs which they showed at dog shows throughout the country. In 1965, they had between twenty-five and thirty dogs. That year there were only three German shepherd champions in the state of Minnesota, and the Pelusos owned two of the three.

In1962, the Minnesota State Medical Association sponsored the first of an annual series of duplicate bridge tourneys. That year, first place went to Dr. Peluso and his partner, Dr. Richard Frey. In 1963, 1964 and again in 1965, the pair repeated their championship play despite determined efforts by others to unseat them.

Dr. Mitchell Pincus

The youngest of the partners in the Robbins, Moehn, Mitchell and Maunder obstetrical practice was Dr. Mitchell Pincus. He came to Minnesota in 1958 from Brooklyn New York, where he was born September 28, 1927. He was one of a number of doctors who knew for his entire life that's what he wanted to be. An uncle was a physician, and he served as a role model for the boy. He enrolled at the University of Michigan for undergraduate work and stayed on there to earn an MS in 1948. He returned to New York for medical school, enrolling at New York Medical College, from which he earned his MD in 1953. He served his internship at Mt. Sinai Hospital in Cleveland and then went on to a residency in obstetrics and gynecology at Akron City Hospital in Akron, Ohio. He helped to finance his education by working summers as a detail man for the Pfizer Corporation. He served in the United States Army between earning his baccalaureate and master's degrees, 1946-1947.

Dr. Pincus and his wife, Katherine, had two children. A favorite family pastime was riding bicycles in the vicinity of their Bloomington home. He and Mrs. Pincus were also devotees of the theater and regular in their attendance at the Guthrie. The family enjoyed sports—swimming in summer and ice skating in winter. Spectator sports, such as baseball and football also rated high with the doctor.

Dr. Carl Rice

Dr. Rice was a general surgeon at St. Barnabas for many years, through the 1940s and 1950s. He was a meticulous surgeon, but one who worked swiftly, believing it was to the advantage of his patients to keep them under anesthesia for as brief a time as possible. He also believed excessive use of narcotic painkillers postoperatively impeded recovery and healing. He and his associate, Dr. Jacob Strickler, were involved with Baxter Laboratories in doing pioneering research on parenteral nutrition and postoperative pain relief. He enticed the then head nurse on 4 Martin, Joyce English, to join his staff in the work on parenteral nutrition. Another member of the staff was medical technologist Jeanne Jensen, who presided over a research laboratory that the team set up on 3 Corridor.

In his spare time, Dr. Rice was a talented artist and cartoonist. He had several oil paintings to his credit. This author is in possession of a humorous cartoon caricature he did of her while he was a patient on 4 Martin, recovering from gall bladder surgery. He and Mrs. Rice were avid bicyclists, riding daily as weather permitted. He also swam daily during summer months. In the fall, he enjoyed hunting and in winter the family would take their ice skates to some of the many rinks available in the area and as time permitted for winter vacations, they could be found on the ski slopes.

Dr. Lawrence Richdorf

Dr. Richdorf was born in our neighboring state of Wisconsin, in Kellnersville, on August 25, 1891. When he was just three years old, the family moved to a farm, where he spent his boyhood. Life on the farm impressed the boy greatly. He helped with all the farm chores as farm boys generally did. His father, though living on a farm, was a veterinarian and the boy was able to observe his father as he practiced his craft. His experiences in treating animals was an influence in helping the boy to decide he would become a doctor of human patients.

He attended the rural schools in the area of their farm and went to high school in Manitowoc, Wisconsin. For the first two years following high school, he taught all eight grades in a country school. Later he got a job assisting the athletic coach at the University of Wisconsin. He entered the University of Wisconsin Medical School in 1913, but took time out during World War I to serve in the armed forces. When he returned to civilian life, he transferred to the University of Minnesota Medical School from which he got his MD in 1921. He continued on at the University of Minnesota, earning a PhD in 1925. He did his internship at Ancker Hospital and the University of Minnesota Hospitals, then secured a fellowship in pediatrics at the Mayo Clinic. He went into private practice, but also taught pediatrics at Minneapolis General Hospital and at the University of Minnesota Medical School. He was on the faculty teaching clinical pediatrics at the University of Minnesota Medical School for thirty-nine years, before becoming emeritus associate professor. He continued seeing patients in his pediatric practice during all this time as well as after retiring from the medical school faculty.

As is true of all college professors, he had several clinical papers published in professional journals. They covered a wide variety of conditions which affected children. In addition to the clinical papers, he wrote biographical stories on two early pediatricians, Dr. Abraham Jacobi and Dr. Julius Parker Sedgewick.

Dr. Richdorf joined the medical staff at St. Barnabas in 1940 and for years after, St. Barnabas was the hospital to which the majority of his patients were admitted. He helped to plan the first pediatric unit in the old Pavilion building.

In addition to his professional activities, Dr. Richdorf was heavily involved in community programs such as the Catholic Boys Home and the Phyllis Wheatley Clinic. He was one of the founders of the Minnesota Heart Association. The interest from a fund he was instrumental in establishing through the American Legion was used for years to pay the salary of the director of the University Heart Hospital. He also worked tirelessly to help eradicate tuberculosis in children, giving every Friday afternoon of his time to a clinic working with children who had tuberculosis.

When he found a child who had no one to care for him, Dr. Richdorf would step in and give a helping hand. He adopted two sons and became guardian to a girl who was like a daughter to him. The Minneapolis Pediatric Society honored him in 1960 and two years later a surprise party for him was sponsored by friends and parents of his former patients. There were expressions of thanks from all in attendance and as a tangible gift of thanks they presented him with a color television set.

Dr. Owen F. Robbins

One of the longtime members of the medical staff at St. Barnabas was Dr. Owen Robbins, who joined the staff in 1938 and continued through the 1940s, 1950s and 1960s. Dr. Robbins was born in Colorado in 1907 and lived in that western state until he had completed his first two years of college. He chose the University of Minnesota Medical School for his medical education, earning both undergraduate and a graduate degree before he got his MD. He interned at Minneapolis General Hospital and stayed on there for a residency in obstetrics and gynecology. In addition, he served a residency and a stint as a teaching fellow at the University of Minnesota, where he would later become an instructor in the medical school.

Dr. Robbins's father was a physician, so it was not unusual for the boy to dream of a career in medicine as well. As was fairly common at the time, he was allowed to accompany his father when he made rounds to his patients, some of whom lived on a Navajo Indian Reservation. It was an interesting experience to observe his father at work on an Indian patient who might also at the same time be under the care of the medicine man or shaman.

Dr. Robbins wrote frequently for professional journals. He participated actively in the Hennepin County Medical Society, serving as its vice president in 1958. The Minneapolis Academy of Medicine elected him their president. He was also an officer on the St. Barnabas medical staff, serving several times as chairman of the obstetric and gynecology section of the staff. He was a member of the Board of Directors of the Sister Kenny Foundation as well as a member of the board of the Minneapolis Boys Club. And he also served on the Board of Directors of the Golden Valley State Bank.

During his days of internship he met his wife, Marjorie. The couple raised a family of two girls and one boy. The boy, Tom, followed his father and grandfather into the practice of medicine.

In his leisure time, Dr. Robbins could often be found tending his tanks of tropical fish. Ultimately, the interest in tropical fish gave way to a stronger interest in travel. As any one knows who has kept fish, it can be a very confining hobby. Whereas a dog or cat owner can board a pet to take a long trip, it isn't that easy with fish in tanks. During their travel days, the

Robbins saw Europe more than once and in 1956, they made a trip to the Orient. Other hobbies included a love of opera and a foray into the art of sculpting. And like a true Minnesotan, or Coloradoan for that matter, he liked to just go fishing.

Dr. Arthur B. Roelke

Dr. Arthur Roelke arrived in Elk River, Minnesota, as a young man in 1923. He set up an office on the second floor of a drugstore in downtown Elk River and went into general practice there. Fourteen years later his practice had increased to the point that he was joined by a colleague, Dr. Gordon Tesch. The two continued to practice in the second floor office until 1941 when the state highway department took the property to build Highway 10 from the Twin Cities through Elk River. At that time, the two doctors built a new clinic building from which they continued their practice that extended to people in the area for miles around. Patients requiring the services of specialists were referred to St. Barnabas for care. By the late 1940s, most of their patients requiring surgery were being referred to Dr. Carl Rice. Drs. Roelke and Tesch also joined the staff of the Princeton Community Hospital when that hospital opened in 1947.

Dr. Wesley G. Schaefer

For forty-six years, beginning in 1927, Dr. Wesley Schaefer, general surgeon, was a familiar figure around St. Barnabas. He first came to the hospital as an intern, then stayed on to join the medical staff. He served as chief of staff in 1941.

Dr. L. Raymond Scherer

Dr. Scherer spent most of his life in Minneapolis. He graduated from Macalester College in St. Paul in 1925, then went on to the University of Minnesota Medical School for his medical degree. He earned his MD in 1928. Next came internship, then a residency both at Minneapolis General Hospital. Later he took postgraduate courses in internal medicine in Philadelphia with Dr. Henry Jump and at the Mayo Clinic. He was on the faculty of the University of Minnesota Medical School, rising to the position of associate clinical professor of medicine. He joined the medical staff at St. Barnabas in 1937, first on visiting staff, then later, in 1942, on the active staff. He was highly regarded by both patients and colleagues, many considering him one of the top internists in the Twin City area. He made several contributions to medical literature with his papers on heart disease and diabetes.

For relaxation Dr. Scherer turned to the world of botany. He was one of the fortunate few to have his own small greenhouse attached to his south Minneapolis home. He and Mrs. Scherer enjoyed raising colorful camellias, azaleas and fuschias in their greenhouse during the bleak cold days of a Minnesota winter. In summer they turned to gardening on the outside of their home. They maintained a lovely garden in their yard which often served as the background for summer cookouts when the doctor would work his magic on the barbeque grill.

The Presbyterian Church was one of Dr. Scherer's special interests. He served as both a Trustee and as an Elder in his church. He and Mrs. Scherer raised a family of three sons. When grandchildren came along, he had developed an interest in fishing at the Scherer summer home on Lake Minnetonka and he enjoyed teaching the young ones the art of being still and having success at hooking a fish.

Dr. Lloyd Sherman

Dr. Sherman graduated from the University of Minnesota Medical School in the mid 1930s. He served his internship at Minneapolis General Hospital, then went into private practice at Siren, Wisconsin. During World War II, he served for three years in the United States Navy, First Marine Division, which saw action primarily in the Pacific theater. When he returned to civilian life in 1946, he served a residency in general surgery at Minneapolis Veterans' Hospital. Studies in the specialty of proctology followed at Temple University in Philadelphia. While at Temple he also served as associate professor in proctology. Always interested in teaching, he joined the faculty of the University of Minnesota Medical School when he returned to Minneapolis to set up a practice in proctology. Dr. Robert Tenner joined him in his practice.

Dr. Sherman was one of the driving forces which led to the establishment of the Joint Medical Education Program at St. Barnabas and Swedish. He served as chairman of that joint program. Later, he and Dr. Tenner, working through the St. Barnabas Hospital Research Foundation, worked together on a project focusing on cancer of the colon.

A talented speaker and writer, Dr. Sherman had many papers published in professional journals and he was in demand to speak on several of the topics about which he wrote

Dr. Sherman and his wife Ruth lived in a home with their daughter Cindy, in Excelsior, right on Lake Minnetonka. Their leisure time activities tended to be associated with their proximity to the lake—fishing, water skiing, swimming. Dr. Sherman was a vestryman at St. Martins by the Lake.

Drs. Archie and John Smith

A father and son team of physicians practicing from their Edina office were Archie and John Smith. Dr. Archie joined the staff of St. Barnabas in 1942, serving as chief of staff in 1953 and again in 1964. Terminology changed, but Dr. John held the same position in 1968 except by that time he was called president of the medical staff. Both doctors were born and raised in Minnesota and both attended the University of Minnesota Medical School, but in different generations. Dr. Archie received his MD in 1929 and first practiced in Thief River Falls, Minnesota. In 1937 he moved his family to Minneapolis where he practiced family medicine for the rest of his life. He and his wife, Eileen, had four children, two daughters and two sons. In 1964, the two daughters were still living at home, but both sons were married and son John had finished medical school and had joined his father in practice. Both men served at different times as the health service physician for the nursing school. Both also were active in their Episcopal church. Dr. Archie served for a time on the advisory council for the nursing school.

Dr. Joseph Spano

Had nurses and/or patients been polled and asked to name the kindest, most loving doctor on the staff at St. Barnabas, the name of Dr. Joseph Spano would certainly have been on the list during the 1930s, 1940s, 1950s and beyond. He said to this author one day that he hoped never to retire for he couldn't imagine his life without his beloved practice of medicine. He got his wish, for he was able to practice even beyond normal retirement, until a heart attack took him unexpectedly. He was one of the few doctors on the staff who made hospital rounds twice a day. He came on morning rounds as was usual with most, but he was also back about 8:30 in the evening to check on his patients and to say goodnight to them.

Dr. Spano was the oldest, or one of the oldest, in a large, poor family from northeast Minneapolis. In spite of being poor, all were able to get college educations because of an agreement among them whereby only one would attend college at one time. Each one knew that when he or she received that coveted degree, it was his or her responsibility to provide financial assistance as needed for the next in line. A younger sister, Frances Spano, graduated from St. Barnabas Nursing School in 1940. This speaks volumes of the family values inculcated in the good doctor from an early age. His patients came from the same Italian northeast neighborhood as he did. Some were his relatives and many were poor, but they loved their doctor. His office in northeast Minneapolis was always crowded and one sometimes had to wait for quite a long time to be seen, even with an appointment. He always had time to listen to each person and to reassure them in his comforting, low key manner.

Dr. Spano first joined the medical staff at St. Barnabas in 1930 as a visiting staff member. By 1935, he had joined the active staff where he remained a loyal member for the rest of his life. He once said to this author that he considered it remarkable that he, a devout and practicing Roman Catholic, could be so well accepted in an Episcopal hospital.

Joseph Spano was born 5 September 1905 in South Bend, Indiana. Later he moved to Minnesota, attending the University of Minnesota where he received both premedical and medical education. He interned at the University of Minnesota Hospitals in 1929-1930. At various times, he returned to the university and to Cook County Graduate School of Medicine in Illinois for graduate studies. He served as an instructor at the University of Minnesota and at Minneapolis General Hospital from 1930-1942. He served in the United States Army Medical Corps from 1942-1946, performing more than seven hundred major surgical operations during his overseas years with the army.

He was a Fellow of the American College of Surgeons as well as the International College of Surgeons in addition to memberships in the American Medical Association, the Minnesota Medical Association, the

Hennepin County Medical Society, the Minneapolis Surgical Society and the American Association of Abdominal Surgeons.

Dr. Spano and his wife, Margaret lived on Stinson Boulevard in northeast Minneapolis. They had two sons, Wyman and Joseph.

Writing for the *Voice of St. Barnabas* in March 1965, an interviewer said, "What does he do for outside interests? He has an enthusiastic interest and zeal for assisting, counseling and advising those in need—a confidant and Good Samaritan to those in his family, his medical practice and his church. He devotes a great amount of energy and money to his interest in The House of Charity."

Dr. Marvin J. Stewart

Dr. Stewart graduated from the University of Minnesota Medical School in the 1930s. As so many others did, during World War II he served in the armed forces, Pacific Theater. Returning to private practice after the war, in 1948, he decided to specialize in anesthesiology, attending the University of Minnesota for the advanced training he needed. He had a pleasant, ready smile that tended to put people at ease and this was a definite advantage for an anesthesiologist. He joined the staff at St. Barnabas in 1953 as chief of the anesthesia department.

Dr. Stewart was married and had a son and a daughter.

Dr. Jacob H. Strickler

Dr. Jacob Strickler came to St. Barnabas originally as a surgical resident in 1946. He had served two years during World War II in the United States Army Medical Corps, European theater. While he was a resident, he became interested in a research project recently begun by Dr. Carl Rice. In 1950, having completed his residency, he joined Dr. Rice in practice and together the two, with the sponsorship of Baxter Laboratories, continued in their quest for better parenteral fluids, especially those regularly used on postoperative patients. Dr. Strickler understood better than most physicians at the time, the effect of electrolytes on the human body. This was a pronounced advantage in determining what the content of parenteral fluids should be under various patient conditions.

During his leisure time, Dr. Strickler enjoyed a good game of bridge and, in fact, he and his wife were perennial high scorers in bridgeramas sponsored by the auxiliary. He also enjoyed sports—swimming, boating and water skiing in summer and in winter, ice skating and snow skiing.

Dr. Gordon Tesch

Dr. Gordon Tesch spent his professional life in general practice with Dr. Arthur Roelke in Elk River, Minnesota. The two joined forces in 1937 when Dr. Tesch entered the practice that Dr. Roehlke had already established in Elk River. During those early years together, they expanded the practice several miles north of Elk River since Princeton at that time had only one doctor, who found it nearly impossible to see all the patients who needed his services. So several Princetonites turned to Elk River for medical care and even after Princeton obtained the services of other doctors following World War II, the Princeton patients remained fiercely loyal to Drs. Roelke and Tesch. With the retirement of Dr. H. E. Cooney in the late 1930s (Princeton's only doctor for a period of time), the hospital he owned, Northwestern Hospital, closed its doors. For the next nine or ten years, Princeton patients requiring hospitalization went usually to St. Cloud, to the University of Minnesota Hospitals or to Northern Pacific Hospital in St. Paul. Princetonites who were patients of Drs. Roelke and Tesch were more likely to be hospitalized at St. Barnabas.

Dr. William T. Walsh

Dr. William Walsh was a graduate of the University of Minnesota Medical School. He interned at St. Barnabas in 1938-39 and joined the medical staff immediately after completing his internship. During World War II, he served three years in the United States Army Air Corps, Pacific theater of operations. Following the war he returned to Minneapolis to resume his practice and rejoin the medical staff. He served as chief of staff in 1957.

Dr. Donald S. Weatherhead

Dr. Weatherhead was born in 1924 in Winnipeg, Manitoba, Canada. He graduated from the Manitoba Medical College in 1947 and interned at St. Boniface Hospital, St. Boniface, Manitoba. He was in general practice in Saskatchewan before coming to the University of Minnesota to study anesthesiology. In 1958, following five years of study and research in anesthesia at the university and one year in private practice, he joined the staff at St. Barnabas as an anesthesiologist. Prior to settling on anesthesiology for his specialty, he gave thoughtful consideration to internal medicine and to pediatrics. He was torn in his choice of specialty, but the consensus of those with whom he worked was that he made an unusually empathic anesthesiologist utilizing the bedside skills he had developed while studying internal medicine and pediatrics. The following quotation comes from an article written about Dr. Weatherhead in the April-May 1962 issue of the *Voice of St. Barnabas*. "Those of us who have approached the ingress to the operating suite as patients realize the awe and apprehension one experiences. It is not until you have passed through those swinging doors and have been placed on a litter outside another closed door, that the full impact of your emotions is felt. It is at this point that you may be greeted by a soft-spoken, bespectacled, twinkle-eyed man in white who will say, 'Good morning, I am Dr. Weatherhead of the anesthesia department.' From then on confidence in everyone returns, you feel that here are people who really do care."

From 1955-1957 Dr. Weatherhead served as an instructor in anesthesiology at the University of Minnesota. He was a diplomate of the American Board of Anesthesiology.

In 1964, he delivered a paper at the meeting of the International Congress of Anesthesia, held in Las Vegas, Nevada. He was well known professionally for he authored several papers for professional journals.

Dr. Lloyd Ashley Whitesell

Dr. Whitesell was born January 22, 1907 in the little town of Browerville in Todd County in north central Minnesota. He went to school in Long Prairie and after high school graduation he turned to the University of Minnesota for premedical and medical education. In 1933 he received his MD from the University of Minnesota Medical School. He was a member of the AOA Honor Society and in 1933 received the Minnesota Medical Prize. He was a member of the American Association of General Practitioners and was certified in 1948 by the International College of Surgeons.

He interned at Minneapolis General Hospital from 1933-34. A residency in surgery at Minneapolis General followed internship. During his years of residency he served as an instructor in surgery at the University of Minnesota. He also served as instructor in gynecology at Minneapolis General, an appointment made while he was still a resident, but one which continued for years after that. In 1936 he joined the medical staff at St. Barnabas as visiting staff and in 1939, following completion of his surgical residency, he went on active staff.

In his early adult years, he was involved in all kinds of sports. This came to an end after severe injuries in a car accident. His interest then turned to aviation and he became a pilot of small aircraft. He bought a Navion plane and flew it all over the North American continent, including both Canada and Mexico.

Another of his passions was hunting. He felt he owed his interest in hunting to having been from a family of pioneers who settled first in Pennsylvania, then followed the wilderness trail through West Virginia and Kentucky. His airplane enabled him to fly to many choice hunting grounds in North America. But he didn't limit hunting to just this continent. He hunted wild boar in Hawaii and all kinds of exotic animals in Africa.He was interested as much in hunting with his camera as in hunting for the kill, so sometimes his trophies were in the form of film rather than the traditional animal head.

Dr. Whitesell married in 1929. He and his wife, Charlotte, raised a family of two sons and a daughter. One son followed his father into medicine. As of 1966, he was practicing in Buffalo, Minnesota.

Dr. Arthur A. Zierold

Dr. Zierold was one of those physicians who began professional life in another discipline. He obtained his dental degree in the early years of the twentieth century and practiced dentistry for a few years in Minneapolis. Later he changed his focus to medicine and used his dental degree to earn the funds to finance his education at the University of Minnesota Medical School from which he graduated in 1919. Then followed a fellowship in surgery at the Mayo Clinic in Rochester and ultimately he also earned a PhD in surgery.

Dr. Zierold was a member of the American Medical Association, the International Society of Surgery (American Branch), and the American College of Surgeons. He founded the Minneapolis Surgical Society and was a professor of surgery and finally professor emeritus at the University of Minnesota.

Dr. Zierold joined the visiting staff at St. Barnabas in1938 and in 1942 became a member of the active medical staff. In 1963, he was the recipient of the St. Barnabas Bowl award.

These then represent the medical staff at St. Barnabas, particularly through the 1930s, 1940s, 1950s and 1960s, the years some would term the heyday of St. Barnabas. As can be seen, they were young and old and had varied interests in addition to their profession. Most were from the Midwestern United States and most earned their MDs at the University of Minnesota. With a very few exceptions, most served in one of the armed forces either during World War II or during the Korean conflict. A majority served internships at public hospitals, particularly Minneapolis General Hospital, and many held teaching positions at the University of Minnesota Medical School. All of this speaks well for their qualifications. For leisure time activities, most got some kind of physical activity through sports or gardening. In this they were, perhaps, ahead of their times for the fitness revolution had not swept the country at that point, but they saw the value in exercising the body as well as the mind. They, along with nursing and supporting staff made St. Barnabas what it was, a hospital of which to be proud.

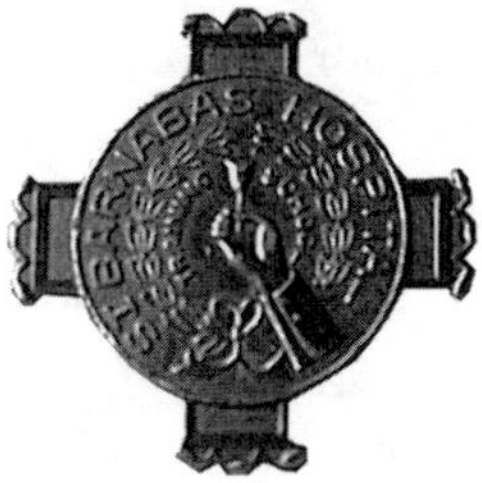

Chapter 13

St. Barnabas Bowl

An award called the "St. Barnabas Bowl" was established in 1952 by Charles Bolles Rogers who had been president of the hospital board from 1937 through nine months of 1944, and 1946 through 1951. It was introduced by Mr. Rogers at the nursing school graduation, September 1951. Presentations of the award were made at nursing school graduations in1952 and 1953. Thereafter, the award was given at the annual meeting of the Hennepin County Medical Society.

The award was administered through the Hennepin County Medical Society as trustees. Each Minneapolis hospital had the right to nominate a physician whom they saw as worthy of the honor. They were to choose a doctor who had excelled in some way in his profession whether through research, some special medical achievement or through leadership of his peers. He or she was to be considered outstanding in the qualities being evaluated for this award. Nominations from the hospitals went to the Hennepin County Medical Society, whose members then selected the best candidate from those nominated.

The award was usually presented annually, but some years may have been skipped because it was stipulated that the award was to be given only when a suitable candidate had been recommended.

The award got its name from a large silver bowl that was passed on with each presentation to the next recipient. On one side of the bowl was the St. Barnabas Hospital seal, while on the opposite side, the name of each recipient and the year of the award was engraved. When St. Barnabas and Swedish Hospital merged to form Metropolitan Medical Center, the name of the award was changed. In 1972 it became known as the Charles Bolles Bolles-Rogers Bowl.

Doctors chosen to receive the award may or may not have been on the staff of St. Barnabas. In point of fact, only seven were St. Barnabas staff members. All the rest were on staff at other hospitals in Hennepin County. Interestingly, all the recipients were men. Whether or not any women ever were nominated is not known. After 1953, the award was presented at the annual meeting of the Hennepin County Medical Society with the president of the St. Barnabas board participating in the ceremony. After 1970, the president of the Metropolitan Medical Center participated representing the hospitals.

Doctors who received the award represented many different medical and surgical specialties. The first winner, not a St. Barnabas staff member, was a cardiologist, Dr. S. Marx White, who earned the award in 1952.

Dr. Silas C. Anderson was the first St. Barnabas staff member to receive the award. His presentation came in 1958, just two years before his death. He had practiced medicine in Minneapolis since 1924 and had played an active role in both the county and the state medical societies.

The next St. Barnabas staff member to receive this recognition was thoracic surgeon Dr. Arthur A. Zierold, winner of the 1963 award. He had been on the staff at St. Barnabas since 1942. Originally, Dr. Zierold was a dentist, graduate of the University of Minnesota Dental School. He changed careers by working his way as a dentist through the University of Minnesota Medical School from which he graduated in 1919.

Two St. Barnabas pediatricians were award winners in different years. Dr. Lawrence Richdorf, 1971 winner, joined the staff at St. Barnabas in

1940. He was also a faculty member of the University of Minnesota Medical School where he taught pediatrics for thirty-nine years. Dr. Richdorf was active in civic affairs in the city and did much charity work in the county. The other pediatrician from St. Barnabas was Dr. Tague Chisholm, winner in 1976. Dr. Chisholm shared the 1976 honor with Dr. Lyle French. Dr. Chisholm is remembered by scores of parents of babies born with harelip and cleft palate. He became an expert in repair of these birth defects and often, years later, it was difficult to see that a defect had ever occurred, so skillful was the surgical repair.

Dr. Carl O. Rice, general surgeon and participant in early research on enhancing the nutritional value of parenteral fluids, was a winner in 1968. Dr. Rice and his long-time colleague, Dr. Jacob Strickler, established their research program at St. Barnabas in the late 1940s under the sponsorship of Baxter Laboratories. They employed one medical technologist in their little laboratory on 3 Corridor. They also enticed Joyce English to leave her position as head nurse on 4 Martin to join their research team. She worked with them in their office, keeping careful records on all the patients who received the experimental mixtures of fluids and additives such as absolute alcohol and intravenous vitamins. She also made daily rounds with them, visiting their hospitalized patients to observe first-hand the progress of patient recovery. Because of the alcohol in the fluids they received, patients of these two surgeons were often able to go through a postoperative recovery with a minimum of other analgesics for pain. The doctors postulated that patients who received little in the way of drugs for relief of pain healed faster than those who were heavily sedated postoperatively.

Dr. Thomas Lowry, 1965 winner, was an internist who had been on the St. Barnabas staff since 1947. Dr. John Moe, orthopedic surgeon on the St. Barnabas staff, was the 1980 award winner. Dr. Moe came to Minnesota from North Dakota, where he earned his undergraduate degree. He went on to medical school at Northwestern University in Illinois, later serving internship and residencies at the Illinois Research and Education Hospital in Chicago, San Joaquin Hospital in Stockton, California, and Gillette State Hospital in St. Paul, Minnesota. He was a clinical professor at the University of Minnesota Medical School in addition to his private practice in orthopedic surgery. At the time he received the Bolles Bolles-Rogers award in 1980, he was director of the Twin Cities Scoliosis Center as well as director of the Savannah Scoliosis Center in Georgia. He was on the staff at a number of hospitals besides St. Barnabas and later Metropolitan Medical Center including Gillette Children's Hospital, Veterans' Hospital, Fairview Hospital, Hennepin County Medical Center, St. Mary's Hospital in Minneapolis, and St. Joseph's Hospital of Savannah, Georgia.

Other winners, not a part of the St. Barnabas staff, included Dr. George E. Fahr, 1957 winner, who is remembered particularly for his work with the Minnesota State Health Department. Dr. Thomas J. Kinsella, winner in 1964, had suffered from tuberculosis early in his life. Years later, as an MD, his area of specialty was treatment of tuberculosis. Dr. Leonard A. Lang, obstetrician and gynecologist on the staff at St. Mary's Hospital, won in 1967. He also served on the faculty of the University of Minnesota Medical School. Dr. Herman E. Drill, in general practice, was the 1970 winner. He was the city health officer for Hopkins and active in the Minnesota Medical Association. He was given the Outstanding Achievement Award by the University of Minnesota in 1960.

Another of the University of Minnesota Medical School faculty members to receive the St. Barnabas Bowl was Dr. C. Donald Creevy, urologist. He won in 1972. He pioneered the treatment of prostatic cancer with transurethral resection. He served on the medical school faculty for thirty years. He was also active in medical politics, being a member of no less than fourteen different medical organizations. He was known as an exacting taskmaster, but also one who was scrupulously honest. The president of Metropolitan Medical Center in presenting the award to him included this personal description: "Honesty, sense of justice and his insistence on one standard of quality care for every patient" regardless of the patient's status in life.

Dr. Orwood J. Campbell, 1966 winner, held a PhD degree as well as his MD. He was a surgeon, long active in county, state and national medical associations. Dr. Cecil J. Watson, an internist on the staff at Northwestern Hospital, was another of the doctors who served on the faculty of the University of Minnesota Medical School. He began his service at the Medical School in 1934 and was highly regarded all over the state.

Dr. Ragnvald S. Ylvisaker, 1975 winner, was also an internist, also on the staff at Northwestern. He had earlier received the Harold S. Diehl Award for his contributions to Minnesota medical practice.

Lastly, Dr. Reuben Berman was an internist and cardiologist. He won the bowl in 1977 for his work in heart research at Mount Sinai Hospital. At one time he had been editor of Minnesota Medicine.

From these few biographical sketches, it is easy to see that the winners of the St. Barnabas Bowl were drawn from a broad spectrum of the doctors living in Hennepin County. Several, but certainly not all, were active in medical politics. And several were associated with the University of Minnesota Medical School. But there were also many who did not have that connection.

A complete list of all the winners can be found in the Appendix at the end of this book.

Chapter 14

A School of Nursing Is Born

In 1947, Helen Hayden wrote an article in the *Voice of St. Barnabas* in which she included this unascribed quotation: "Nursing is Christianity with its sleeves rolled up." We don't know the source of this bit of wisdom, but it is something we can imagine the good Dr. Knickerbacker would have said. Though he did not live to see the graduation of the first nurse from St. Barnabas Hospital School of Nursing, we believe he would have been pleased to hear nursing described in this way.

With the opening of the Martin building in 1894, St. Barnabas began a giant stride toward the hospital that Alumnae and former employees still living today would recognize. An earlier attempt to begin a nursing school was begun in the early 1890s but abandoned when the decision was made to close the hospital for a period of time to clear the land and build the new Martin building. In the city of Minneapolis at that time, several other hospitals had begun opening schools of nursing. Northwestern Hospital, a few blocks south of St. Barnabas, opened the first school of nursing west of the Mississippi in 1883, just 12 years after St. Barnabas came into being as the old Colonial Hospital, the first hospital in Minneapolis. Minneapolis General Hospital, two blocks to the west of St. Barnabas, opened its doors in 1887; Swedish Hospital, just across Seventh Street, south of St. Barnabas, opened its doors in 1898 and St. Andrew's Hospital, over across the river to the east, opened in 1912.

For most of these hospitals, opening the institution also involved the opening of a nursing school since student nurses almost always provided nearly the total staff for a new hospital. A matron, who may or may not have been a nurse herself, would be hired to be in charge of the nursing department, and she may have had one or more graduates working as supervisors under her direction. Since there were no standards yet governing requirements for a nursing school, anything went that was considered possible and reasonable by those in the business of deciding whether a hospital would be established and who would staff it once it came into being.

Because there were no preparatory programs for nurses west of the Mississippi before Northwestern opened its school, it follows that few trained nurses were available for hire in this relatively new city. The objective for most hospitals in establishing these schools was not so much the development of a pool of graduates as it was to satisfy the immediate staffing needs of newly opened hospitals. One factor mitigating against standards for nursing schools was an absence of a body of knowledge that could be identified specifically as Nursing. There was also not a very clear idea of what was entailed in properly caring for the sick and injured.

During the 1950s or 1960s, a paper meant to be humorous made the rounds of several people in the nursing department at St. Barnabas. It listed two pages of remedies that often were used during the mid nineteenth century to treat injuries and illnesses. Some from that list were included in the chapter of this book on organization of the medical staff at St. Barnabas. Others not included in that chapter were the kind of thing which may have passed as nursing in those days. Some of those measures included the following:

- For corns on the feet, wrap the toe with a blade of fodder;
- for croup, wet a wide strip of heavy flannel with heated turpentine and tallow and wrap it around the neck;

- for earache, soak cotton in hot sweet oil or laudanum and place it in the ear;
- for neuralgia, make a warm poultice of bear-grass root and sweet milk;
- for pneumonia, until the doctor comes, place a poultice on the chest made of pine tar, mustard seed and vinegar;
- for a teething baby, rub gums with a silver thimble, then wrap a nutmeg in a cheese-cloth and pin it inside his shirt.

People in those days must have had tough skin to enable them to tolerate some of these treatments. But in areas where people were isolated from medical care, they had to learn to care for themselves and often developed measures like this in the belief they were routing out whatever evil was causing the problem.

From the time of the Crusades onward, in Europe, there were religious orders of men or women who took on the responsibility of caring for the sick and injured. The study of medicine was still rudimentary, but small steps were being taken in that field under the religious orders. With the religious revolts and the Thirty Years War in sixteenth-century Europe, medicine moved from the monastery to the university. Since universities of the time were all male institutions, the religious women who had been providing much of the nursing care, such as it was, were not welcome as scholars, and so the practice of medicine was divorced from the practice of nursing. The period from 1500-1860 was termed the "Dark Period" in nursing. Most respectable women stayed in the refuge of the home, so except in hospitals operated by religious orders in predominantly Catholic countries, the only women left to staff hospitals were the immoral, the illiterate and the drunken. In short, people who had no other options for supporting themselves. The stigma attached to the practice of nursing after that was difficult to dispel.

Florence Nightingale, who lived from 1820-1910, is recognized as the one person who did most to establish nursing as an honorable profession to be practiced by decent, God-fearing women. She was the daughter of wealthy British parents who were visiting Italy at the time of her birth, so she was named for the Italian city in which she was born. Her father was a well-educated man who doted on his daughter. Under his tutelage she received an education comparable to or exceeding that available to men in universities of the time. She was an apt student and readily absorbed and applied all that she learned at the knee of her father.

She was also a devoutly religious person and declared that she had been called by God, in a vision, to spend her life in ministering to the sick and poor. Though her father had provided the education that nourished the mind of this remarkable lady, he didn't anticipate how she would use that education. Her parents wanted for her what all proper parents of the day wanted, that she would marry well and live happily ever after. She was an attractive girl and there were many suitors, even proposals of marriage, but she wanted none of it. Over the strenuous objections of her family, she pursued her interest in care of the sick.

From the beginning, she considered compassion and commitment necessary in a nurse, but as time went on, she came to realize that intelligence and training were equally important. She kept journals of her ideas, later published as Notes On Nursing in which she outlined all she felt should be included in nursing practice and training. Along Miss Nightingale's journey of preparation to follow her dream, obeying the call of God as she felt it had been revealed to her, she learned of an institution in Germany which was providing training for nurses. She resolved to go there to learn all she could. But again, her family objected and refused to allow her to go. Finally, on the guise of visiting relatives on the continent, and with the cooperation of these relatives who were sympathetic to her cause, she did spend three months at this place, the Deaconess Institute in Kaiserwerth, Germany.

The institute had been founded in 1836 by Pastor Theodor Fliedner and his wife, Fredericke. It began as a refuge for discharged women prisoners. Later, the Fliedners added an orphanage, a normal school and a hospital. They developed a nursing program in the hospital to answer the need for trained and compassionate women to care for their patients. They spent a good deal of effort in influencing better classes of women to enroll in their nursing program to become "deaconesses" as they termed their nurses. Their deaconesses took no formal vows, but they did promise to spend their lives working for Christ. The philosophy followed by the Fliedners at Kaiserwerth appealed to everything Florence Nightingale felt about nursing. The secret three months she spent at Kaiserwerth were the only formal training she ever had in nursing, but what she learned validated all the feelings she had developed since she first experienced that vision of God calling her to care for the sick.

Florence Nightingale is regarded as the founder of modern nursing because she developed and implemented a plan for training laywomen to become nurses. She believed nursing services should be available to all and that the public should be responsible for paying for nursing care. During the Crimean War, she took a band of volunteer nurses to serve at the British military hospital in Scutari in what we know today as Turkey. With the greatest of difficulty, she was able to bring about drastic reforms at that hospital with the result that men treated there had much higher survival rates than had been known previously in British military hospitals. The grateful men who were her patients at Scutari nicknamed her the "Lady with the Lamp" because of her practice of making rounds through the night to the bedsides of all in need of her care and observation. She returned to England a heroine when the war ended.

She spent the rest of her long life working to insure that schools be developed to educate women to become nurses. St. Thomas Hospital in London was the site chosen for the development of the first nursing program based on the Nightingale principles. The fact that school flourished through the twentieth century is testament to the soundness of the ideas put forth by Miss Nightingale.

In the United States, the first attempt to organize a nursing school was made by the Nurse Society of Philadelphia in 1839. They set up a program that provided a period of elementary instruction in nursing. The successful student was given a certificate. Since there was no body of knowledge identified as "nursing" at that time and since there were no training programs around for nurses, one is led to wonder who made up the membership of the Nurse Society of Philadelphia, and what did they teach in their certificate program? Be that as it may, at least it was an attempt to provide some sort of training for those who would care for the sick.

The first nursing schools in the United States that we would recognize today came in 1872 and 1873. The work of volunteer caregivers in military hospitals during the Civil War brought the idea of training programs to the attention of the public. The New England Hospital for Women and Children in Boston attempted to establish a school during the Civil War, but failed in that attempt. In 1872, the school was reestablished along the lines of the

Nightingale principles. Bellevue Hospital in New York City established its nursing school on May 1, 1873. They were to go on to produce many nurses who in the next century became leaders in the profession. In the 1950s St. Barnabas had one of their alumnae, Dorothy Merrell, at the helm of nursing service and nursing education at the hospital. She was an inspiration to many who had the privilege of knowing her and working with her.

Both the New England Hospital program and the one at Bellevue were established on Nightingale ideals, as were many other nursing schools established in the country during the last quarter of the nineteenth century. Unfortunately, a chronic problem with these schools established with such high purpose was insufficient financial backing. So over time the schools were absorbed by hospitals and the educational purpose was subverted to the needs of nursing service. The schools and their students were simply exploited as sources of free labor. Even at best, the schools that did try to maintain an academic rather than a service approach to nursing tended to teach the "how" of nursing with little regard for the "why." Student assignments were made up on the basis of the amount of work that needed to be done with little regard for the kind of experience the student needed or already had learned.

Teaching was usually done by doctors on the staff of the hospital and in some cases supplemented by whatever the director or superintendent or matron (or whatever she might be called) had time to teach. The value of a broad variety of experiences was not considered, so many hospitals with as few as thirty daily average patient census established nursing programs. And single purpose hospitals, such as mental hospitals or tuberculosis sanitaria, also established programs even though they could offer just that one kind of experience to students. The number of nursing programs established proliferated. There were only four hundred schools in 1900 and by 1920 there were over three thousand schools throughout the country.

In the early years of the twentieth century, state boards of nurse examiners were being established. Minnesota's board dates back to 1907 and a St. Barnabas graduate, Eleanor Hamilton, class of 1898, served on that first board. But the focus of the state board at that time was on examination and licensure of graduates of nursing programs. It took another twenty years or so before the boards were also charged with setting standards for nursing schools.

A hospital in the nineteenth century and the early twentieth century too, was looked upon as a last resort for recovering from illness or a place to provide care for those who had no one at home to care for them. It was considered by many people to be a disgrace to send a relative to a hospital for recuperation. For this reason, there were not great numbers of potential students waiting in line to enroll. At St. Barnabas for the first ten years of the school, only two to eight students were graduated each year. Opportunities for graduates to work in the hospital were limited. As a matter of fact, once the school at St. Barnabas got going to the point where there were upper class as well as beginning students, the few supervisors who had been on the staff were replaced by upper class students. The 1916 booklet about St. Barnabas lists only three nurses who worked on nursing floors in the hospital. In addition, there was the superintendent of nurses, an assistant superintendent, a night supervisor, an operating room supervisor, an assistant operating room supervisor, a chief anesthetist and two assistant anesthetists. This apparently was the total nursing staff of the hospital which at that time, according to a Board of Nursing report, had a daily average patient census of one hundred fifty. Only four of the nurses listed were not St. Barnabas graduates. Seven graduates from St. Barnabas came from the classes of 1899, 1906, 1909 and 1915.

From information available today, we can conclude that the school established at St. Barnabas probably followed the Nightingale principles fairly well. A summary report concerning St. Barnabas Hospital School of Nursing was prepared at the Minnesota Board of Nursing and made available to me in the early 1970s. The report lists all of the chief nurse administrative officers of the hospital from the beginning of the school. Only the first of these, Eleanor Weston, did not have in her resume, schooling from one of the large eastern schools operating on Nightingale principles. She was a graduate of Indianapolis City Hospital School of Nursing. Harriet Hartry, the second nursing superintendent listed by the Board, was a graduate of Brooklyn Hospital School of Nursing in New York. The board report indicates she was replaced by a St. Barnabas graduate, M. Dorothy Rhodes, but Miss Rhodes' education was not limited to what she had gotten at St. Barnabas, for she had done postgraduate work at Boston Floating Hospital, another of the acknowledged leading hospitals at that time in nursing education.

A booklet prepared in 1964 to commemorate the seventieth anniversary of the founding of the school, listed the following requirements for admission: "Three letters of recommendation, one a statement as to the prospective student's health by her family doctor, the other two character references, one of which was to be written by her pastor…"

Students were accepted almost entirely on the basis of character evaluation as supplied by these letters with relatively little academic training considered necessary. It must be said, however, that many of the girls had high school training while a meager minority boasted from two to four years of college work.

Requirements listed in the Board of Nursing report indicate that in 1905, two years of high school education were required. It was not until 1920 that high school graduation was made a requirement.

In the early days of the school, there were several older students who came with prior experience in another career field, usually schoolteaching. One student from that first class, Ella Gibson, was only sixteen years old when she entered the school, but the usual student was much older than that. Age requirements apparently were not in effect until 1922, when according to the Board of Nursing, applicants had to be between the ages of eighteen and thirty one. In 1935, the minimum age was raised to nineteen, but reduced again to eighteen in 1943. According to the board report, the age requirement was changed again in 1944 to seventeen and one half years minimum age. At that point, one hundred eight of the one hundred nine students in the school were enrolled in the Cadet Program, designed to increase the supply of nurses for the armed forces. Lowering the minimum age by one half year was possibly done to increase the pool from which prospective students could be drawn and to increase the possibility for more young women to enlist in the Cadet Corps as their contribution to the war effort. A 1948 bulletin from the school listed the minimum age as seventeen. School bulletins from the 1960s make no reference to either minimum or maximum age requirements for admission.

There was a requirement by the Board of Nursing for several years that a candidate for licensure had to be nineteen years old when writing licensure examinations, so in practice, the minimum age on entrance to the school actually was seventeen or older in order to meet the age requirement for writing boards.

In the early 1960s, the faculty accepted three women into the program who were in their upper thirties, married and had children at home. None of the three lived in Whitney Residence, but commuted from their homes and their homemaker responsibilities. All three were excellent students. Two, Muriel Hegg and Milka May, graduated in 1965, and Erene Gross, graduated in 1966. They were unusual women, to be sure. Muriel had five children ranging in age from a son who would be entering kindergarten the fall after Muriel's graduation, to another son who graduated from high school at nearly the same time as his mother was graduating from St. Barnabas. Milka had a tragic past, having been a survivor of the Nazi Holocaust and a death camp where several members of her family died. She, too, had children at home. And Erene was also the mother of children still at home. All three handled the multiple roles of wife, homemaker, mother and student very capably.

Later in the 1960s, men were accepted as students for the first time in the history of the school, and they proved themselves to be capable students as well.

Some history of nursing texts, in describing entrance requirements for the early schools, stated effort was expended to recruit as plain-looking women as possible, the theory being, apparently, that these women likely would not marry and therefore would stay with the profession of nursing. There is no indication this was ever a consideration at St. Barnabas, and looking at the graduation pictures on the racks in the Historical Library, one is impressed by the fine looking group of women who went through the school. Just out of curiosity, the marriage rates for graduates from the early years were computed. Only two of the six graduates from the first class married after graduation. There were only two in the second class and neither ever married. In the third class, only two of eight married. But the ladies of the fourth class, in 1900, broke the pattern when three of four in the class married after graduation. Several in those first three classes were older and possibly already career oriented when they entered the school, and this may have had more to do with their marriageability than their appearance did. During the 1960s several St. Barnabas students were elected queens in various beauty and personality contests, further debunking the idea that a nurse should be as plain looking as possible.

A doctor's evaluation of the prospective student's health was reflected for years in the references submitted by high school counselors even into the 1960s. Many included in their references that the student had a strong back and good feet!

As for clothing and equipment which the student was to bring with her to the school, a document dated 1915 and entitled "Instructions for Probationers" listed the following:

- 1 pair of ground gripper shoes, fitted with rubber heels.
- 1 pair of rubbers to fit shoes." (A parenthetical note then explained the shoes and rubbers could be purchased after arrival in Minneapolis from John Girard, 133 South Seventh Street.)
- A watch with a second hand.
- A fountain pen.
- An inexpensive umbrella.
- Four plain dresses as near like the sample as possible. (Apparently a drawing or picture of the dress was enclosed with a note that the blue chambray from which the dress was to be made could be purchased at Dayton's in Minneapolis. The description of the dress went on to specify that it was to be made in one piece, "sleeves to button so that they may be rolled up over elbow; seven gored skirt with a six inch hem…when finished to be two inches from the floor; front yoke to be fine tucked to form a pointed yoke; uniform to button down the back with buttons extending down to the skirt." Further it specified the buttons must be white pearl, 3/8 inch in diameter and that the material should be shrunken before it was made up. Lastly, there was to be "a plain standing collar attached to the waist."

Next the requirements listed:

- Six sets of plain, strong underclothing made without ruffles or trimming." (The underclothing was to include three petticoats of plain blue or other washable material.)
- Eight narrow hemstitched turnovers. These may be made from the hems of hemstitched napkins." (This author hasn't the foggiest notion of what a turnover was or how it was used!)
- Two laundry bags marked with name; these to be made of sheeting 1.25 yards square when finished.

- One smaller laundry bag of smaller size, to be made of sheeting, twenty-seven inches square.
- Eighteen outing flannel toilet napkins.
- One shoe bag with five compartments.
- One pair of blunt pointed scissors.
- One napkin ring with name engraved.

The pamphlet suggested that every washable item be labeled with Cash's woven names. Students on through the years, probably right to the end of the school, bought Cash's woven names. They were readily available at Dayton's for many years. An address for the Cash Company, J & J Cash, Ltd, of South Norwalk, Connecticut, was supplied as was the price for the labels, $2.00 for twelve dozen.

The last line on the requirement list read, "Unmarked laundry will not be returned from the laundry."

The School bulletin dated 1946 stated that an applicant who was in the upper one third of her high school class or who had successfully completed prior college work would be given preference in admissions. Health requirements were spelled out as follows: "She should be within normal limits as to weight and height. Remedial physical defects such as enlarged tonsils, carious teeth and defective vision must be corrected before entrance. Accepted applicants must be immunized by their personal physicians for typhoid, smallpox and diphtheria before entering the school, unless they have been so immunized within the last year."

By 1948, academic entrance requirements had been specified which would meet standards for admission to the University of Minnesota, since students would be taking science and social science courses at the university during the first two quarters at St. Barnabas. The courses a student had to have prior to admission were four years of English, two years of social science or foreign language, two years of physical and biological science, one year of history, two years of mathematics and five electives. At that point, one or more years of college work were also mentioned as desirable. Students were also required to obtain a satisfactory score (not specified) on the pre-entrance nursing aptitude test battery. And by that time, a personal interview had also been added to the requirements for admission.

Early on in the school, students were paid monthly stipends, the first recorded by the Board of Nursing being three dollars per month in 1916. The report includes a notation that this amount appeared to have been given in years prior to 1916 as well. By 1923, the stipend had been increased to five dollars per month beginning after successful completion of the probationary period. In 1925, students were having a one-month experience of twelve-hour special nursing duty for which the patient paid the hospital five dollars per day. The board report does not stipulate how much of that five dollars per day went to the student. By 1935 the stipends had been discontinued.

In 1937 the school began to charge tuition. Fifty dollars was listed as the tuition for that year, thirty-five dollars of which went to the University of Minnesota. The next year, tuition had been increased to one hundred seventy five dollars, part of which went to the University of Minnesota, and mention was first made of the availability of a loan fund. In 1939, they didn't list tuition as such, but indicated that one year in the nursing school would cost approximately five hundred dollars. From 1942-1945, the federal government subsidized the education of students in the Cadet Corps, which included almost every student enrolled in the school. Tuition fees returned in 1946 then two hundred thirty dollars for the year. Tuition increase again in 1947 to three hundred dollars along with the first mention of availability of scholarships. In 1948, tuition was four hundred dollars and by 1951, five hundred fifty dollars. The University of Minnesota affiliation for basic and social sciences was discontinued and the program at Macalester College substituted in its place. Tuition to Macalester alone was four hundred dollars. By 1953, the cost to the student for the entire program was six hundred thirty nine dollars.

At this point, student service to the hospital was being given a dollar value, offsetting the cost of education. Service given by a first year student was valued at sixty cents per hour; service given by a second year student was valued at one dollar eight cents per hour and that of a senior student was valued at one dollar thirty-seven cents per hour. In 1956, the out of pocket expense to the student was seven hundred twenty six dollars and by 1957, seven hundred seventy five dollars. The bulletin for 1964-1965 showed a dramatic increase in fees due to the addition of board, room and laundry fees, which had not been charged during the years that student clinical hours were controlled by nursing service. After 1962, the nursing school was split entirely from nursing service and the hours of clinical experience were those deemed necessary to learning a given part of the curriculum, so credit for service given by students to nursing service was no longer honored. Up to 1962, student service to the hospital was considered replacement for board, room and laundry. Fees in 1964-1965 were three hundred seventy-five dollars tuition for the first year, plus a fifty dollar health fee, four hundred twenty dollars board, two hundred twenty dollars room and fifty dollars laundry. Second year fees were three hundred twenty dollars tuition, fifty dollars health fee, three hundred fifteen dollars board, one hundred sixty five room and thirty-seven dollars and fifty cents laundry. Board, room and laundry were less for second year students because the second year was the year they were away on affiliations, so not using board, room or laundry at the hospital. The third year had been shortened by one quarter, so students paid two hundred forty dollars tuition for the third year, a fifty dollar health fee, three hundred fifteen dollars board, one hundred sixty five dollars room and thirty seven dollars and fifty cents laundry. At that point there were a multitude of scholarships available plus a revolving loan fund to help the student who was unable to pay the increased costs.

A school bookstore had also been opened to offer both convenience and cost saving to students on textbooks. Uniforms were purchased by the student directly from the uniform company and came to a total cost of one hundred one dollars for the three years.

There was also a work program available whereby second and third year students could be employed as unlicensed practical nurses during off-duty hours. Qualification to work as an unlicensed practical nurse depended on the student having completed the course of study related to the place she was being asked to work. First year students, lacking the clinical experience to work as practical nurses, could be employed as nurse aides. After the licensure law for practical nurses became a mandatory law, students were prohibited by law from employment as practical nurses.

In the early years of the nursing school at St. Barnabas, students were accepted at different times of the year. So although we refer to the class of 1897 as the first to graduate, actually they did not all finish at the same time because each of the six in that class entered the school at a different time. It sounds as if instruction was either very individually oriented, or there was very little instruction other than on the job training. It appears the answer concerning those first six students was "both."

Throughout the history of the school, all students entered as probationers, though in later years, much less emphasis was placed on probationary status than in the beginning.

The expectation by the later years was that every student who was accepted in the program had the capability to complete it. In the early years, black stockings and the plain blue chambray dress distinguished the probationer from other students. The probationary period started at two months' duration, then was increased to four months and later to six months. After the affiliation with the University of Minnesota for sciences and social sciences was begun, the end of the probationary period coincided with the completion of the two quarters of university studies. The same applied when Macalester College was used in place of the university and again when Video Nursing Education replaced the Macalester affiliation.

To mark the end of probation, early students were capped and allowed to wear the blue check uniform of the school. When the Cadet Nurse Program came to the school in the early 1940s, the blue checks gave way to white dresses with a patch on one pocket indicating the individual was a student. The class which graduated in 1951 was the last to wear the white student uniform. Blue checks with white aprons came back with the class of 1952. Students began wearing the school uniform only a few weeks after they entered the school, at a time when they had progressed sufficiently in nursing arts that they could be assigned to the clinical areas. Capping services came after successful completion of the college courses in basic and social sciences. Many can recount how much longer it took to dress for duty after capping. Somehow, it was difficult to learn how to pin that cap so that it would stay in place through a full shift on duty. The author recalls missing breakfast on several occasions after capping because by the time she got to the dining room for breakfast, students were lining up for the mandatory trek to the chapel for chapel service before going on duty at 7:00 A.M. One member of the class of 1949 was particularly fond of coming to a student's table, picking up the breakfast tray and saying "Time for chapel, freshman."

Capping services were held at Gethsemane Episcopal Church for several years. About 1950, St. Mark's Cathedral became the site for both capping and graduation services.

Perhaps as class sizes increased, the smaller Gethsemane church did not offer enough seating for school services. The class of 1951 was the last to be capped at Gethsemane, though their graduation service was at St. Mark's. The cap had multiple purposes and its use for nurses went back probably to the days when religious orders provided the nursing care given. The cap may have been a vestige of the veil worn by the sisters in the religious communities. It was symbolic of professional status, but it was also a way to keep the hair in place. For years long hair was frowned upon unless it could be braided, pinned up or otherwise kept under control.

Washing and starching the St. Barnabas cap and then folding it properly was a problem for many. For years there was a woman at the hospital who would wash and starch a cap for a small fee and most felt it worth the money to have her do it, though they were on their own when it came to folding it. There was a session held with each class about to be capped during which a bit of the history of the cap was given and all were shown how to properly fold it. The back section of the cap was to be folded to resemble a candle. The brim then was folded just to the seam line so that the halo of the candle would show above the brim. Students wore plain white caps. A black stripe was added at graduation and worn thereafter. The only difference between the 1894 cap and the twentieth century version was that the 1894 cap was worn higher on the head, covering more of the hair. The St. Barnabas cap was distinctive and designed for use only by St. Barnabas students and graduates. This was the prevailing custom for all schools at the time.

The pin given to each at graduation was also distinctive to the school. It was crafted of sterling silver. The design was done at Tiffany's in New York and pins were ordered from there at first. Later, Hudson's in Minneapolis carried the pins, making it much easier for the unlucky graduate who wanted to replace a lost pin to do so. The pin was in the shape of a Greek cross, signifying the religious origin of the school. There was a laurel wreath, the Greek symbol of honor, surrounding an up-stretched hand which held a communion cup, referring to the honor of serving as well as to the religious origins of the school. Each nurse's name was engraved on the back of the pin. For years, representatives of the Women's Board pinned the pins on new graduates at graduation. Later, in the 1960s, a faculty member or an alumnae member did the pinning.

Minnie Paterson was the first St. Barnabas graduate. She was twenty-six years old when she entered the school. She had been a schoolteacher prior to that time. After she graduated from St. Barnabas, she went to New York for postgraduate education. Completing that, she moved to Chicago where she joined the Visiting Nurse Association in that city. She returned to Minneapolis in 1907 to organize the first Visiting Nurse Association (VNA) here. She held the position of director of the VNA until 1922. During those years, she was also active in the Red Cross, being a personal friend of Jane Delano, organizer of Red Cross nursing services nationwide. It was Minnie Paterson who organized the first Red Cross nursing service in Minnesota and she served as its first director in 1913. During the influenza epidemic of 1918, Red Cross nurses gave yeoman service in caring for the flu victims. Red Cross nursing service was also particularly important during World

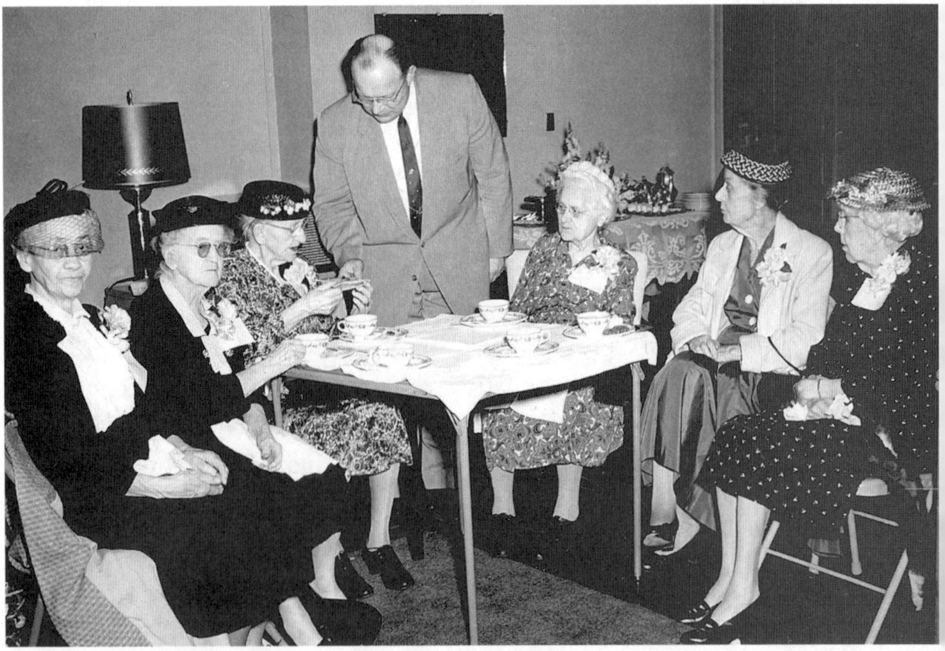

Minnie Paterson returns her pin to the hospital, May 1956. Left to right are Louise Briggs (class of 1904), Charlotte Roberts (1898), Minnie Paterson (first graduate, 1897), Robert Bachmeyer, hospital director, Minnie Eggleston (1899), Maud Trageser (1902) and Caroline Rankiellor (1901).

War I because it was through the Red Cross that nurses were recruited for military service.

In 1922, Minnie moved to Aberdeen, Washington, where she worked for eighteen years. In 1940, she moved to Santa Rosa, California and in 1944 she returned to Minnesota for retirement. In 1954, at a tea given at the Minneapolis Society of the Blind, she was awarded the Jane Delano award in recognition of her contributions to Red Cross nursing in Minnesota. She must have been very proud, having known Jane Delano personally back in the early days. In May of 1956, a tea was held at Knickerbacker Residence, honoring the living graduates of the first ten years of St. Barnabas Hospital School of Nursing. Minnie was there that day, along with six others from those first ten years. On that day, she gave her school pin back to the hospital. Mr. Robert Bachmeyer, then hospital director, received the pin on behalf of the hospital. Later Miss Paterson wrote a very touching note of thanks to me as president of the alumnae, thanking the organization for the lovely day and recounting her pride at being a St. Barnabas graduate. She died in 1957, at the age of eighty-seven years.

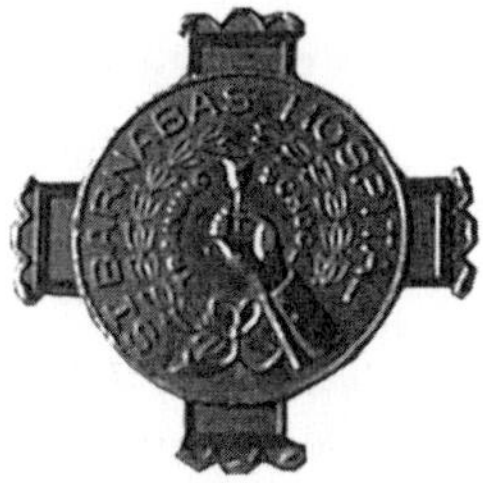

Chapter 15

From Apprentice to Student of Nursing

There likely was no curriculum as we would identify it today in the nursing school which opened at St. Barnabas in 1894. There was no practice that could be identified solely as nursing at that time and it is likely the teaching done was on the job type "how you do this" teaching. For example,"How to encourage a sick person to eat when he didn't feel like eating, how to make a bed without moving him out of it, measures that might make a bedridden person more comfortable," and so on. It would have been the kind of thing that a mother or a family member would do for someone sick in bed at home.

It took time to develop what became the practice of nursing. At the same time, the practice of medicine was also in a relatively primitive state. It was more the art of medicine than the science of medicine at the time and this, too, was reflected in what the nurse might be asked or encouraged to do for a patient.

Even though the Minnesota Board of Nurse Examiners had come into being in 1907, at that point they were not involved with establishing quality nursing education in nursing schools, but rather with identifying and credentialing with licenses, nurses who possessed the minimum skills needed to practice nursing safely. Inspections and evaluations of nursing programs came several years later at the board. The first indication recorded by the board of hours of instruction being given at St. Barnabas was in 1916. Board records indicate students were on probation for eight weeks after admission to the school. During those eight weeks they had six hours of class and two hours of on-duty time each week. The classes they took at that time included twelve hours of bacteriology, sixteen hours of hygiene, chemistry, though the number of hours taught is not given, theory of nursing, again no hours given and "Demonstrations," though the report doesn't indicate what was being demonstrated. After probation, students were paid three dollars per month. Their schedules included mainly duty time, with classes scheduled either at 4:00 P.M. or 7:15 P.M., which would have been quiet or bedtime hours for patients. They were allowed twenty-one hours per week for recreation and three weeks of annual vacation. The hours of instruction in 1916 totaled two hundred five, including the classes listed during the probationary period plus thirty two hours of anatomy, sixteen hours of dietetics and cooking, twenty hours of materia medica, sixteen hours of bandaging, sixteen hours of analysis of urine, nine hours of nursing in general medical diseases, ten hours in surgery, ten hours in gynecology, thirteen hours in obstetrics, six hours in infants and children, thirteen hours of infectious and contagious disease, four hours in nervous and mental conditions and twelve hours of eye, ear, nose and throat. There was one instructor in 1916 who earned fifty dollars per month plus board and room.

In 1920, the school reported it was offering two hundred fifty two hours of instruction over the three years the student was enrolled. The school also reported to the board they had one instructor whose responsibility was to insure these two hundred fifty-two hours of instruction were given. She was a St. Barnabas graduate, Lulu Saunders, from the previous year, 1919. Five other nurses, all St. Barnabas graduates, were listed along with Lulu as the faculty of the school. They were Amelia Peterson (Gunderson), class of 1916, operating room supervisor, Katherine Reid, class of 1909, operating room head nurse, Zelma Moores (Farnham), class of 1920, operating room supervisor (it isn't clear whether there were two operating room supervisors or whether she replaced Amelia Peterson some time during the year. Amelia did become a nurse anesthetist, so perhaps that occurred in 1920 with Miss Moores replacing Amelia.) Effie Newman, class of 1917 was night supervisor in 1920 and Rebeka Johnson, class of 1909, is listed as obstetrics head nurse. The pictorial booklet published in 1916 listed Anna Armitage, class of 1906, as supervisor in maternity. Perhaps she left teaching to Rebeka.

Experience hours listed in the 1920 report included eight weeks of medicine, sixty four weeks of surgery, eight weeks of child care, sixteen weeks of obstetrics, eight weeks of diet kitchen, two weeks of tuberculosis, sixteen weeks of operating room, sixteen weeks of eye, ear, nose and throat. Eight weeks of charge nurse experience were also listed in 1920. Apparently this was considered a well-rounded curriculum for the time. A November 27, 1922, letter from an unknown source to Clara Noyes of the American Red Cross is quoted, "The school in connection with St. Barnabas Hospital is considered one of our best schools."

In 1923, the school listed just one instructor as the faculty, that being a Miss Margaret Younglove. She was a graduate of Asbury Hospital and earned a salary of one hundred dollars per month. The record does not indicate whether she also got board and room.

In 1925, the school had a waiting list for admission to the program. The probationary period, by that time being termed "preclinical period," had been increased to four months. Two classes of student nurses were accepted each year, in September and March. By 1925 they had increased the hours of instruction to five hundred ninety, adding classes in ethics and professional problems. Students who failed State Board Examinations at that time were allowed to rewrite the examinations after a suitable period of tutoring. The 1925 report also included the first reference to a one-month experience in "special nursing," which appeared to be an experience in which the student was assigned just one patient for daily twelve-hour shifts, much like a private duty nurse would have practiced. For this special nursing the hospital collected five dollars per day from the patient, but it isn't clear whether any part of the five dollars was shared with the student who provided the care.

Hours of instruction were noted again in the 1927 report to the board, but that year, the hours were reduced by thirty-three, though there is no

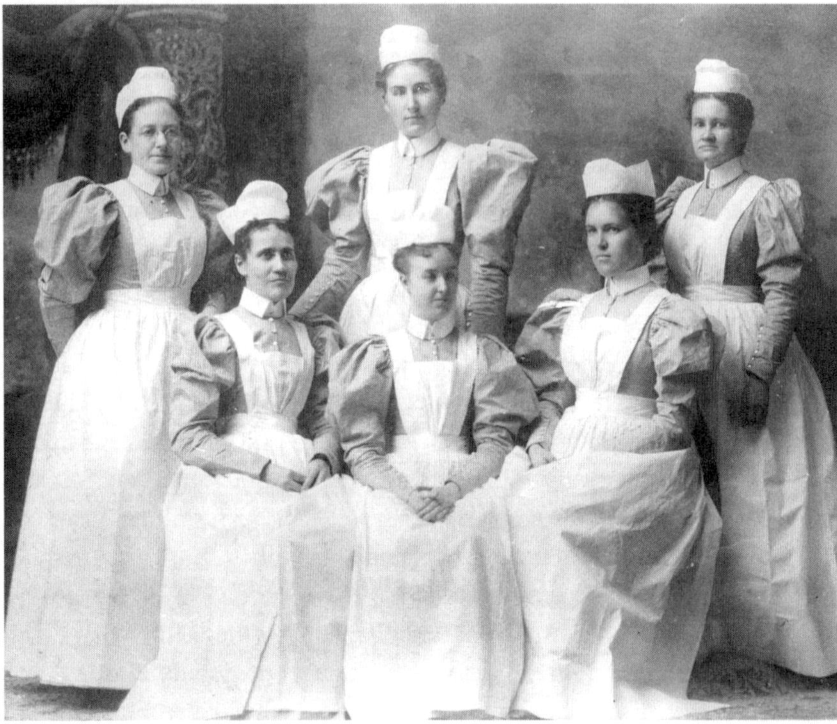

Original school uniform, class of 1897.

indication what happened to those thirty-three hours. That year the school also reported they were offering public health experience at the Minneapolis VNA to the student who had the highest scholastic average in the school. The reader may recall from the last chapter that the Minneapolis VNA had been established and was directed for years by the first graduate of St. Barnabas Hospital School of Nursing, Minnie Patterson. She may well have had a role in encouraging this experience for St. Barnabas students.

In 1932 the board made five suggestions to the school as follows: 1) That students not be held responsible for verbal orders 2) That students be required to wear special aprons or gowns in the operating and delivery rooms; 3) That case records be kept for students with diagnosis noted; 4) That case studies be added to the special diet experience; and 5) That a bulletin outlining the course in nursing be made available to every applicant for admission to the school.

The next report, in 1935, referred back to progress made on the five suggestions made by the board in 1932. The report indicated the following: 1) Not much change; 2) Satisfactory; 3) Greatly improved. (Interesting that case records still referred to medical diagnoses rather than to nursing measures used.); 4) Improved, but few special diets. Whether this was a comment on a small number of case studies involving special diets or whether it was questioning why few people were on special diets was not clear; and 5) No change. There had not been a school bulletin since 1922.

In 1935, 32% of the graduating class failed state board examinations and as a result, the board placed the school on probation and forbade them to admit any new students during the one-year period from mid 1935 to August 1936. The challenge given to the school was to spend that one year without new students improving the quality of education to be offered at the school. The specific recommendations given to the faculty by the board included: 1) Formation of a school advisory committee to make recommendations regarding improvement of the program; 2) More supervision of students be accomplished by hiring more faculty; 3) More clerical assistance be made available to the director of the school; 4) More maid service be provided so students wouldn't have to spend so much time cleaning; 5) Better living, study and teaching facilities be provided—they observed, "the nurses' home is gloomy and mattresses on which students sleep are thin and hard"; 6) Everyone on the faculty should study Nursing Schools Of Today And Tommorrow; and 7) Add affiliating courses to round out experience in the diet kitchen and in medicine.

A January 1936 notation in the file states the school was still not allowed to admit new students. The recommended advisory committee had been formed, but it had not met. An affiliation had been arranged at Glen Lake Sanitarium for tuberculosis and further diet kitchen experience. The school library was very poor. Classrooms were still inadequate, but student living accommodations had improved.

The accomplishments to which the faculty could justifiably point with pride when the board revisited the school in mid 1936 included the appointment of an advisory committee to work with the school on curriculum improvement. The committee included representatives from the community, particularly in education in the community, representatives from the hospital board, from the medical staff and from the alumnae. The advisory committee had met since the January visit of the board. The school had begun an affiliation with the University of Minnesota for teaching of basic and social sciences during the preclinical period of the program. The preclinical science and social science courses were offered over two school quarters, or six months; The Whitney building was under construction at the time and more classroom space was made available to the nursing school as a result of that construction. Improvements were also made in the already existing school facilities. Addressing the need for more faculty members, for the first time head nurses and supervisors were designated "assistant clinical instructors" of the school. Effort was made to hire more graduates to work as staff nurses, thus relieving the service burden on students, at least to some extent. The board had asked also for improvements in the school library, but it was still two more years in the future before steps were taken to satisfy that request.

The first affiliation to be offered to St. Barnabas students was a three-month long pediatric experience at Gillette State Hospital in St. Paul. Pediatrics was not at that time a regular part of the curriculum, but this experience was offered on an elective basis for students who might be interested in that field of practice. In 1937, that affiliation at Gillette State Hospital was made a regular part of the St. Barnabas curriculum, so every student was assigned at some point to that three-month affiliation. Also added to the curriculum in 1937 was another affiliation, this one a forty-two day experience in tuberculosis nursing at Glen Lake Sanitarium. One of the many accomplishments of Minnie Patterson, St. B's first graduate, was a role in bringing about the opening of Glen Lake for the treatment of Hennepin county victims of tuberculosis, a prevalent communicable disease of the time. The 1937 faculty at St. Barnabas could boast of a substantial increase in hours of instruction to 1,047 hours over the three years of the program.

Apparently the work done by the faculty during that one year of board probation was bearing fruit. Unfortunately, as often happens, the plans which began so enthusiastically with board prodding rather fell by the wayside as time went on. The advisory committee aforementioned existed for one year, then stopped. It was reactivated again in 1938 and from that time to the close of the school it was a regular part of the school operation. The tuberculosis experience started at Glen Lake in 1937 was not available to

St. Barnabas in 1938 and for a few years after. It was picked up again in 1945, then replaced in 1947 with a ten week affiliation in communicable diseases at Minneapolis General Hospital. The Minneapolis General course had two obvious advantages in that it covered all communicable diseases which were occurring in Minneapolis at the time and Minneapolis General Hospital was only two blocks away from St. Barnabas, so there was no transportation problem for students and no need for them to relocate from their St. Barnabas dormitory rooms during the affiliation. The communicable disease affiliation was later shortened to six weeks and eliminated entirely in 1957.

At the same time the communicable disease affiliation was established at Minneapolis General, a four week affiliation in outpatient nursing was also established at Minneapolis General. The outpatient course remained at Minneapolis General for several years until General notified St. Barnabas it needed all of its outpatient facilities for their own students. This was in the early 1960s and the new affiliation which replaced the one at Minneapolis General was at the St. Paul Outpatient Center. At that point a new course, Community Health Problems, had been developed at St. Barnabas. It was designed to supplement the outpatient course and effort was made to coordinate the two as much as possible.

The school, heeding the earlier advice of the nursing board, in 1938 opened a school library. The opening was a meager one, to be sure, since the total holdings of the library when it opened was thirty-six volumes, but at least it was a start.

The momentum toward school improvement continued with another increase in hours of instruction to 1,310 hours in 1939. Helen Platt was appointed nursing arts instructor August 1, 1939. She continued in that position until she was made director of nursing in May of 1943.

The time given over to hours of instruction began backsliding in 1940 and by 1945, more than three hundred hours of instruction had been lost. The figure was down to 1,003 hours that year, the lowest it had been since the reorganization of the school after coming off of board probation. There is no explanation for the reduction. One can speculate that it may have been related to the shortage of nursing personnel during World War II, lack of time and personnel for teaching, and the use of students for service during some of the hours that had been given over earlier to instruction.

A bright spot in the school's report to the board in 1945 had to do with the library. The thirty-six volumes reported in 1938 when the library was established, had grown to five hundred sixty volumes by 1945. A 1945 addition to the school curriculum was a three-month affiliation course in psychiatry, offered at St. Peter State Hospital. The affiliation had been offered for the first time in 1943, but only on an elective basis at that time. The 1945 change made the course a regular part of the curriculum for all students. In 1946, the affiliation was moved to Moose Lake State Hospital where it stayed for two years, then back to St. Peter for ten years and back once again to Moose Lake in 1958.

In 1946, the decline in hours of instruction reported to the board was reversed again and this time, there was no further backsliding. Each time the hours were reported, the number had increased. The school bulletin published in 1946 listed twenty-three "officers of instruction" for the school. A closer look at the list revealed that only three of the twenty-three had fulltime responsibilities in the school. A fourth person was the director of the school, but apparently she reported to the director or superintendent of nurses. Marion Dunn, appointed director of nursing education on 1 February 1946, was the first person listed by the school to have a title indicating her responsibility was full-time in the school. It is not clear whether she still reported to the director of nurses or not. She stayed only a little over one year, then was replaced by Blanche Ostlund, who also stayed only a little over one year. Miss Ostlund was replaced by Gertrude Braun, St. Barnabas graduate, class of 1942, who was hired in an interim capacity until a fulltime director could be hired.

The list of twenty-three "officers of instruction" in that 1946 bulletin included eighteen people who were head nurses or supervisors. It is significant to note their nursing service titles were listed first followed by "assistant clinical instructor". A nineteenth person among the twenty-three was the head dietitian, Elvera Spotts. Obviously, all nineteen of these people had rightful priorities which came before the education of nursing students.

In 1948, a new school bulletin was published which listed twenty-six people called the "faculty of the nursing school." Basically, it was the same list as the one labeled "officers of instruction" with a few changes. The 1948 list included not only the head dietitian, but also a teaching dietitian, but the teaching dietitian reported not to the director of the school, but to the head dietitian. The 1948 list still only included three instructors and a director in the school and the school director still reported to the director of nursing. On the next page in the 1948 bulletin, was a list of twenty-four physicians labeled "members of the hospital instructional staff." Reading through the course descriptions, it was apparent the doctors did the bulk of teaching. There was a nurse instructor assigned to each course, but she had basically a coordinating role and she might teach one or two hours at the end of the course on "nursing care of the patient with ___________." You could insert any diagnosis. Not only that, the nursing measures tended to be pretty general and the reasons for using these measures were usually not covered. According to that 1948 bulletin, one nurse instructor was responsible for seven of these physician-taught courses. Only in operating room, pediatrics and obstetrics did an instructor carry responsibility for only one course. But those instructors were first supervisors of their departments and second instructors.

In 1948, Esther Lucille Brown, financed by the Russell Sage Foundation, conducted a study of nursing education programs nationwide and reported her findings as well as her recommendations for improving the quality of nurse education in the country. One of the needs she identified in her study was the "need to study and analyze nursing functions." In other words, to determine why we do what we do for patients. Without that "why" piece of the course, it was difficult to determine what value nursing procedures would have for the patient. The preparation being given to most nursing students through excessive reliance on physicians for teaching (this was a widespread practice, not just something at St. Barnabas) was more on the level of "junior doctor" than nurse. The information the physicians included in their lectures, interesting as it was to most students, was more watered down medical education than nursing education. Some doctors enjoyed the teaching and were good at it, while others did it more as an obligation than an activity they enjoyed. And of course all of them had first priorities which did not include teaching students. They were there first and foremost to care for the patients who came to them. One by-product of the system was greater interest of staff doctors in the nursing program and the students they taught. Many looked upon the nursing students as "their girls," and there was a closeness between students and physicians which was lost after the doctors stepped out of the nursing classroom role.

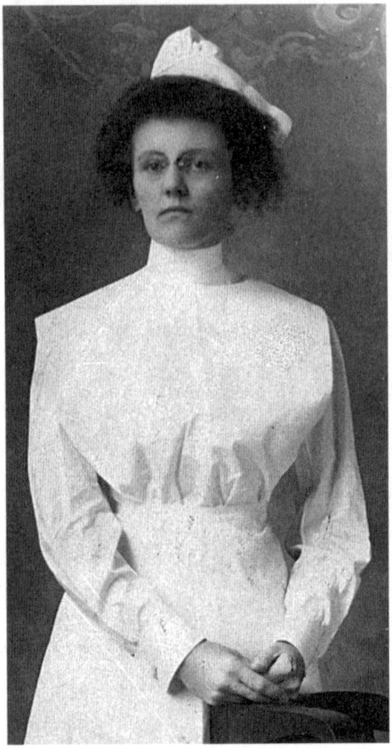

Graduate uniform 1909
Alice Kickenapp Davis

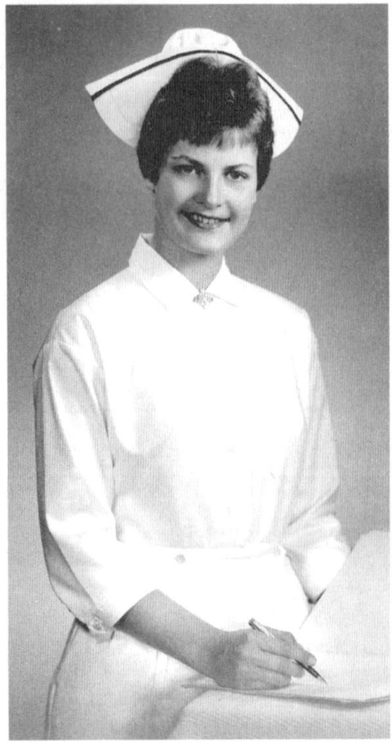

Graduate uniform 1962
Leona Kots

In 1940, St. Barnabas opened its first pediatric unit. There was the hope that some day students could get all of their pediatrics at St. Barnabas, but because this early unit had only sixteen beds, it was decided to keep an affiliation for pediatrics. The difference was that in 1940, that affiliation was moved from Gillette State Hospital to the University of Minnesota. Four years later, in 1944, the St. Barnabas pediatric unit had expanded sufficiently to accommodate an eight-week course in pediatrics for all students. The eight weeks at St. Barnabas were supplemented by four additional weeks at Sheltering Arms, which at that time was serving as a hospital for children with polio and other crippling diseases. Sheltering Arms and St. Barnabas had a close relationship through the Episcopal Church dating back to the very beginnings of the hospital.

The establishment of another affiliation, this one in obstetrics also began in 1944. It was offered at Hamline Asbury and was three months in length. The original Asbury Hospital had been in the building that in 1943 became

Knickerbacker Residence. The new Asbury was on the south side of Elliot Park, making it, like the affiliations at Minneapolis General, a convenient one for St. Barnabas students who could easily walk to Asbury, eliminating the need for relocation from the school dormitory during that course.

In 1946, the nursing board noted the hours of clinical teaching at St. Barnabas were minimal and that the bulk of teaching was being done by physicians rather than nurse instructors.

The event, which more than all others, moved the St. Barnabas curriculum to the modern era was the appointment on July 15, 1950, of Dorothy Merrell as director of nursing at St. Barnabas. The system of keeping school and service together under one director continued, to be sure, but Miss Merrell came to St. Barnabas with a rich background in both nursing service and nursing education. She received basic nursing education at Bellevue Hospital School of Nursing in New York, class of 1937. Like many nurses of her time, she served in the military during World War II, seeing action in surgical units of military hospitals in Africa, Sicily, Italy, France and Germany. After the war, she enrolled at Western Reserve University in Cleveland, Ohio, earning a baccalaureate degree in nursing administration in 1949 and a Master of Arts in Education in 1950.

Hours of instruction at St. Barnabas had increased to 1,402 by the time Miss Merrell was appointed and the number increased steadily during the eleven years she spent at St. Barnabas. In 1950, "ward classes" were being scheduled on all units to supplement the specialty courses students were taking. At that point, a student's class assignment and her clinical assignment were not necessarily concurrent. So, for example, she might be learning obstetrics during the fall quarter because everyone in the second year class took it together, but she might not actually have any experience on the maternity unit until six or perhaps even nine months later. The ward classes did help to fill that gap if it existed. They also provided an opportunity for discussion of particularly unusual or interesting cases which were on the unit at the time.

Under Miss Merrell's guidance, more clinical instructors were hired, so they could be more readily available on the units to guide student experiences. Duty hours and patient assignments were still done by the head nurse. The rule of thumb was assignment of students to forty hours of combined duty and class time. As recently as 1946, it had been forty-eight hours combined duty and class time. That changed to forty-four hours in 1948 and forty hours in 1950 and thereafter until the school was split from nursing service in 1961.

Another 1950 achievement was the hiring of a fulltime librarian. She spent most of her time in Staples Memorial Library, the school library named in honor of Mrs. Loring Staples, but as school librarian, she was also responsible for Grimes Memorial Library, which was the doctors' library. Being familiar with the holdings in both libraries was an advantage to both students and faculty. Sometimes, when a desired reference was not available in the Staples Library, the librarian could get it from Grimes Memorial Library, though neither faculty nor students were allowed otherwise to use the Grimes Library. The original librarian hired at St. Barnabas stayed only four years. She was replaced by Silvija Kupchs, who came in 1954 and stayed on to retirement sixteen years later. Silvija's story is included in the chapter on displaced persons.

In 1951, the preclinical science and social science affiliation at the University of Minnesota was replaced with a similar program, at Macalester College, two semesters (nine months) in length in place of the two university quarters (six months).

By 1953, there were six full-time instructors on the faculty, all of them with baccalaureate degree preparation. The hours of instruction had increased to 1,582 including 182 hours of ward classes. The library also continued to expand, having six hundred eighty nine titles in 1953. In addition, the library also included a number of professional periodicals. National League for Nursing achievement tests were being given on a regular basis at that time. They covered eight major clinical courses which students were learning. In 1953 the board report noted there had been only three failures on state board examinations in the prior eight years, a record to be proud of and a far cry from the 1935 experience of 32% failures in one class.

In 1951, St. Barnabas joined with three other Minneapolis nursing schools to form the Central Teaching Program. The three schools were Abbott, Northwestern and Eitel. Eitel closed its school soon after that, leaving just Abbott, Northwestern and St. Barnabas. These three continued the program and their close relationship for several years. The primary objective in establishing the program was to provide concurrent classroom instruction with clinical assignments. The clinical courses were taught more than once each year to a class composed of students from all three schools. Assignment of classroom space was made so that each school hosted each course once during the year, providing an even distribution of the burden of traveling to class at one of the other hospitals. The three schools were all within walking distance of each other or on bus lines so students were responsible for getting to class on their own. There were approximately the same number of students from each school each time the course was taught.

At the time the Central Teaching Program was established, the preclinical program at the University of Minnesota, in which all the schools had been participating, was replaced by the program at Macalester College. Students from all three schools attended the classes together at Macalester, so from the time they entered their nursing programs, they had contact with one another. Over time interschool friendships were established and they even scheduled some extracurricular activities together, one of them being the annual Tri-School formal dance.

One desirable outcome for faculty of the central teaching program was the opportunity of working with faculty members from the other two schools, networking and learning from each other. For example a primary mentor for me, when I was a young instructor in 1953, was a much older, more experienced instructor at Northwestern who took me in hand and provided lots of guidance and suggestions to improve teaching. Joint faculty meetings of faculty from all three schools were held quarterly.

Dorothy Merrell was a key person in the whole central teaching program. She had close collegial relationships with the directors from the other two schools, but in addition, she was looked upon by other faculties as a leader. At the time of her resignation from St. Barnabas in 1961, she was a member of the Minnesota Board of Nursing as well as a member of the Board of Review of the National League for Nursing Accrediting Service. She moved from Minnesota to California and there, in her retirement, she married a California artist, Chester Engles. At the time of this writing, she is widowed, but still living in her home in California.

National League for Nursing accreditation became a reality for St. Barnabas in 1951 with the granting of temporary accreditation. A school seeking NLN accreditation for the first time was given temporary accreditation, then visited two years later to insure that standards achieved when the temporary designation was given were being maintained. St. Barnabas

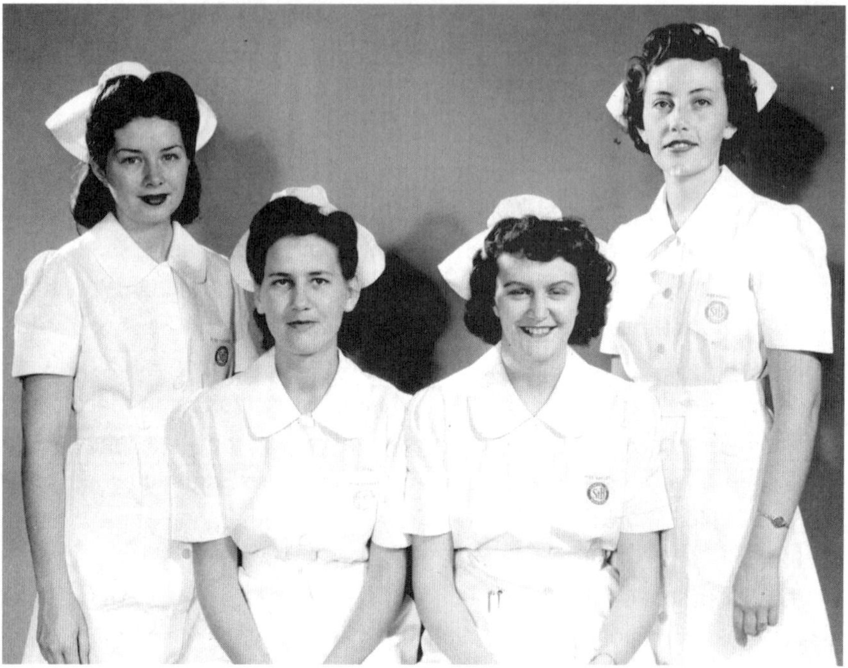

Student uniform worn 1942 to 1951. Members of the class of 1945 pictured.

received its full accreditation in 1953. In 1961, there was a resurvey visit for accreditation and that time the school didn't fare as well as in 1953. At the time of the resurvey, many changes were in progress, but few results of those changes were evident to the visitor. Accordingly, the NLN board of review gave only provisional accreditation following the 1961 visit and scheduled another full-scale review with another visitor in 1963.

In mid 1961, when Miss Merrell resigned, nursing at St. Barnabas was divided into two departments, Nursing Service and Nursing Education. Each of the two had full department status in the hospital organization and each had its own director. Grace Terry, St. Barnabas class of 1951, was named the new director of nursing education. Prior to my appointment to this position, I served on the faculty for five years as a clinical instructor. Following graduation from St. Barnabas I had earned a Bachelor of Science degree in Nursing Education from the University of Minnesota.

In 1962 the three schools of the CTP were notified by Macalester College that the nursing program at the college was to be dropped from their curriculum. Through the Directors' Conference Group of Third District

Minnesota Nurses' Association, the three central teaching program directors learned of two other Twin City nursing schools which were searching for a new preclinical college affiliation. The other two schools were Mounds-Midway School of Nursing in St. Paul and St. Mary's Junior College in Minneapolis. Directors of these two schools joined the CTP three and together the five combed the Twin City area for a new college program for their preclinical students. But it was to no avail. There was no college in the area willing to replace the Macalester affiliation.

Ultimately the five schools turned to educational television, at that time a relative newcomer to higher education in the Twin Cities. Dr. Lois Anderson, who prior to earning her doctorate at the University of Minnesota, had served on the faculty at Mounds-Midway, was engaged to work with the five directors in establishing the Video Nursing Education program. The group was breaking new ground for no nursing school anywhere in the United States had done anything like this before. Dr. Anderson recruited and hired distinguished, well prepared faculty to teach each of the science and social science courses previously taught in the college affiliations. The steering committee, composed of the five school directors, reviewed credentials and had a voice in the hiring of faculty.

Production assistance was provided by Delores Paul, who was hired to work with instructors in adapting their courses to the medium of television. Television receivers were obtained by each school. The directors were briefed by Dr. Anderson on screen size, the number of receivers they would need given the number of students enrolled in each school, the distance students should sit from the receivers and seating arrangements which would provide optimum viewing for every student. (At St. Barnabas, the auxiliary stepped up and paid for the television receivers and stands needed.)

With the video nursing education program, freshman students took science, social science, pharmacology and communication classes in a classroom in their own school. The program was a cost-saver (though that was never a factor considered in developing it) both in terms of time and dollars. Students no longer had the long commute-time to and from St. Paul for classes at Macalester and the school no longer had to pay for bus transportation for the students. Students did miss the social interactions with students in other disciplines which they had at the college, but most compensated and met other students on their own.

Arrangements were made for the television instructors to come to each school to meet face to face with students on a regular basis and to explore their questions. In hindsight, this may or may not have been necessary. Twenty first century Distance Education students complete whole college degrees without ever having face to face meetings with either the instructor or fellow students, though they communicate with each other regularly by email. Perhaps the VNE students would have done as well without the face to face sessions, but the medium was new to nursing education and members of the steering committee were anxious to insure students would get the same quality of instruction they had gotten previously in the college setting.

The 1963 school bulletin for St. Barnabas listed 3,194 hours of instruction given over the three years. The length of the school program had been shortened to thirty-two months rather than the thirty-six months of previous years. Since the school was a separate department from nursing service at that point, student experiences in the hospital were under the total control of faculty members who had full-time appointments to the school.

In 1963, the NLN Accreditation Service scheduled another full-scale visit to the school. During the two years between visits, the faculty concentrated on implementing all the plans that had been only on paper in 1961. Few changes were made from those original plans, but during the 1963 visit all faculty had worked with the changes and all were comfortable in relating to the visitor what they were teaching. The result was most gratifying in that the school was granted full accreditation and even commendation on a job well done.

One new course, Community Health Problems, had been developed, but again, the instructor had gone through the course with two different groups of students and at the time of the visit was confident in her explanation of what the course was all about. As. school director during the visit, I learned later that the NLN visitor, a director of nursing from Nebraska, was keeping two notebooks during her visit. She was so impressed with the new Community Health Course that she made notes for her own faculty to consider in establishing a similar course. After the board of review met and the outcome of the visit had been voted upon, she called me to ask if she might make a return visit to St. Barnabas to learn more about the Community Health course. During that second visit, she told me that St. Barnabas was

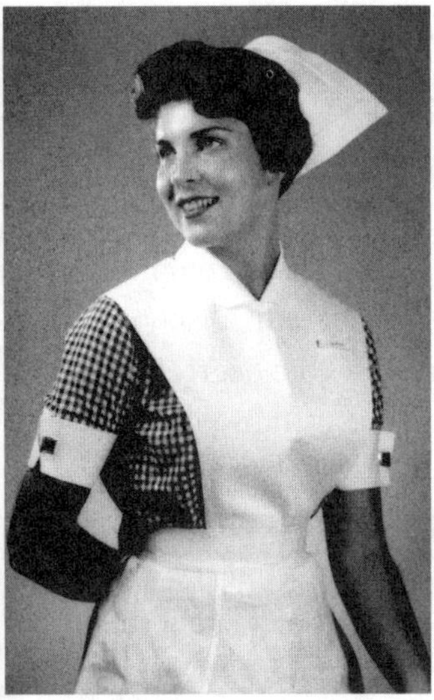

1950s student uniform, French cuffs, starched aprons.

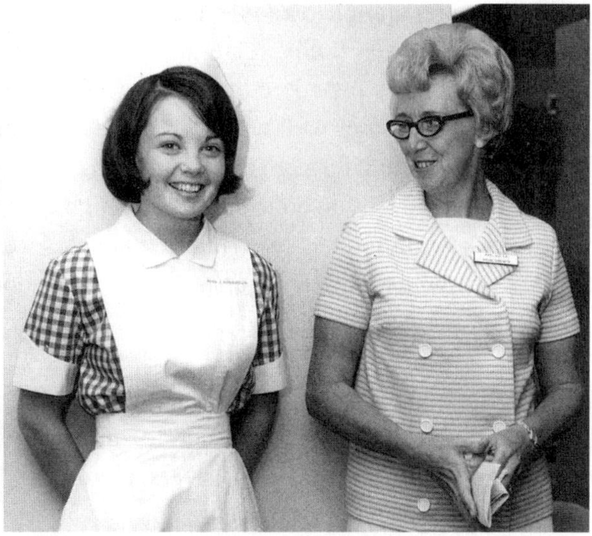

A 1960s uniform, wash and wear fabric with self cuffs, larger checks than in 1950s. Student is Judith Anderson. Muriel Hegg, on the right, is the only student to graduate from the school with five children under age 18 at home. In this photo, taken in 1968, Muriel is the supervisor of the new psychiatric unit.

only one of two schools who got full accreditation at that meeting of the board of review, though there were several schools up for resurvey visits. She also said that on the evening after the board met, she and Dr. Eleanor Lambertson met to toast St. Barnabas and the successful outcome for the school. Dr. Lambertson had spent one long weekend in Minneapolis serving as a consultant to the school prior to the resurvey.

A few words seem in order here about National League for Nursing accreditation and why having it was important to a nursing school. First of all, though accreditation and approval sound as if they are synonymous, when applied to a nursing program, there is a distinction in meaning. The state board of nursing grants approval to operate a nursing program. Without that approval, the program cannot exist. The state board regulations are in effect the law of the state relative to a nursing program. The National League for Nursing Accreditation was a voluntary thing and receiving that accreditation was a stamp of quality or a hallmark of excellence for the program.

The advantages in having NLN accreditation were threefold: 1) the public; 2) the school; 3) the student. The public benefited because the persons graduated by the school were going out into the world equipped with the best preparation available in the profession. The school benefited in two ways—there was public relations value in having this mark of excellence. The school also benefited in that the accreditation process itself forced the faculty to consider well what they were doing and to make improvements in the curriculum through this evaluation exercise. The student benefited by getting an education considered to be high quality. Prospective employers often gave preference in hiring to graduates from an accredited school. A graduate who wished to go on for further education and higher degrees found that higher education institutions also gave preference to those graduates from accredited schools.

The accreditation given by the NLN lasted for a maximum period of six years. The school was asked to submit a written report at the end of three years. At the end of six years, there would be another written report plus a visit from a representative of the National League for Nursing. The visitor would prepare a report on findings during the week-long visit to the school. That report, along with the written report prepared by the school was turned over to a board of review that would study both reports and determine whether or not criteria for accreditation had been met. They might choose to deny accreditation or withdraw it from a previously accredited program, to place an already accredited program on probation for a period of time, or to grant accreditation for a period less than six years. Basically, if the period was less than six years, the period of time until the next visit really was a probationary time. This last option might be utilized if the school had promising looking plans on paper, but had not yet implemented those plans. This was the case with the 1961 visit to St. Barnabas.

I resigned in 1965. We had our first child while I was director of the school and were hoping to have a second child. The responsibilities at the school were just too heavy to allow me the time I wanted to spend with my husband and our children. I also hoped to add a master's degree to my resume before a second child joined the family.

I received the master's in late July of 1966 and our baby son eight weeks later. I then became the first executive director of the Minnesota League for Nursing, a part time position at that time. After six years with the League, I was appointed associate executive director of the Minnesota Board of Nursing, a full time position. In 1975, my husband, Ken Terry, took a position with the Department of Army. The new job included a requirement for mandatory rotation, so when our family left Minneapolis in 1975, we embarked on a twenty-year odyssey which found us stationed in five different states and Japan. Ken retired in 1995 and we returned to McAlester, Oklahoma, one of the duty stations to which he had been assigned years earlier. He died here in 1997. I continue to make my home in McAlester.

My replacement at St. Barnabas was Ruth Weise, an old friend and former instructor from the University of Minnesota. Ruth was hired several months before my resignation to teach Community Health Problems and to become familiar with the school. She was an immediate favorite with students, who were delighted to have her take over the directorship of the school in September of 1965. She capably guided the school through the last eight years of its existence. No better person could have filled that difficult role, but she did it well and the school closed as one of the strong nursing programs in the state, a distinction it had held for many of the years it existed. Ruth stayed on with Metropolitan Medical Center, serving as director of educational services. She lives today in Bloomington, Minnesota, and though an octogenarian, she keeps busy with volunteer work at Gillette State Hospital and in her church. Dr. Knickerbacker would have liked Ruth just as those who know her today like her. I am sure of that.

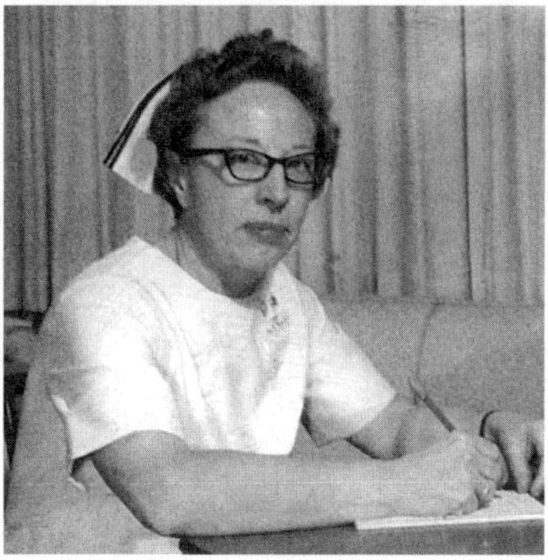

Ruth Weise

When St. Barnabas and Swedish Hospitals merged on October 1, 1970, to become Metropolitan Medical Center, both schools of nursing were required by law to close their doors since the parent corporations of both schools no longer existed. The classes admitted to both St. Barnabas and Swedish in 1970 were the last to enroll at both schools. The board of Metropolitan Medical Center could have opted to open a new hospital school, but by that time it was apparent that the collegiate schools were going to replace hospital schools in producing the professional nurses of the future. Instead of opening a new school to replace the two that were closing, the new center chose to open its facilities for affiliations with collegiate programs. South Dakota State University came first, occupying the school quarters in the Whitney building as well as using the clinical facilities in the hospital. In 1979, St. Olaf College moved its third and fourth year students to MMC on affiliation. In addition to St. Olaf, in 1979 MMC had affiliation agreements with the University of Minnesota School of Nursing, Gustavus Adolphus College and the College of St. Catherine, all among the leaders in baccalaureate education for nurses in Minnesota.

St. Barnabas graduated its last class on March 23, 1973, 102 years after the founding of Cottage Hospital, forerunner of St. Barnabas, and seventy-nine years after the first student entered St. Barnabas Hospital School of Nursing.

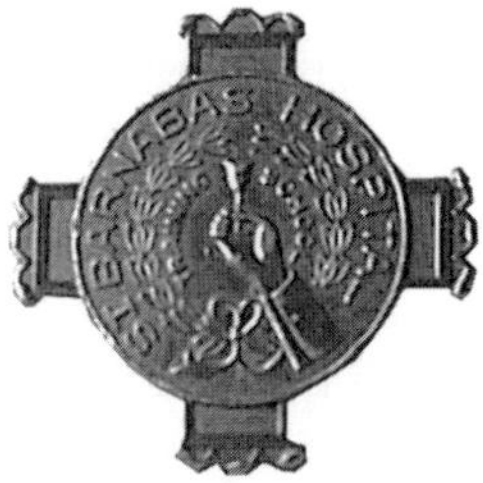

Chapter 16

On Being a Nursing Student at St. Barnabas

Students entering St. Barnabas Hospital School of Nursing often came with idealized images of the nurses they hoped to become, though for most the image they carried in their minds changed during the three years they spent in the school. During the years he served as hospital chaplain, the Reverend F. D. Tyner asked each freshman student to write a paper on "Why I Want to Become a Nurse." He read every paper, then ranked them and at Capping he presented a silver candleholder to the student who wrote the winning paper for the year. During preadmission interviews with students, faculty members usually asked the candidate to state why she wanted to become a nurse. Most indicated a desire to help people or some variation of this theme. But often they were a bit fuzzy about how they would help.

There were those who came to the school with more realistic impressions of the work done in hospitals. Several had worked as nurse aides. Beginning with World War II, hospitals were forced to consider and develop means to supplement their short supply of registered nurses since many RNs had joined the armed forces as their contribution to the war effort. Practical nursing schools, as a separate kind of preparation for nursing, did not come into being until after World War II, so there was not a large supply of LPNs available to fill the gap. Nursing staff needs in the civilian sector had to be met in other ways. Women who left nursing earlier to raise families were encouraged to return to practice. Another way to increase available staff was to hire and provide on the job training for ancillary people who could do some of the routine tasks previously done by nurses. The nurse aide, later called nursing assistant, became a permanent part of the nursing staff during and after the war. Prospective nurses often chose working as a nurse aide as a means of "testing the water" or learning more about work done in the hospital in order to help them decide whether or not nursing was for them. As freshman students, they came with a better understanding of what they might be asked to do as registered nurses.

Another group, smaller than the nurse aide group, who probably had more realistic images of nursing, were those who had family members who were graduates of St. Barnabas or other schools. For example, Margery Stone, class of 1951, had an older sister who was a graduate of Northwestern Hospital School of Nursing. Hazelle Lundell, graduate of St. John's in Red Wing, had a younger sister who enrolled at St. Barnabas, though she dropped out during her first year in the school. There were a small number of students who fell into this category.

The appendix for this book lists several sets of sisters who graduated from St. Barnabas—there were several twosomes and six groups of three among graduates of the school. The Haas sisters and the Muetzel sisters are two groups of three who would be remembered by those living in this first decade of the twenty first century. Leona, Marcella and Marie Haas all graduated in the same class, 1926, though they were not all the same age. Leona, known as "Lohni" by most people, spent her whole career in private duty nursing. She worked private duty for many patients hospitalized at St. Barnabas in the 1940s and 1950s and she always took time to get to know the students assigned to the same unit as her private patient. She never married, but both of her sisters did. Marcella McConville did not work at St. Barnabas during most of the years her sisters did, but she was active in the alumnae association and she met students and new graduates through that means. Marie Winslow, the third sister, worked part time for years as a float or sometimes as a regular staff member of a particular unit. All three sisters were active members of the alumnae and all were steadfast supporters of student activities. They went the extra mile to get to know students.

The Muetzel sisters all graduated in different years, starting with Wilma, who graduated in 1949. Verlaine was in the class of 1960 and little sister Dianne, 1963. All were excellent students, usually ranking near the top of their classes. Their father, bringing Dianne to enroll in 1960, commented about his great pride in having all three of his daughters become St. Barnabas nurses.

A third group of three from one family were the Watts—a mother and her two daughters, all St. Barnabas graduates. Florence Robinson Watts graduated in 1928. Some years later, she found herself a single mother with three children—a son and two daughters—to raise. She was still living in Minneapolis at the time, so she returned to St. Barnabas and worked there until she retired thirty-three years later. Along the way during those years, she remarried and would be remembered by many as Florence Buck, head nurse for years on 5 Pavilion and later in the new building as head nurse on 3B. Her first daughter, Joanne, graduated from St. Barnabas in 1951 and married a doctor, Jorge Torres, who had done his residency at St. Barnabas while she was a student. Joyce, the younger daughter, married while still a student. After she graduated in 1953, she and her husband remained in the Minneapolis area and like her mother before her, Joyce Dudley worked at St. Barnabas for some time.

As nursing programs proliferated in the state following World War II, competition to attract students to the school increased and recruitment programs were developed to take St. Barnabas out to high schools throughout the state. In the 1950s, teams composed of one student, one faculty member and one alumnae member, traveled to career day programs throughout the state. Serving on the board of trustees at the time was Ray Mithun of Campbell-Mithun Advertising Company. He served as an advisor in establishing recruitment programs. His advice could best be summed up in one sentence, in his own words, "You sell soap where you know people buy soap." In other words, he advised the most productive use of time would be to revisit schools that had already sent students to St. Barnabas. The tactic worked.

There were almost always students from the southwestern part of the state, Tracy, Pipestone, Slayton, all towns that had been visited by recruitment teams more than once. Over time the counselors in these schools would notify the nursing school of upcoming career day programs and invite St. Barnabas participation. Later, the Minnesota League for Nursing, working with high school counselors, developed the "Nursing Education Directory" which listed comparable information about every nursing school in the state. I had the privilege of chairing the committee that developed the directory and of receiving the thanks from counselors who found it a very useful tool. Episcopal churches throughout the state also referred students to the school, though for most years, Episcopal students were still in the minority in each class. When Jean Houle was hired as the first community relations director, she took over the recruitment program. Working in concert with the school administration she took teams of students out to present more structured recruitment programs than the earlier teams had presented. For example, the program she developed for 1960 was entitled, "Have Uniform—Will Travel." Each year she would develop a different program to use for all the visits she and her student teams made that year. When she resigned, the program was continued by her successor, Betty McTaggert, as Jean had established it.

In the early years of the school, the age of an entering student was quite variable. Some had earned college degrees in other disciplines, particularly in teaching, and had decided to pursue nursing careers after trying another profession for a while. By contrast, the youngest student ever to enroll in the school was only sixteen years old. She was in that first class, graduating in 1897. Her name was Ella Gibson. She was born in Canada of English-born parents. She was orphaned at age ten, but by that time her parents had moved with her to Minneapolis. She attended Wilder College before enrolling at age sixteen in the nursing program at St. Barnabas. Though she had no parents, fellow classmate, Minnie Paterson, took her under her wing. Minnie was several years older than Ella and acted as a big sister to her. The other four members of their class followed Minnie's example and tried to be the family Ella no longer had. They nicknamed her "Gibbie," the name by which she was known to them for the rest of their lives. Four years after graduation, on February 12, 1901, Gibbie married Herbert L. Birum, a man she met years earlier when both were students at Wilder College. The couple had a daughter, Beth, who always regarded Ella's friends from St. Barnabas as her adopted aunts. The Birums moved to Montana to live shortly after their marriage. They were married for more than sixty years when Herbert died in November 1961. Gibbie made a trip back for a visit to St. Barnabas after that. Needless to say, she was impressed by the difference in St. Barnabas Hospital then as compared to the St. Barnabas she had known so many years before.

At the time Gibbie graduated, there were no state regulations regarding the practice of nursing. Later, after licensure became a reality, age requirements were set for one to receive a license. In 1922, St. Barnabas required applicants for admission to the school be from eighteen to thirty one years of age. In 1935, they raised the minimum age to nineteen, but kept the maximum age at thirty one. In 1943, possibly because of participation in the Cadet Nurse program, the minimum age on entrance to St. Barnabas was lowered to eighteen and the next year, 1944, to seventeen and one half. Later, the faculty paid little attention to the age of an applicant and when three married students enrolled in the 1960s, all were over thirty-one. Meantime, the state had placed an age limit in law, requiring that a graduate must be nineteen years old in order to write state board examinations. In practice, most girls, and much later boys, who enrolled at St. Barnabas were at least eighteen years old. The following is quoted from an email which I received from Carol Jensen Scanny, class of 1961: "I came to St. Barnabas a very young seventeen-year-old, from rural Minnesota. St. Barnabas was one of the few schools that accepted seventeen-year-olds (then). That put me up on the floors practicing my nursing skills on real LIVE patients before I was eighteen! The first time I took a blood pressure I had the arm all pumped up, and found the stethoscope was still at the nurses' station!"

Carol goes on in her email to describe some of her impressions as a new student at St. Barnabas. She says,

> When we toured (the hospital) before beginning school in the fall of 1958, we were in the oldest part of the hospital (visiting) some offices, including Miss Merrell's. I think the chapel was on the first floor and I remember being impressed by that area—though it certainly was not what one would call "a bright and cheery place."

> Our food at St. Barnabas always seemed very good to me. I can remember having cottage cheese topped with pomegranate seeds—something I had never seen before. (Don't they say keeping military personnel fed well is one way to keep them happy?) There is a word I will never forget and every so often bring it up in (medical) conversation—"scrofula." A patient, in a teasing way, accused me of causing that disease in him because I was so late with his morning bath. I do believe the word can describe a generally unclean condition and skin deterioration...He was such a nice guy and I can almost see him yet—one remembers those patients with fondness.
>
> I remember so well the dorms and the older sections of the hospital, "Pav" and Wellesmere. Our second and third years were spent in the remodeled section of the old hospital—behind the serpentine wall, complete yet with housemothers! There seems to be a movement afoot to rename the persons medical people take care of as "clients." I have always stood firm in my belief that I would want to be a "patient"; somehow a client just doesn't ring well—there is a special sense of caring in "patient care."

Like so many other facets of the nursing program, the orientation for new students evolved over time. Prior to the establishment of the affiliation with Macalester College, students had attended two quarters at the University of Minnesota, taking basic sciences and social sciences. Orientation for new students then was limited to assignment of a Big Sister for each incoming student. The Big Sister was to be on hand to greet her Little Sis and then to show her around, making her more comfortable with the school. Over time, the Big Sis' developed some initiation rites, but they were never official and for the most part, were not known to faculty!

There was no counterpart orientation to the University for nursing students. Most walked to classes at the University from St. Barnabas. It was possible to get there by streetcar, but there were often delays. And besides the streetcar cost money, while walking was free! June Lundin entered with the class of 1951. She dropped out along the way to be married, so did not graduate with them. June was Canadian, from Regina, Saskatchewan. She came to school with a fur coat that was the envy of all who walked to the university during the cold winter months. I remember seeing June, perfectly comfortable, walking across the Washington Avenue bridge with icicles hanging around the hem of her fur coat!

Anatomy lab was always in the morning, then students would walk back to St. Barnabas for lunch and afternoon nursing classes (complete with struggle to stay awake after the long morning walk and the excessive amount of fresh, cold air!) Standing in line at the cafeteria, Marge Elmen, class of 1951, invariably called back, "Cadaver hash again today. Take lots so they can't feed it to us tomorrow!"

The attrition rate during the first year was very high during the university days. For example, the class of 1951 entered with forty-seven students, but lost eleven after the first quarter in the program. From this, a rather bizarre (and cruel) requirement arose. Before going home for the Christmas holidays, all freshman were required to pack up, in boxes, everything in their dorm rooms. That way, when the university grades came, if a student didn't pass, her belongings could be sent home without having her return to the school. There was a strange, almost unreal feeling for students when they returned to find the boxes of a loved roommate were gone, knowing that person would not be back to school again. That practice seems to have ended when Dorothy Merrell took over direction of the school.

When the university affiliation was changed to the Macalester affiliation, orientation programs also changed. The Big Sis-Little Sis program at St. Barnabas continued as before, but in addition, students were encouraged to participate in orientation-week activities of the college.

When the Macalester affiliation was dropped and the Video Nursing Education Program was developed, another change in orientation activities occurred. Supplementing the Big Sis-Little Sis program was a full week of orientation at St. Barnabas. Some social activities were planned to allow freshmen and their upperclass sisters to become better acquainted. One of the highlights of the week was a visit to a theater performance or to a first run movie downtown. One of the early years of the Guthrie Theater found the whole freshman class in attendance at a performance there. Another year, the year *It's a Mad, Mad, Mad World* came out, all the freshmen attended that movie together. And still another year, the movie was *West Side Story*. Once the preclinical period was completed, the student was ready to receive her school cap. Folding the cap was an art in itself. Most students tried to keep the cap as clean as possible in order to avoid folding it more often than necessary. Most also learned that the most secure way to hold the cap in place was to use a hat pin on each side of the middle section of the cap.

Early capping ceremonies apparently were held in the hospital chapel. As transportation modes improved, making it possible for more families to attend the ceremonies, the chapel was not large enough to accommodate everyone. Capping services then were held at Gethsemane Church, the parish to which St. Barnabas owed its beginnings. The class of 1951, capped in 1949, was the last class to be capped at Gethsemane. Graduation services by that time had already been moved to St. Mark's Cathedral, and capping ceremonies were moved there too. The much larger nave of St. Mark's accommodated the larger family groups which gathered for this moving ceremony.

Students were introduced individually by one of the nursing arts instructors as each came forward to the communion rail to have her cap placed by a member of the Student Government Association. And for every capping and graduation ceremony there was the processional with students and faculty processing by twos to the strains of "Pomp and Circumstance" played on that marvelous pipe organ in the cathedral. The recessional, leaving the nave, was always "The St. Barnabas Hymn," composed by St. Barnabas's own, Dr. Frederick Tyner.

More than half a century later, hearing that tune brings back a flood of memories. The April-May 1962 issue of the *Voice of St. Barnabas* carried the comments of three newly capped students. Cheryl Griffen said, "Capping to me is a symbol of completion and beginning. A mark of achievement for our first months here and a goal for the ones to follow." Bonnie Rosevold commented, "Capping is the occasion that makes the trials and doubts of the present year seem trivial and an inspiration to strive harder for a cherished goal in the years to come. It is the turning point long awaited for, and never to be forgotten." And according to Barbara Grinde, "It is the fulfillment of a year of preparation to become an RN. When we receive our caps, we feel that now we are a real part of the nursing program. Like any award, it takes work to realize it, but the work seems minor when compared to the privilege of wearing a St. Barnabas cap."

During the 1940s and 1950s, George Grim wrote a column, "I Like It Here," for the *Minneapolis Morning Tribune*. His column from a day in 1945 or 1946 carried a story written by a Mary Jean Thompson, freshman student at St. Barnabas. The roster of graduates of St. Barnabas does not include a Mary Jean Thompson, so either she dropped out of the school before graduation or she used a fictitious name in writing to Mr. Grim. It appears the story may have been one of those Dr. Tyner assigned freshman students to write in his Ethics class. Regardless, the story was good enough not only to be published in the newspaper, but it also was printed in the 1946 Bulletin of the school.

Mr. Grim wrote the following:

> Last week—at one in the morning—Mary Jean Thompson sat in her room, trying to write. Mary Jean, from Stillwater, is a spring freshman at St. Barnabas hospital—preparing for a career as a nurse.
>
> She was thinking about her job and her future. Suddenly, she started to write a story—called "Mary Smith, RN."
>
> Picture the new patient in 237. A doctor, new to her, has taken her to this strange hospital to have an operation in the morning. This patient lies alone in 237, overcome with a feeling of apprehension and helplessness.
>
> Upon whom can she depend in this strange place? Is her doctor as good as they say he is? Will the anesthetic be hard to take? Do they really care about her?
>
> As Mary Smith walks down the corridor, she knows she has a duty to perform far greater than the usual pre-operative work. She will go into 237, and making a guess at the patient's personality, try to establish confidence in the doctor, point out the success of that type of operation, casually mention how easy modern anesthetics are to take, and she will show this patient that she is not caring for her just for a monthly salary alone.
>
> Mary Smith closes the door, leaving the patient alone again. Only this time, the patient does not feel alone. She is able to go to sleep,

rested, because she has found a friend and knows that tomorrow someone will be there, keeping her life for her, someone who really cares.

After Mary Smith's work is done in 237, she goes into 231 to sponge off the perspiring face of a dying man, perhaps breathing a prayer between her lips, keeping time with his loud respirations. Then into 230, where she tries her best to satisfy a selfish, fussy patient while listening to his long line of scolding and complaints.

Many times, Mary Smith, RN would like to scream at all those green lights above the door and say, 'Get it yourself,' move away and never come back. Many times she has cramped a muscle in her tongue to stop herself from hurting an ungrateful patient.

But no one knows this side of Mary Smith, RN, no one but the four walls of her room, her pillow and her God. No one knows because Mary Smith is a nurse. She is a servant created by God to nourish the sick in body, mind and spirit. She acquires her technical skill from her instructors, she receives her skill in common sense and patience from her God.

Today, Mary Smith is a success in the nursing profession. She is repaid for her work in many ways besides happiness, satisfaction, popularity and health.

Whenever she hits a rough spot in her life, she finds the will to carry on because she holds back in her mind a little quotation her chaplain used in ethics class: "You can accomplish anything you wish in this world if you work for it, pray for it and honestly believe you will get it!"

Perhaps Mary Smith, R. N., isn't fictional. Perhaps her name is really Mary Jean Thompson of Stillwater. Who understands.

Another story, apparently written by a freshman student, though there is no byline, is this one that appeared in the *Voice of St. Barnabas* in January 1958.

Tension had been mounting for days, and finally the time arrived for us to have our first experience on the hospital services. November 14 had been encircled on each of our calendars for about a month and we all were excited and anxious to meet our first patient.

The night before, each of us had painstakingly tried to iron out the seemingly permanently embedded creases in our white bibs. But slowly things began to take shape and by Thursday morning, precisely 5:30 A.M., we bounded out of bed after the simultaneous ringing of all alarm clocks and started the tedious process of dressing in our unfamiliar uniforms. It was certainly surprising how wide awake everyone seemed even though the night had been one of continuous tossing and turning! After taking several flashbulb pictures, we were all practically blind but that did not affect our appetites at all, for the next thing we agreed upon was having breakfast.

We all went to the cafeteria together and for the first and probably the last time, no one wanted to be first in line.

We were expected to be on our specific stations by 7:00 and we were determined to be prompt at least for our first day.

Then came a series of disappointments. Several girls had been ill with colds and sore throats and they were not allowed to have a patient. They could just stay for the orientation to the floor and then they had to go back to the dorm. This certainly came as a 'low blow' and it took some time to recover from the shock.

Most of the girls did have patients though and it seemed like each thought that her patient was the nicest. Judging from the girls' comments, everything ran smoothly and before they knew it, time was up and their first day on the floor was at an end.

I suppose you are wondering if we are all still determined to be nurses after one day of real experience. I can only quote what one of the girls was overheard to say at lunch that day—"When do we get to go back on the floors again? I can hardly wait!"

Written by Miss Disappointment, who spent her first day in the dorm with one of "those" colds.

Evelyn Lewison, class of 1932, wrote, "We had strict head nurses. Uniforms had to be perfect—no holes in stockings."

Another student from the 1950s was admonished about the sad condition of her shoes. She answered, "I'm waiting to buy new ones for graduation." This response came from the instructor who admonished her in the first place, "It beats me how you can be so optimistic about those shoes when you are so pessimistic about everything else!"

One of the first school activities the new student would be introduced to was the school choir. State board records indicate the school choir was organized in 1948. However, Evelyn Lewison, class of 1932, said they had a choir when she was in school. And the 1946 school bulletin has a picture taken at choir practice, labeled, "The student choir, sponsored by the Women's Board and conducted by Mr. Ylvisaker, is a popular activity." By 1948, the choir was a going concern that sang at all capping and graduation ceremonies. In the 1950s and 1960s they sang at several places throughout the Twin Cities, including several church services and Christmas appearances at shopping centers such as Southdale, Brookdale, Apache Plaza and Har-Mar Mall. They also presented a spring concert for several years in the 1960s. They went caroling through the halls of the hospital one evening close to Christmas each year.

Over the years, there were only about half a dozen directors of the choir. Mr. Ylvisaker was replaced in 1948 by Mr. Gerald Larson, who was a senior medical student from the university, working as a junior intern at St. Barnabas. Later Jerry would go into private practice in Cambridge, where he lived until retirement. After his graduation from medical school, he was replaced as choir director by Mr. Herbert Hoover, an undergraduate student at the university and a relief orderly at the hospital. Mr. Hoover joined the navy with the outbreak of the Korean War and he was replaced by Dr. Byron Armstrong. Dr. Armstrong was an intern at St. Barnabas at that time. He was replaced later by Mr. Howard England, who was a salesman at Dayton's Department Store and director of a church choir in the city. The choir grew in size during the fourteen years Mr. England was its director. His last year with the choir, there were sixty-six members in the organization. He was replaced in 1964 by Mrs. Loni Lindholm, also a church choir director and a member of the Carillon Singers, a semi-professional group led by Mrs. Edith Byquist Norberg. Loni was a young mother, even having one maternity leave during her tenure as choir director at the school. In 1968, she was replaced by a Mrs. Kingsley, who served for the rest of the years the school existed. For the last graduation service, there were few students left to sing in the choir, so faculty members joined with them to expand their numbers enough to sing the music requested for the occasion—and they did a very creditable job of it!

Another activity to which students would have been introduced soon after enrolling in the school was Student Government Association. Referring again to state board records, 1938 seems to have been the year that student government was organized at St. Barnabas. In 1951, a student council was formed to act on behalf of student government. 1951 also saw the first involvement of students in the Minnesota Student Nurse Association. Over the 1950s and 1960s, several students were actively involved with MSNA, attending local meetings, but also the state and national conventions of the student association. In 1954, St. Barnabas students were elected to the three top offices in the Third District of the Minnesota Student Nurse Association. 1955 class member, Judy Morris, was elected president of the association, Julie Clark, vice president and Jo DuFour, secretary. Jo and Julie were also members of the class of 1955. Several members of that class were regular in attendance at district meetings as well as attending both state and national conventions.

Margie Mac Donald wrote a report for the *Voice of St. Barnabas* on the 1954 national convention in Chicago. Her report included the following:

> Eight St. Barnabas students spent the week of April 25-30 at the National Student Nurse Convention in Chicago, Illinois. They reported having a marvelous time and even the meetings were fun.
>
> Minnesota presented a half hour program called "Midwest Harvest" which represented the midwestern states and we were honored to have our own St. Barnabas quartette (Jan Johnson, Joy Lessard, Carolyn Johnson and Jan Lundborg) sing their original "Prisoners in White." They were declared a big success.

> The other four students who attended the convention were Judy Morris, Sally Stafford, Julie Clark and Jo DuFour. Miss Morris was chairman of the committee for Minnesota's display at Chicago. The students at each school of nursing in Minnesota dressed small dolls in their student uniforms.
>
> These dolls, with a drawing of the Mayo Clinic as a background, represented Minnesota.
>
> Minnesota was well represented by students and came back with what we think is the highest honor—a member of Minnesota Student Nurse Association was elected president of the National Student Nurse Association for the coming year. This student is Phil Halvorson of the University of Minnesota. Miss Halvorson was honored at a tea on June 10 by the Third District MSNA. We certainly wish Miss Halvorson lots of luck as president.

Thirteen years later, St. Barnabas had fourteen students in attendance at the National Nursing Student Association convention in New York. Note the slight change in name of the association, reflecting the latest philosophy of nursing education. The topics discussed at that convention included "real" nursing, health and legislation, students and economic security, and human relations. As always, the student association conventions were held in the same city and nearly the same time as either the American Nurses Association Convention or the National League for Nursing Convention. The 1954 student convention cited above was held in conjunction with the ANA convention in Chicago while the 1967 student convention was held the four days preceding the NLN convention in New York.

Diane Carlson, class of 1967, wrote a story for the winter 1967 issue of the *Voice of St. Barnabas* about St. Barnabas student involvement in a program of MNSA.

> Several St. Barnabas students are taking part in a "one to one" program with children of minority groups. This is part of Third District Minnesota Nursing Students Association Human Relations Project.
>
> The students work through area settlement houses and social workers and are matched individually with a child referred by his school

or the caseworker. The students participating in the program have found it very rewarding.

Another human relations project has been the presentation of nursing career panels to junior and senior high school students. Audrey Kreitlow, Iris Staubus, Judy Erickson and Diane Carlson presented panels throughout the day at Buffalo, Minnesota, this fall.

In February, Nancy Taft and Patti Holmes joined students from Abbott, Fairview and Northwestern in giving a series of panel discussions at Bryant Junior High. The girls discussed salaries, job availability, postgraduate work, nursing programs and dormitory life. The junior high students visited St. Barnabas later and toured through the building and school to learn about actual hospital life.

Our student nurses are finding much satisfaction in the sharing of promoting better community and human relations through these programs.

A poem which appeared in the May 21, 1965, issue of *Chat From Checks*, the student newspaper, illustrates how students of 1965 viewed the role of a nurse.

To Be A Nurse

To be a nurse is
To walk with God
Along the path that
The Master trod;
To soothe the achings
Of human pain,
To faithfully serve
For little gain.
To lovingly do
The kindly deed,
A cup of water
To one in need.

Chat From Checks also carried these reminiscences of a senior concerning her first year in the school:

> September 7, 1962, found forty two frightened girls entering Whitney Residence. Much to our amazement the first week was survived, with the help of Big Sis's, Cinerama, the Patio-party, Initiation, and West Side Story, and with the hindrance of homesickness, fire drills, etc. Next came T.V. classes with Mrs. Coe and Professor Bentley, bus rides to Macalester and Dr. Reuther and Mr. Shawnee. And then at least a million more and equally exciting memories...Open house and our carnival theme with Pam as our artist; Emily; slumber parties with no sleep; Sue Rogowski's bugle at 6:00 A.M. Marg, Jackie, Judy and Sally playing cards; races to the phone, Jan Meyer and Colleen Connor at frat. parties; decorating for Christmas; Janeen finding an interest at Mac; yelling at the interns and getting yelled at by Mrs. Lau; prowlers; hours of studying (???) the night before finals; the first day on the floor and one scared frosh using a mattress pad for a bath blanket; capping and finally feeling like a nurse; first injection on April fool's day and Miss Lundell's horror at the novel way of marking off the quadrants; Elaine's phone calls and contemporary cards; raids and sleeping in the hall the night before graduation. These marked our freshman year and what a year it was!!!

A freshman student's impression of the school may well have begun with her assignment to a roommate and a room at Wellesmere. When Wellesmere was new in 1906, it was the only residence of its kind in the city. By the 1950s, facilities were much older and what was considered top of the line in 1906 seemed dark and dreary according to mid-century standards. House rules, too, at mid-century were a shock to some of the girls who had been allowed greater privileges while living at home. All students were to be in by 10:30 P.M. during the winter months and 11:00 P.M. during summer. They could have one midnight curfew per week providing they weren't scheduled to work the next morning. They were allowed two overnights per month or could take a midnight curfew in lieu of an overnight. And if they arrived back at the residence before midnight, they could finish that late leave in the recreation room providing the student hostess on duty was notified.

The hostess was obliged to be properly dressed until all guests were out of the residence and the door was locked. Students were required to sign out and in when leaving the residence. The hostess was responsible for assuring that all who signed out for the evening had also signed back in before she went off duty. One rule which must have raised some questions read, "Nurses will choose their friends and places of recreation with discretion." There were many other rules listed, but most had to do with consideration for the rights of others when living in a dormitory.

After graduation each year, rooms would be reassigned based on one's class. Second year students lived on the third floor of Knickerbacker with some overflow, if needed, on the first floor. Second floor at Knickerbacker was for seniors. They too, might have some overflow in first floor rooms depending on the size of the class. When a student was on affiliation at St. Peter or Moose Lake, she may have been asked to vacate her room at Knickerbacker, meaning there was no place for her to stay should she want a weekend back at her home school during that psych affiliation. Again, class size and availability of rooms dictated whether or not the student had to vacate her room.

The spring 1960 issue of the *Voice of St. Barnabas* had an article on the razing of Knickerbacker and the memories of a nurse who once lived there. Part of that article is quoted below:

> "Knicker"—although patched and a little worn in spots—was dear to most of us. No one cared too much if we pounded a nail in the wall to hang our favorite pin-up fellow or casually admired singer. It was OURS and it was HOME…Remember the porch steps? They were cracked.
>
> And then there was that l-o-n-g one near the top, where, when one watched, one could always tell the juniors just moved in from the seniors by the way they stumbled a bit on that one step. The porch where so many good-byes and hellos were exchanged…and maybe important decisions by young lovers were made there! If it could

only talk, what a story of charming, twining young love, smiles, and—yes, maybe—heartbreaks....our precious little 'backyard' where we basked in the summer sun on one side, while our washing waved merrily in the breeze on the other..... Knickerbacker may be gone, but we will always think of it being a part of us and St. Barnabas.

There was the senior student who awoke during the middle of the night to a scratch-thump-scratch-thump noise and turned on the light to investigate. In the middle of the floor was a mouse, trying to drag a cookie he had found heaven knows where. He was so greedy he would not leave the cookie to flee, but just looked at the student, sitting petrified in the middle of her bed. She threw something at the vicious beast, then grabbed her alarm clock and slippers and ran off to the safety of a bed whose usual occupant was on night duty. The next morning she reported to Annie Smith, the maid, about her nocturnal visitor. So Annie went to the housemother to ask that an exterminator be called. The housemother replied, "Oh, that girl just has an overactive imagination. No need to call an exterminator for that." Annie set a trap near the door of the room where the beast was last seen and when she caught it, she took it to the housemother saying, "Here is Miss Kornmann's imagination."

And there were the water fights on third floor. That seemed to be one class's way of blowing off steam. A student, returning to the dorm after a weekend off, and accompanied by her sister, was greeted with water cascading down the steps from the third floor to the tower level on the southeast side of the building. The sister was horrified that such things went on—the student just ran to her room to get her camera to catch the action!

And there was the night that Carol Rugland was visiting Joyce Bissell in Joyce's third floor room—on the west side of the building, near the fire escape. Joyce was sitting with her back to the window and Carol, facing the window, looked up to see a man peering in. She got excited and ran into the hall to call for help. What formed in her mind as "Help, there's a man peeking in Bissell's window" came through her panicky lips as "Help, there's a man pissing in Beekel's window." Fifty plus years later, Carol is reminded at every gathering of her class of the night her tongue got disconnected from her brain!

The junior-senior banquet was a highlight for both classes each year. Receipts from the pop machines in the hospital went to the junior class and the banquet each year was paid for from that money. The juniors were responsible for all the planning, making reservations at a restaurant, or sometimes a country club, choosing the theme and the menu, and arranging for entertainment and a speaker. It was not a formal affair, but every girl dressed in her Sunday best. Often a new dress was purchased or sewn for the occasion. After the move to the new hospital in 1958, there were more machines and more money, so other things might also be paid from pop machine receipts. New Singer sewing machines were purchased from that fund for the sewing room set up in what had been the doctors' dining room when Whitney and Pavilion were still being used as the hospital.

There were picnics and the annual swim picnic at the Lake Minnetonka home of a board member or a women's board member. In the early 1950s, it was at the Sweatt home and in later years at the home of the Newell Weeds. There were athletic teams and league play through the YMCA or the park board for those interested in softball or baseball during summer months and in volleyball or basketball in winter months. Opponents for the games were teams from other nursing schools in the city. There were formal dances, usually one a year. And various fundraising events for causes chosen by the students.

One of the projects for which fundraisers were held was the school yearbook. The first one was published in 1963, named *Sabarho* after a paperbound similar publication from years long past. There was a yearbook published from 1963 every year until the school closed in 1973. Sharon Krampitz, class of 1963, had the monumental task of editing that first yearbook. The product they produced was excellent and the yearbook became a traditional part of every year after that. (There was a maxim among faculty that "If you do anything two years in a row, it becomes a tradition.") The editor each year was a senior student, Pat Warren in 1964, Mary Jo Bixby in 1965 for example.

Beginning with the 1964 yearbook, there was a dedication page, always planned as a closely guarded secret, to be revealed only at Honors' Day. Hazelle Lundell, that much- loved fundamentals instructor to whom reference has been made several times in this book, was the first to be so honored. The next year, 1965, it was Dr. Emil Schleicher and then, of course, after that it was a tradition. Evelyn Dressel, Mabel Christiansen and Ruth Weise were some of those to whom the yearbook was dedicated.

The dedication of the last yearbook, in 1973, was particularly interesting to me for two reasons. In the first place, the dedication was to an idea, rather than a person. The dedication read: "The Sabarho staff chose to dedicate the book this year to an idea instead of just one person, and that idea was freedom. Freedom to be what we are, to realize man's potential, and to be free to strive toward a goal, whatever that goal may be."

Sculptor Paul T. Granlund captured freedom in his sculpture, "Sprites," located in the courtyard of the Metropolitan Medical Center. Mr. Granlund said, "For me, sculpture is a celebration of being alive. In 'Sprites' I hope to give shape to the feeling of exuberance, the spirit of well-being." The second reason that dedication was so interesting to me is that Mr. Granlund was the reason I chose nursing as a career. He was a blonde, curly haired, apple-cheeked young man, a freshman at Gustavus at the same time I was also a freshman there. My goal in those days was to become an artist, but after spending one semester in art class with Paul Granlund and observing his great talent, it was apparent to me that I couldn't stand the competition, was probably going to starve to death as an artist, and I'd better choose another career that would guarantee three meals a day for me. Paul's wife, Edna, was also a student at Gustavus in those days. She was a nurse, by the way, who earned her baccalaureate in nursing from Gustavus. And that's the "rest of the story."

In order to keep the price of *Sabarho* to a minimum, students scheduled fund-raisers each year to help defray expenses. In 1965, they sponsored a spaghetti dinner. In 1966, they put on a variety show, "St. B. Au-Go-Go" which went great! They raised four hundred dollars with that one event. Hospital staff, school staff and faculty and even some of the doctors contributed talents to that show and similar ones held in other years.

In 1958, the *Voice of St. Barnabas* added a regular feature to that paper. Beginning then there was always a page entitled, "Checkerboard," which was about happenings in the school of nursing. Contributors to that page were students, faculty and school staff, such as long-time registrar, Elma Ann Lyon. It was a good way for all hospital staff, patients and visitors who read the *Voice* to become more familiar with the accomplishments of students and staff in the school.

In 1963, students developed their own little publication, *Chat From Checks*. It was a folksy kind of paper, entirely the brainchild of students and geared to the things students wanted to say and read. Some of the comments were "in" things that really had little or no meaning to outsiders who read it, but were meaningful to students. Mrs. Christensen, then a residence receptionist, became the advisor to the editorial staff. She also ran off the copy on the school mimeograph machhine. That first year, there were co-editors, Susan Kuklish and Lois Buhl. The next year Lois was editor, and like the *Sabarho*, the editor was always a senior student. Mrs. Christensen continued to be the advisor year after year. Most of the work on that paper was done during the evening hours when Mrs. Christensen was on duty at the reception desk. There was more than adequate space to work in the reception area and storage space below the counter to stack paper supplies as well as materials in progress for publication. *Chat From Checks* provided a great vehicle for students to freely express feelings about anything. The guidance of Mrs. Christensen helped them to keep their writings in good taste. Faculty who wanted to know what was going on in student conversations always read *Chat From Checks*.

In the nineteenth century, new schools of nursing were particularly interested in recruiting healthy, strong women, preferably as plain-looking as possible. The idea, apparently, was to insure that young men would not be interested in pursuing romantic relationships with plain-looking girls and therefore these would be the girls who would stay with nursing. More than one hundred years later, this seems to be curious thinking. We know today that many men were attracted by just the idea that a girl or woman was a nurse, a potential wife who would know how to do a good job in managing a home and raising children. And we also know that marriage and family did not preclude the possibility of success in nursing. Many found they could have both and many did have both.

As for students being plain looking, the number of beauty queens among St. Barnabas students attests to their pulchritude. To list just a few, there was Zola Koster, elected by MNSA, October 20, 1958, as centennial queen. That same year, freshman student, Mara Ziemelis, was elected by hospital personnel to represent St. Barnabas in the Miss Flame Contest October 6-

10, Fire Prevention Week. Another St. Barnabas student elected by fellow members of MNSA was Pam Loza, who was Miss Student Nurse in the 1963 Aquatennial queen competition. Tri-school formals were mentioned in the chapter on curriculum. A queen was always chosen for that formal. Glenna Thoreen, class of 1959, on April 11, 1958, was queen of the Tri-School Formal. In 1962, the formal was held earlier in the year, in February, and the queen elected for that one was their Queen of Hearts, Rose Velde. Beverly Nelson and Carol Timmer, both members of the class of 1961 and recipients of Darling Freight scholarships, were pictured as "Christmas angels" on the 1958 and 1959 Darling Freight Christmas cards. So much for plain looking women and nursing!

All references to students so far have been to girls. For most of the history of the school, its graduates were girls or women. Beginning in 1967, men were admitted as students. There had been sporadic interest from men inquiring about admission to the school, but most years, the interest would be from just one man. Faculty had discussed the issue and decided it would be a disservice to both the man and the school to admit just one as the first ever admitted to the school. Some were returning service men who had served as medical corpsmen and wanted admission with advanced standing on the basis of their experiences. Challenge examinations were developed in some schools to allow recognition of previous learning, but blanket advanced standing was not considered acceptable in most schools because the experiences these men had lacked the breadth that was generally required to grant advanced standing. A corpsman usually had wide experience in caring for trauma patients, but none in caring for elderly or new mothers or children. Finally, in 1967, there were three young men, all qualified in every way and they were admitted as members of the class of 1969. They were Miles Beckstrom, James Kluxdal and James Cavers. All continued on to graduation from the school.

In 1973, Kenneth Terry, then a graduate student at the University of Minnesota and a part-time employee of the Minnesota League for Nursing, wrote a term paper for a psychology course entitled "The Male in Nursing." He interviewed several male graduates and students as well as directors of nursing programs that had admitted male students. Ruth Weise, then director of the school at St. Barnabas, was among those he interviewed. Following are some quotes from his paper:

> From all conversations, a fairly clear picture of a "typical" male nurse emerges. As far as background is concerned, most men entering nurse's training are on the older side. Many or perhaps even a clear majority, have served in one of the various branches of the military as medics, corpsmen or aides. In most instances, there is solid (family) background in the health field.

Mr. Terry goes on to cite one man whose mother had been an LPN for years and whose brother was a nurse anesthetist. He finished that paragraph with, "In all cases that I observed, no matter what the background, there was a strong desire and need to serve and help other people." Further on, he states,

> One particular hospital area in which male nurses are extremely effective is in pediatrics…It was generally felt by all the interviewees that the males filled a very real need on the part of the children. At a most traumatic time for them (sick, away from home, strange environment, etc.) the man represented a substitute father for them and they made the transition from home to hospital and recuperation periods much easier and more enjoyable. The men too, generally felt that the "peds" experience was a highlight of their education.

He explored the possibility that some women may refuse to be cared for by a male nurse. He cited the experience of one man he interviewed who said in all his three years in training, only one woman refused to have him care for her. She was a Philippine-born woman and he felt the cultural difference was the deciding factor there, rather than any personal animosity toward male nurses. This same young man said that one day, a female MD said, rather sarcastically, to him, "What's a man doing in nursing?" He responded to her, "What's a woman doing in medicine?" It cleared the air and after that they had a good working relationship.

Mr. Terry went on:

> This example does bring up a point that Mrs. Lee made regarding the male being more aggressive than the female student. A reply such as he made would probably never have been made by a female.

In the same vein, Miss Weise related an episode that brought about some changes in teaching at St. Barnabas. In a demonstration by a faculty member of a particular piece of equipment, the males wanted to know not only what it was for, but also how it worked and the instructor was at a loss to explain since no student had ever asked that before. Needless to say, the instructor made it her business to get the answer in order to be prepared should the issue arise again.

A point of interest for Mr. Terry was the acceptance of the male students by the female classmates who greatly outnumbered them. He stated,

> Generally, it was found that there were very few problems. Miss Weise did cite heavier drinking as a difference, but attributed this to the males being older and from different life styles (service backgrounds etc.). It was mentioned by three of the interviewees that upon entrance into the training program there was a distinct male-female separation into like groups. However, after a time both were amalgamated and they became not male and female nursing students, but just nursing students, period....the director asked one of the fellows if there was any illicit behavior going on in the dorms (males and females in the same building). "Hell, no," he said, "It would be like incest."
>
> Mr. Terry made four conclusions based on this limited survey:
>
> 1. Males in nursing are not the feminine, gay types that popular opinion would have us believe. They are dedicated and able persons working in an area they feel best qualified in.
>
> 2. The number of males in nursing is increasing and they are able to compete equitably with their female counterparts and in some areas of nursing, they are superior.
>
> 3. Males are generally well accepted by their female co-workers, fellow students, patients and medical staff.

4. In training programs, their grades are no better or worse than females.

An Honors Day program was inaugurated at the school in 1963. Previously, awards had been given at both capping and graduation ceremonies. One award, particularly, gave cause to rethink how the awards were given. That was the Schleicher Award for the best bedside nurse in the junior class. It was given at capping. The award winner was not notified in advance, so she could not alert family to be on hand to share her joy in receiving this important honor. The remarks I gave as the school director at the time at that first Honors Day tell the whole story.

> On behalf of the faculty, let me welcome you to the first Honors Day Program of St. Barnabas Hospital School of Nursing. With this program today, we are inaugurating a tradition which we hope to continue and to develop further in years to come. In setting aside a day such as this, the faculty means to give recognition to all in the school who have extended themselves beyond that which was required—to those who have not been content just to pass, but to strive for the best which a nurse can give.
>
> In addition to recognizing achievement by the presentation of awards, it is also our purpose today to recognize the contributions of students who have given their time and energies to (non-academic) activities of the school. You will note that page two of your program includes a list of class leaders—the officers for each of the classes, the officers of student government and the editors of our school yearbook and school paper. Certainly these people deserve recognition for the effort which they have put forth in organizing and promoting such activities as the junior-senior banquet, the fall open house, the recent open house for high school students, the children's Christmas party, the all school dinner dance, etc.
>
> When the faculty first determined there would be an Honors Day Program, they were thinking in terms of a date near to and preceding graduation. Since most of the awards which are given are designated for graduating seniors, it seemed appropriate to plan

> this program close to graduation day. In addition, it appeared to the faculty that an Honors Day Program could be made even more significant by planning it to fall on a date already important to the nursing profession. And so it was that May 12, the birthday of Florence Nightingale, was suggested and accepted. It was one hundred forty four years ago today that Miss Nightingale was born in the city of Florence, Italy. It would do each of us well to reflect upon the contributions made to our profession by just this one person and the great distance the practice of nursing has come in the one hundred twenty years or so since she first began her work in nursing. Although we can't all be Florence Nightingales, each of us can strive to do the best of which we are capable and in this way each make our own contributions to nursing. It is to recognize just such effort, that we have this program today.

Honors Day became a tradition which carried through for the remaining years the school existed. It was a day to be enjoyed just for what it was, not because it was a part of capping or graduation, but just because it was important to recognize those who worked hard to become the best they could be. Parents were invited and some did come. Hospital administration and nursing service people were also invited. Following the planned program, there was a tea in the Whitney living room. Of course, all students were off duty for the occasion and there were no classes scheduled which might have prevented some from attending.

And so finally came the last week before graduation. For some students, the time had gone by unbelievably fast, while others thought the day would never come. Several were planning post-graduation weddings. Some had succeeded in getting faculty approval to be married before graduation. The marriage policy of the school varied over time. For years students weren't allowed to be married, period. During the 1950s, the faculty relaxed the rule somewhat to allow marriage if the student were achieving well in the school and if she understood there would be no special privileges for her because she was married and living off campus. Having to secure faculty permission to marry and move out of the dormitory seemed punitive to some students, but it was never meant to be so. Faculty saw their primary responsibility to encourage each student to do the best she could do and for some the distraction of a new marriage was seen as the added burden that could prevent a student who may have had scholastic difficulty from acceptable achievement.

Pregraduation antics could be bizarre. For example, some classes had Rip Day. On the last day a student was on the unit as a student, anyone could, and did, rip a part of the student's uniform. Sometimes it got a little out of hand and some students ended the shift having to wear a patient gown or isolation gown over their undergarments because the uniform had been torn away. Fortunately, that tradition died somewhere along the way. And then there was the tradition of dressing the nude statue at Charlie's Café Exceptionale in a St. Barnabas student uniform. Charlie's sat on the corner of Seventh Street and Fourth Avenue South, so it was just a short walk away. Students one year must have alerted the newspaper of their intention to dress the statue, for they were pictured in the next day's edition of the Star Tribune. Another era found students dressing a dummy in a student uniform, then propping the dummy up in the Washburn fountain, in the yard outside of Wellesmere. They also managed to get their picture in the newspaper that time. There was Senior Skip Day—perhaps that was bargained for in lieu of Rip Day! For some there was a little drinking in the dorm. At the root of it all was the need to blow off steam in anticipation of achievement of the goal they had been after for three years.

And then the great night at St. Mark's was there. The women's board, later the auxiliary, provided corsages for each of the graduating students to wear. Wearing a white uniform after three years in checks was a new experience. Prior to graduation, all in the class would agree on one style of uniform, so all were wearing identical white uniforms. Fran Warde, graduating in the class of 1951, designed the graduation uniform for her classmates. Perhaps that had been done before or maybe after. Usually the uniforms were ordered from a uniform company.

At the church, students lined up for the processional—seniors first, then juniors, then freshman members of the student choir and finally members of the faculty. In practice, most of the students in the school were in the processional because most students sang in the choir. They processed from the front of the church back to the narthex on the north side aisle, then through the narthex and in the center aisle all the way to the front of the church and the pews reserved for them. The processional was solemn and

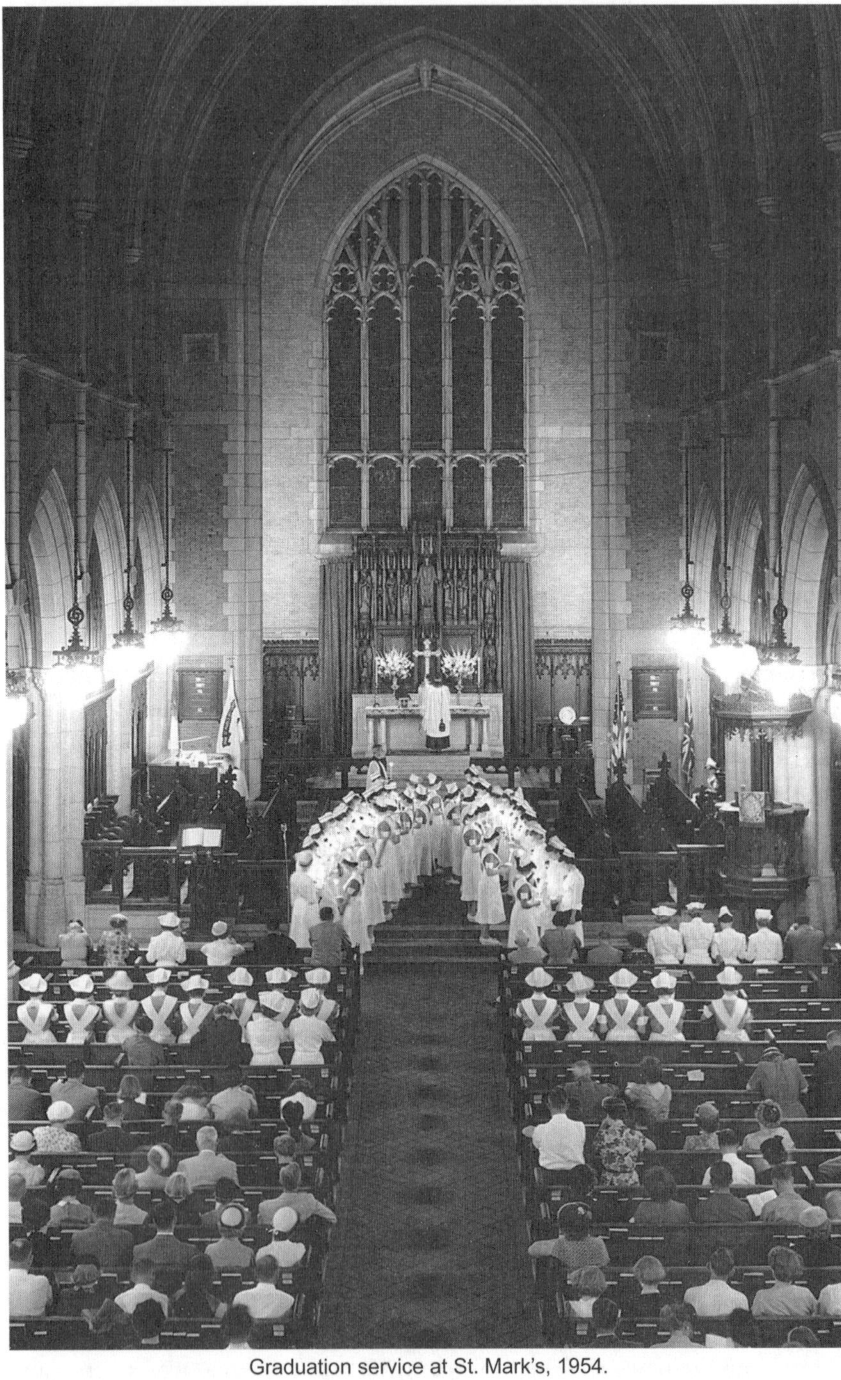

Graduation service at St. Mark's, 1954.

meaningful, but it also provided opportunity for graduates and their families to spot each other as the ceremony was starting. Members of the alumnae always served as ushers.

Earlier in the year, students in the graduating class had decided who they would like to have as graduation speaker. If possible, that person was recruited to do the job. The dean of the cathedral and the hospital chaplain always participated as did the hospital administrator and the director of the school. The president of the board of trustees handed each student her diploma and representatives from the women's board, later the auxiliary, and later still, the alumnae pinned the distinctive sterling silver pin on each graduate.

The Florence Nightingale Lamp Ceremony came after pins and diplomas had been bestowed. It began with all members of the graduating class repeating the Nightingale Pledge. Then each graduate came forward with a candle which she lit from one held by the chaplain, who had lighted his candle from the eternal flame on the altar. After every graduate was lined up next to the communion rail with lighted candle in hand, members of the junior class came forward, each carrying a candle. Each junior was placed facing a graduate and on signal, graduates lighted the candles of their junior, now declared senior, successors. Since there were no underclassmen to whom the light could be passed by the last graduating class, members of that class received the light from the chaplain as in years past, but then passed it to members of the alumnae recruited to attend for that very reason.

There were closing prayers and the benediction, then the graduates led the recessional back out of the church. The auxiliary always provided a reception following the ceremony. There were reunions with family, lots of tears, and lots of flashbulb pictures. Pictures were not permitted during the service in the cathedral, but afterwards at the reception they would be taken.

In anticipation of the graduation of the last class, faculty planned a number of activities in which they participated with students. Every effort was made to deal with separation anxiety, which some feared could be a problem with those who knew they were the end of the line. Three staff members in the school, Elma Ann Lyon, Mabel Christenson and Hazelle Lundell, decided they wanted to do something special as their gift to the class. They began planning and discussing in the fall, soon after school re-

CLASS OF 1955

BENOY, IZELLE
BURDORF, LORRAINE
CARLSON, JOYCE
CLARK, JULIETTE
COOK, PATRICIA
DOCHOW, MARY JANE
DUBEL, MARCIA
DUFOUR, JO
FARRAR, BETH ALICE
FRETHAM, CLARICE
INGSTAD, MARIE
JACOBSON, JANICE
JONES, SHARON
KELLING, SHIRLEY
LUND, DARLENE
MACDONALD, MARGARET
MORRIS, JUDY
NIELSON, ROSE MARIE
OLSON, MARGUERITE
RADEMACHER, AUDREY
RANES, CATHRYN
RAUSTAD, CONSTANCE
SAVRE, ARLA
SKYTTE, JOANNE
STEWART DIANE
STROM, MARILYN

St. Barnabas Hospital School of Nursing

Capping Service

CATHEDRAL CHURCH OF ST. MARK
FRIDAY, JUNE 12, 1953
8:00 P.M.

Capping Service program, Cathedral Church of St. Mark, Friday, June 12, 1953, 8 P.M.

Capping Service

PROCESSIONAL - - - - - - *The Church's One Foundation*
Hymnal No. 396

GREETINGS - - - - - - *The Very Rev. Frederick M. Morris*

SCRIPTURE AND PRAYERS - - *The Very Rev. Frederick M. Morris*

STUDENT CHOIR - - - - - *Mr. Howard Englund, Director*
LAMB OF GOD - - - - - - - - - - *Kalinnihof*
INTO THE NIGHT - - - - - - - - - - *Edwards*

ADDRESS - - - - - - *Rev. P. M. Gillfillan, Hospital Chaplain*

CAPPING CEREMONY
PRESENTATION OF CLASS - - - - - - *Mrs. Marie Meader*
Miss Ann Desich
Instructors in Nursing
PLACING OF THE CAPS - - - - - - - *Student Council*
ST. BARNABAS HOSPITAL PRAYER - - - - *Freshman Class*

GREETINGS TO THE CLASS - - - - - - *Miss Dorothy Merrell*
Director of Nursing

PRESENTATION OF AWARDS - - - - - - - *K. S. Klicka, M.D.*
Director of St. Barnabas Hospital

STUDENT CHOIR
GIVE ME YOUR TIRED, YOUR POOR - - - - - - *Berlin*
THE LORD BLESS YOU AND KEEP YOU - - - - - *Lutkin*

BENEDICTION - - - - - - *The Very Rev. Frederick M. Morris*

RECESSIONAL - - - - - - - *St. Barnabas Hospital Hymn*

RECEPTION IN THE PARISH HOUSE
COURTESY OF THE WOMEN'S BOARD
OF ST. BARNABAS HOSPITAL

Members of the St. Barnabas Hospital School of Nursing
Alumnae Are Serving As Ushers

THE ST. BARNABAS HOSPITAL PRAYER

O Almighty God, who callest thy holy Apostle Barnabas to follow in the steps of thy blessed Son in administering to the sick and suffering, grant to us the same spirit of consolation, that by gentleness and love, through faithfulness and patience, we may serve thy afflicted children. Support us in thy work; endow us with wisdom and skill; give us sympathy for one another; deliver us from temptation, and at last bring us to thy rest and peace; through Jesus Christ our Lord. Amen.

ST. BARNABAS' HOSPITAL HYMN

(Tune—"Go Forward, Christian Soldier"—Hymn No. 553)

Written by the Chaplain for all the workers in St. Barnabas when he was a patient in the hospital and realized how every member of the hospital staff does everything possible to help a patient back to health and strength.

"Go heal the sick and suffering"
It is our Lord's command,
Be patient, firm but gentle
In look and word and hand—
The sick revert to childhood
No matter what their age,
The rich, the poor, the cultured,
The foolish and the sage . . .

When tempted to be angry—
Your patience sorely tried,
Let nothing blight your vision,
He's always at your side
To guide, direct and strengthen
Throughout the night and day,
He never fails the faithful
Who with Him watch and pray . . .

Ofttimes you will grow weary,
Your task will lose its glow,
His strength will give you courage,
His life through you will flow;
In times of tribulation,
In times of doubt and fear,
In times when you are downcast
Be strong, for He is near . . .

Rejoice, then, in His power,
Be thankful for His grace,
We all are His co-workers
And have our special place;
Think not of self or comfort,
Life's struggles never cease—
He fought the fight that we fight—
In Him we all find peace . . .

— F. D. TYNER
Easter Sunday, April 1, 1945

sumed following the summer break. Mabel and Elma Ann took the design of the school pin and worked it into a round silver pendant which could be worn on a chain around the neck or attached to a charm bracelet. Then they ordered enough of the pendants crafted so that one could be presented to every student and every member of the faculty. To finance the project—kept secret, of course—Mabel and Elma Ann spent the fall selling calendars and placemats. Their sales efforts were successful and they raised enough money to cover the entire cost of their gift.

Meantime, Hazelle (labeled "seamstress extraordinaire" in the *Voice*) was at work on a banner to be presented to the hospital in honor of this class. It used the design of the pendant the other two had designed. This was worked in padded silver lame` on a blue velvet background. The pendants were presented at the senior banquet. The banner was displayed at graduation, then hung at Metropolitan Medical Center to be shared with all employees and visitors. It hangs today in the historical library. The three generous ladies received profuse thanks for their efforts, with some telling them the pendant was more meaningful to them than the school pin. "Reactions were beautiful" is the way Elma Ann described the outcome of the project.

There were thirty-one in that final graduating class, making it about average in size for the last thirty years of the school's history. The largest class ever to graduate was the class of 1963, with fifty-six members. The class of 1962 held the distinction of having the highest overall scholastic average in the history of the school. Closing the circle for St. Barnabas, the board of nursing staff member who administered state board examinations to the last class was a St. Barnabas graduate, Grace Terry, class of 1951. One member of the class had given birth to her first child only a day or two before the exams, but she was there to complete those all-important exams.

The alumnae conducted a survey to determine what kind of jobs St. Barnabas graduates had after graduation from the school. They ranged from airline hostess-stewardess to parish nurse to the Peace Corps and volunteer coordinator. A few included special notations on the surveys they completed. Marie Miller, class of 1936 said she had the honor of working with Sister Elizabeth Kenny; Peggy Tremble said she was the first St. Barnabas graduate to become an airline stewardess. Shirley Land, class of 1951, was an airline stewardess before she came to St. Barnabas. She used her earnings from the

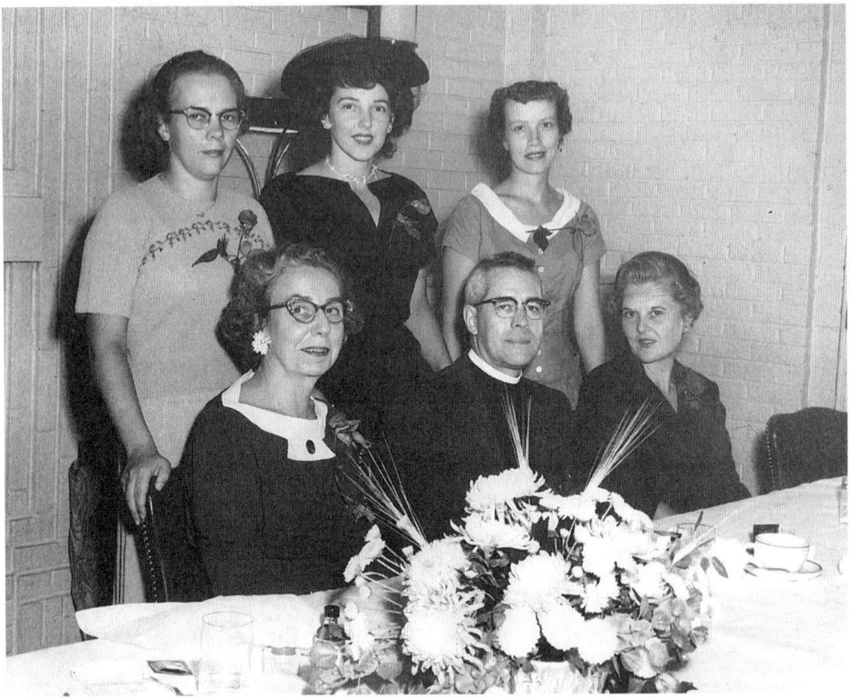

Nurses' Alumnae Banquet, 1957. Left to right, front row: Dorothy Merrell, Chaplain Gilfillan, Irene Sobotka. Back row, all Alumnae members: Marian Westman Nyberg (1948), Norma Vermeer Torvik (1948) and Delores Friedli Holl (1952).

airline to finance her nursing education. Two members of Shirley's class, Joyce Bissell and Janet Erickson, became airline stewardesses after graduation. Neta Kanne Reinecke, class of 1937, served in the U. S. Army Nurse Corps, earning six theater ribbons, five battle stars and a bronze star; Dora Daniels Sanders, class of 1945, was the first St. Barnabas graduate to become a police officer; Grace Tanigawa Traynor was the first Japanese-American officer in the Navy Nurse Corps; Diane Carlson Evans, class of 1967, posed for the nurses statue at the Vietnam memorial in Washington DC.

Judith Anderson Lawson sent a story she wrote entitled "Nurses Make a Difference." It seems an appropriate way to close this chapter.

> It was twilight in the twelve-bed Intensive Care Unit as I began another night shift. The lights were dim, the monitor alarms were set on low, in the background a symphony of cardiac monitors endlessly chirped out the heartbeats of each of our patients as they

rested for the night. I tied up the neck of a patient gown that I wore over my uniform, part of my night ritual, in an effort to stay clean as well as stay warm, as our unit tended to be chilly in the pre-dawn hours. I offered up a silent prayer that the shift would be a quiet one. "Please, God, no emergencies tonight." With that thought, I began my hourly tasks.

I smiled as I recalled the words of a silly tune we used to sing in nursing school. I squatted to drain the hourly output from my patient's foley bag and marveled at the accuracy of our lyrics. Years of study and preparation for this! Ever so precisely, I transferred the straw colored fluid into a graduate. Slowly, I rose from my chore on the floor and met a pair of eyes, round and frightened, looking back at me. My comatose patient was now awake and his eighty year old, massive black body was trembling as he tried to speak.

"Sk…Skuse me, Miss, but…Is you an angel?" he whispered.

My jaw dropped a bit, and I paused an extra second to react to his question.

The blue glow from the monitors, the semi-darkness, and my ridiculous gown, coupled with my patient's cardiac arrest earlier in the day, added up to one likely conclusion. This must be heaven.

Setting aside the hours-worth of urine, I instinctively reached around the huge chest to hug his very alive self and carefully explained the events of the day. He listened to every word and seemed to understand, with a nod and weak smile, that this was a hospital and I was his nurse, not an angel at all!I asked if there was someone I should call to share that he was awake.

Were family members waiting for an update? "No, no missy…no one to call. No family, no one waiting." And he drifted off to sleep.

Each hour as I approached his bedside, he awoke briefly and would share a sentence about his lifetime, a decade at a time. It was as if he prepared a message for me each hour as I tended the other patients and, episode, by episode, I learned the highlights of his existence.

As usual, the last hour of our shift had a quicker pace as we scrambled to prepare for a busy day in the ICU. My new friend slept through his last set of checks. I tried not to disturb him, but wondered what his next message for me might be. I gave his large black hand a gentle squeeze and reported off for the night.

I returned to work for the last night of my "stretch." A shift off was long overdue. Wearily, I listened to report with half an ear, as nothing much had changed from the night before. The evening nurse included a message that the gentleman in bed #8 had expired at 0800…and went on with her report.

From the nurses' station, I looked out over the orderly ICU. My eyes lingered over the very vacant bed #8 as I slowly and deliberately tied up my cover gown. I took a deep breath and wiped away a single tear that slipped down my cheek. "Make sure he's not alone, God," I prayed, "and, please, no emergencies tonight"…and began another set of hourly checks.

Chapter 17

Remembering the Nursing School Faculty

Records were found verifying the employment at St. Barnabas of seventy-eight women whose primary responsibility was the teaching of nursing students. In addition to those seventy-eight, twelve directors or superintendents were identified and they likely had some teaching responsibilities. In the early days, along with their administrative responsibilities, they probably had sole responsibility for teaching students

A board of nursing report for 1916 included the first reference to a person listed as an instructor. The identity of this instructor was not included in the record though it did say she earned fifty dollars per month plus room and board. That report did not include the number of hours of instruction that were being provided. The first instructor identified by name in board of nursing records was Lulu Saunders, class of 1919 at St. Barnabas. She was listed as an instructor on the 1920 board report, which also indicated the school was offering two hundred fifty two hours of instruction over a three-year period. The school continued having just one or possibly two instructors well into the 1940s. The bulk of teaching at that time was done by physicians with supervisors and head nurses on the clinical units carrying out the responsibility of teaching skills that could only be learned or could best be learned in the clinical area.

The following vignettes refer to the twelve administrative officers in the school plus the seventy-eight instructors for whom records were available. It is possible there were some who have fallen through the cracks, but every effort has been made to include as many as possible who served on the school faculty.

DIRECTORS OR SUPERINTENDENTS OF THE NURSING SCHOOL

Miss L. B. Jones

Gibbs and Bachmeyer, writing for the *Bulletin Of The Hennepin County Medical Society* in 1959 stated, "In 1895, it was deemed necessary to systematize the work, and Miss L. B. Jones was appointed matron. She organized and superintended the first training school of nurses." There is no reference to Miss Jones in Board of Nursing records. However, there was no Board of Nursing until 1907 and the two references in which board records identify a chief nurse administrative officer are problematic with regard to time. The board record says Miss Eleanor Weston was the first superintendent of nurses, but that record does not indicate when she was hired or how long she served. It does say she was a graduate of Indianapolis City Hospital School of Nursing, so she may well have been influenced to come to St. Barnabas by Dr. Knickerbacker sometime in the eleven years he served as Bishop of Indiana. Possibly she came as a replacement for Miss Jones.

Harriet S. Hartry

Here there is discrepancy between the Board of Nursing record and the records of the Board of Trustees of the hospital. But remember again, the Board of Nursing record was made after the fact, so most likely the information in Board of Trustees records is the correct information. The Board of Nursing record states Miss Hartry was a graduate of Brooklyn

Hospital School of Nursing in New York. The Board of Trustees did not include that bit of information in their records, but they did state Miss Hartry was employed as superintendent of nurses in 1899 and that she served in that capacity until 1907 at which time she was made superintendent of the hospital, a post she held for twenty three years, until 1930. Alumnae records indicate she was instrumental in encouraging the organization of the school of nursing alumnae, the first such alumnae organization in Minneapolis. In the early years of the American Nurses Association (its forerunner, actually), a nurse joined that organization by referral from her alumnae association, so establishment of alumnae associations was important to the development of professional standards for nurses.

M. Dorothy Rhodes

Miss Rhodes was appointed director of nurses in 1916 and served until January 1938. She was a 1906 graduate of St. Barnabas and had done post-graduate work at Boston Floating Hospital prior to her appointment as director of nurses at St. Barnabas. An entry on the board record indicates Miss Harriett B. Leach was hired to be superintendent of nurses for a six-month period in 1917. There is no indication whether she worked under Miss Rhodes, or perhaps was filling in for Miss Rhodes for some reason. The United States entered World War I in 1917 and possibly Miss Rhodes was on leave to provide service either in that war or in care of influenza victims, since there was a major influenza epidemic at the time. The Board of Nursing record indicates Miss Hartry took over the job of superintendent of nurses in August of 1917, but doesn't specify how long she worked in that capacity. Remember, at the time she was already superintendent of the hospital. At any rate, apparently at some point Miss Rhodes returned and again took up the reins of director of nurses, serving through all of the 1920s and most of the 1930s. When Miss Rhodes resigned, she went to California.

Christine Peterson

In early 1938 when Miss Rhodes left, another St. Barnabas graduate, Christine Peterson of the class of 1911, was appointed acting superintendent of nurses. Since 1928 she had been assistant superintendent of nurses, with primary responsibility for administration of the nursing school. Apparently she turned down the appointment as superintendent on a permanent basis, although academically, she was qualified to serve in that capacity. She had a baccalaureate degree that she had earned from Gustavus Adolphus College in 1901. She taught school for six years, then on January 15, 1908, she enrolled as a student at St. Barnabas.

She graduated from St. Barnabas on January 15, 1911, and thereafter she worked for a time as night supervisor on two surgical wards and one ward for children (thirty patients in all). Those were the days of truly long hours in nursing. Miss Peterson's niece was interviewed for a 1955 article for the *Voice of St. Barnabas*. She stated that she knew of many times when her aunt worked eighteen to twenty hours in a single day, enabling her to keep close contact with the patients in her care. She often maintained these ties after the patient had been discharged from the hospital and in her later years it was not unusual for her to receive ten to twelve letters a day from former patients and former students. Years later, women who had been students while Miss Peterson was on the faculty remembered how she spent many of her off-duty hours helping students to review for state boards. Some felt their passing the boards on first writing was due to her tutelage. Other former students remembered how she gave them money to pay the state board examination fees. Still others remembered how a new dress and shoes might be delivered mysteriously and anonymously to a girl who was invited to an important party and had nothing to wear and no money to buy new clothes.

Miss Peterson was hospitalized at St. Barnabas in the 1950s and at that time she said she had been a nursing arts instructor in the school. Since the record does not indicate she held this position, it is assumed that teaching nursing arts was probably one of her duties during her tenure as assistant superintendent of nurses. Miss Peterson died at St. Barnabas on January 14, 1955, almost forty-four years to the day after her graduation from the school.

Ellen Aird

Miss Aird was the superintendent of nurses hired on a permanent basis after Miss Peterson. She joined the staff on June 1, 1938. She was a graduate of St. Mary's Hospital School of Nursing in Rochester, class of 1923. She also had taken postgraduate work at both the University of Minnesota and

Teachers' College, Columbia University in New York, though the board record doesn't indicate when she did this. It does indicate that she took a one-year leave of absence in 1940 and 1941, then returned to continue service at St. Barnabas until May 1, 1943.

Helen Platt

Miss Platt was hired at St. Barnabas in 1939 originally to teach nursing arts. It was she who filled in for Miss Aird when Miss Aird took her leave of absence. And when Miss Aird resigned, Miss Platt was hired as her replacement. Miss Platt was a graduate of Butterworth Hospital School of Nursing in Grand Rapids, Michigan. Her title as director of nurses differed from Miss Aird's. On February 1, 1946, apparently the position of director of nurses was split, as it would be again in July of 1961. At any rate, Miss Platt was named director of nursing service on February 1, 1946 and she continued in this position until July 1950.

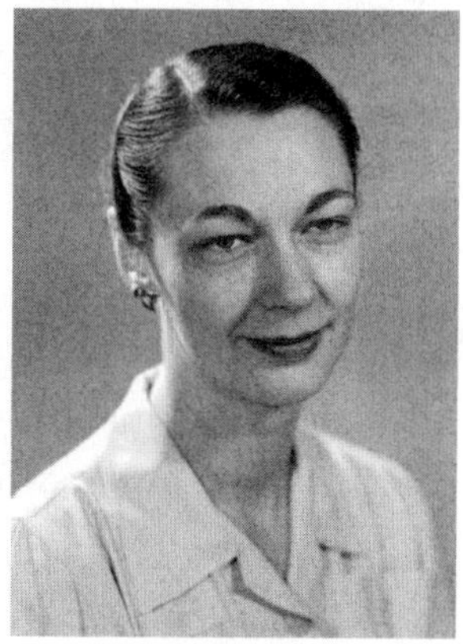

Helen Platt

Marian Dunn

Miss Dunn was appointed director of nursing education at the time Miss Platt became director of nursing service, February 1, 1946. She was a graduate of Asbury School of Nursing in Minneapolis. She stayed at St. Barnabas only a bit over one year, until April 30, 1947. Board of Nursing records do not indicate who was in charge from April to October, when Miss Dunn's replacement arrived. Perhaps Miss Platt moved back to fill both positions on a temporary basis.

Blanche Ostlund

Miss Ostlund joined the St. Barnabas staff as director of the school of nursing on October 1, 1947. She was a graduate of Johns Hopkins Hospital School of Nursing. She held a baccalaureate degree from Gustavus Adolphus College and a master of arts from the University of Minnesota. She, like Miss Dunn, stayed only a bit over one year, resigning in December of 1948.

Gertrude Braun (Sears)

Again, as in 1938, a St. Barnabas graduate was hired on an acting, temporary basis, as replacement for Miss Ostlund. Gertrude Braun was a member of the 1942 class at St. Barnabas and had been serving as the nursing arts instructor and later as a med-surg instructor on the faculty prior to her appointment as acting director. She served for one and one half years in the capacity of acting director. She continued on after Miss Merrell was hired to become the director of nursing, serving as associate director of nursing education until June of 1952. During that time she was married and she traded her faculty position for homemaker, mother responsibilities when she and her husband moved to Granite Falls, Minnesota.

Dorothy Merrell

In Chapter 15, Dorothy Merrell was cited as the one person, more than any other, who brought St. Barnabas Hospital School of Nursing into the modern era of nursing education. Ironically, she was hired as director of nursing, when the two departments, service and school, were reunited under one administrative officer. Perhaps the school just wasn't ready in 1950 to move out on its own. The number of faculty was still very low in relation to the number of students being admitted. For example, in 1952 there were only six instructors and nearly one hundred students in the program. There was a library, but its better days were still ahead. Miss Merrell joined the St. Barnabas staff on July 15, 1950, and served for eleven productive years. Her biographical information is in Chapter 15.

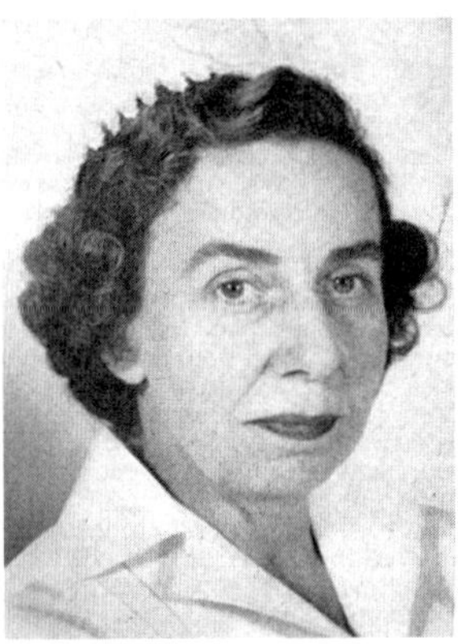
Dorothy Merrell

Grace Kornmann Terry

When Miss Merrell resigned, another St. Barnabas graduate, class of 1951, was appointed director of nursing education. A counterpart, Miss Virginia Schmidt, was appointed to be director of nursing service. Splitting the nursing department again was an idea whose time had come in 1961, though this had not been the case years earlier. I asked to be appointed on an acting basis for three months, at which time a decision could be made by either party, me or hospital administrator, whether or not to continue. I had worked for five years under Miss Merrell and had been a student during part of Miss Merrell's tenure. I regarded her as a mentor and held her in very high esteem. I was not certain I could or wanted to be a replacement for so great a lady. Ultimately, I did decide to stay on as director of nursing education, dropping the acting part of the title in October of 1961. My biographical information is also included in Chapter 15 of this book.

Ruth Weise

My replacement was Ruth Weise, who took over the position of director of nursing education September 1, 1965. She was a native of Park Ridge, Illinois. She received her nursing education at St. Francis Hospital School of Nursing, Evanston, Illinois. She took postgraduate education at Yale University and earned a baccalaureate degree in nursing education from the University of Minnesota where she also earned a master of arts in educational psychology. She was an instructor at the University of Minnesota School of Nursing when I was a baccalaureate student there in 1952. She also had post-masters education at the University of Washington before returning to Minnesota in 1965. Prior to her appointment as director of nursing education, she served for nearly a year on the faculty at St. Barnabas teaching Community Health Problems. Further biographical information on Ruth can be found in Chapter 15.

Many instructors stayed at the school for periods of only one to three years. The majority were young and several were married to university students. When the husband finished school and found employment, often elsewhere, the wife would resign to follow him. Some left to pursue further education and some left to raise families. A small minority left to explore other parts of the world.

Instructors in the school are listed below in alphabetical order rather than in numerical time sequence.

Betty Aasland

Betty was hired in 1968 to be a part-time instructor in pediatric nursing. She graduated from the University of Minnesota with a bachelor of science in nursing and a master of education. She had worked as a staff nurse at Hennepin County General Hospital and as an instructor at Swedish Hospital

School of Nursing. In addition, she had been an assistant professor in the department of nursing of Jamestown College, stationed at their clinical affiliation, North Memorial Hospital in Robbinsdale.

Marian Anenson

Marian came to St. Barnabas first in 1954 as an assistant instructor in nursing arts and later as the instructor for that course. Then she became a med-surg instructor, serving in that position until 1962, when illness forced her to resign. In 1963, with her health restored, she returned as an assistant instructor, serving part-time in pediatric nursing and part-time in maternity nursing.

Lois Barnes (Overland)

Lois was a clinical instructor in the late 1940s. A graduate of the University of Minnesota School of Nursing, she married while on the St. Barnabas faculty and resigned some time later.

Josephine Barrow

Josephine joined the faculty as a med-surg instructor in 1962. She was originally from Philadelphia, Pennsylvania, and had received all of her nursing and academic preparation in Pennsylvania. She was married and the mother of four children. The family relocated from Pennsylvania to Minnesota because of her husband's job. She brought a mature outlook as well as a different cultural outlook to the faculty that at that time had several young instructors and only one other from Mrs. Barrow's age group.

Mary Ellen Andrew Baxter

Originally from Tracy, Minnesota, Mary Ellen was a 1961 graduate of St. Barnabas. She took advantage of the school arrangement with Macalester College and after completing the program at St. Barnabas, she enrolled to complete a bachelor of science in nursing from Macalester. She was married and had a child 15 months old when she joined the faculty at St. Barnabas in July of 1965. She served as a part-time instructor, assisting with teaching maternity nursing. She had worked as a float in nursing service prior to moving to the faculty position.

Phyllis Becker (Burke)

Phyllis was one of the first instructors added to the faculty in the early 1950s after the appointment of Dorothy Merrell as director of nursing. She was a graduate of the College of St. Teresa in Winona. At St. Barnabas she was the clinical instructor assigned to teach medical nursing and to supervise students on 2 Whitney and 2 Pavilion. She married a University of Minnesota engineering student while she was at St. Barnabas. After he completed his education, the couple moved in 1955 to Ponca City, Oklahoma, where Bill was employed in the oil industry.

Jeanne Bergfald

Jeanne was employed in 1952 as the clinical instructor on 3 Whitney, 4 Martin and 5 Pavilion. She was a graduate of Swedish Hospital School of Nursing and held a baccalaureate degree from St. Olaf College. She had previously served on the staff of Naeve Hospital in Albert Lea. Jeanne stayed only one year. In 1953 I replaced her at St. Barnabas.

Gretchen Blau

Like Mary Ellen Baxter, Gretchen was a 1965 addition to the St. Barnabas faculty. She grew up in Melrose, Minnesota, and was a graduate of the University of Minnesota School of Nursing with a bachelor of science in nursing. She worked in pediatrics at the University of Minnesota Hospitals for one year before coming to St. Barnabas. During that year she married her husband, then a pediatric resident at the University of Minnesota Hospitals. At St. Barnabas, she taught med-surg nursing.

Alice Bradee

Alice was born and reared in Milwaukee, Wisconsin, and graduated from high school in Waukesha. She enrolled at Marquette University from which she received her bachelor of science in nursing in 1958. She did six months of staff nursing at St. Luke's Hospital in Milwaukee before moving to Minneapolis. She was appointed a staff nurse in nursing service at St. Barnabas in April 1959, moving to a faculty appointment as a surgical clinical instructor on September 1, 1959.

Susan Woodard Broberg

An eastern import to the St. Barnabas faculty was Susan Broberg. She was born in New York City, graduated from Horace Greeley High School in Chappaqua, New York, and Skidmore College in Saratoga Springs, New York. She was a chemistry major at Skidmore before she became interested in nursing and ultimately she received her bachelor's degree in nursing. Her student experiences at Skidmore included one month of operating room nursing at Albert Schweitzer Hospital in Haiti, West Indies. After college graduation, she went on to work in the operating rooms at New York University Hospitals and later moved to Minnesota for appointment in ICU, gynecology and general surgery at the University of Minnesota Hospitals. Her husband was from Waconia, Minnesota, and was attending the University of Minnesota Law School in 1963 at the time Susan was appointed operating room instructor at St. Barnabas.

Sheila English Cadwallader

Sheila came to St. Barnabas in 1961 as a staff nurse on 4B. She was from Fargo, North Dakota, and a graduate of Deaconess Hospital School of Nursing in Grand Forks. After only a few months on staff, she married Gary Cadwallader, a salesman for IBM computers. In 1962 she joined the nursing school faculty as a clinical instructor on 4A. During the last half of 1963, three of twelve members of the school faculty were pregnant. Sheila was the first to have her baby, followed by Lillian Ramsey in late 1963. My baby was the third to be born on January 9, 1964. We all took leaves of absence. When Sheila returned after the birth of her son, she worked part-time as an assistant instructor in maternity nursing.

Miriam Cameron

Miriam joined the St. Barnabas faculty in 1967 as an instructor in pediatric nursing. She held a bachelor of science degree in nursing from the University of Minnesota and had worked as a staff nurse at the heart hospital, University of Minnesota, and in pediatrics at University of Minnesota Hospitals. She also had done a stint as head nurse at Fair Oaks Nursing Home in Minneapolis.

Arlene Carlsen

Arlene was a 1965 addition to the faculty, assigned to med-surg nursing and a clinical instructor spot on 4A. She was born in Brooklyn, New York, and graduated from Fort Hamilton High School in Brooklyn. She came to Minnesota for college, earning a bachelor of science degree in nursing from St. Olaf College. She returned home after graduation from St. Olaf and worked for a time at Yale Medical Center in New Haven, Connecticut. Later she returned to Minnesota and to employment on the faculty at St. Barnabas.

Lois Carlson

As if to confuse everybody, I hired two Carlsons for faculty spots during the same month. Two differences, besides their clinical areas, separated them. Arlene was Carlsen with an "e" and she was Miss Carlsen, while Lois was Carlson with an "o" and she was Mrs. Carlson. Lois was appointed clinical instructor in the operating room. Like Susan Broberg, the instructor whom she replaced, Lois was married to a university student, Erik Carlson, who was a junior at the University of Minnesota Medical School when they married. Lois came to Minnesota from Bismarck, North Dakota, where she graduated from Bismarck High School. She attended the University of Minnesota, graduating with a bachelor of science degree in nursing.

Elvera Carlton

Vera Carlton was no stranger to St. Barnabas when she was appointed to the St. Barnabas faculty as a teaching dietitian in 1962. As Elvera Spotts, she had been the head dietitian preceding Ethel Haga. She received her degree in nutrition from the University of Minnesota and served a dietetic internship there before coming to St. Barnabas the first time. She was married at that time, but later divorced from her husband and dropped the Spotts name at the time of her divorce. She served as a therapeutic and teaching dietitian at Glenwood Hills Hospital immediately preceding her appointment to the St. Barnabas faculty. Her son, six years old at the time of her faculty appointment, was her great pride and joy and stories of his exploits made the faculty break room discussions, along with the stories of Hazelle Lundell's nieces and nephew. After January 1964, we three who had been pregnant all at the same time, added the latest on each of our babies. One might say we were a family-oriented group!

Mary Takamura Chapus

When I left St. Barnabas in 1956 for employment with the Department of Army in Germany, my replacement as med-surg clinical instructor on 3 Whitney, 4 Martin and 5 Pavilion was Mary Chapus. Mary was Nisei, from a Southeast Minneapolis family. She had previous experience in teaching before coming to St. Barnabas. She was newly married in 1956, to a Frenchman who was studying engineering at the University of Minnesota. She resigned to have their first child in 1959, just about the time that I, recently married, returned from Germany, so I stepped back into the position I left when Mary was hired in 1956. After the birth of their daughter, the Chapus moved to Teheran, Iran, where Edmund was employed. Later they moved back to his hometown of Grenoble, France.

Ann Desich

An early 1950s appointee to the faculty was Ann Desich, who came as an assistant instructor in nursing arts. She was a graduate of Kahler School of Nursing in Rochester. Her replacement in 1954 was Marian Anenson.

Evelyn Dressel (Tollefson)

Evie, as she was known to all her friends, was from LeSueur. She was a St. Barnabas graduate, class of 1950, and a graduate of the University of Minnesota with a bachelor of science in nursing education. Following nursing school graduation, she worked on 2 Whitney while setting aside funds to pursue her degree at the University. Though assigned as a staff nurse on 2 Whitney, she also participated in teaching nursing arts. When she completed her degree, she returned to the faculty as a med-surg instructor. She later married the brother of a fellow St. Barnabas graduate, Janie Tollefson, class of 1951. The couple had one son.

Betty Eichenlaub

Over the years there were just a bare handful of nurses at St. Barnabas who wore the dainty little organdy caps from the older eastern nursing schools. Blanche Ostlund was the first in memory of those living today, although Miss Hartry probably also wore one. Dorothy Merrell wore her cap from Bellevue with pride. Jeanne Scanlon, OR instructor, wore one and so did Betty Eichenlaub. Betty was from Toledo, Ohio, and graduated from a Toledo high school and the University of Toledo, where she earned a bachelor of education degree. She got her nursing education at Johns Hopkins School of Nursing in Baltimore. She was appointed to the St. Barnabas faculty as maternity nursing instructor in August of 1963. She was married to a doctor, who was on the staff at University of Minnesota Hospitals. The couple had five children, ranging in ages from six to eighteen at the time of her appointment to the St. Barnabas faculty.

Margaret Elvin

Margaret was a 1940s appointee to the St. Barnabas faculty. The 1946 school bulletin lists her as the med-surg Instructor, but by 1948 she was teaching nursing arts. She was married and left St. Barnabas around 1949 or 1950 to have a child.

Linda Fezler

Linda came to St. Barnabas as a med-surg instructor in 1966. She was a graduate of St. Olaf College department of nursing and had staff nursing experience at Fairview Hospital prior to her appointment to the faculty at St. Barnabas. She was an active member of the young adult group at Central Lutheran Church.

Yvonne Gorecki

Yvonne was hired in October of 1962 as a clinical instructor on 4B. She had obtained a bachelor of science in biological sciences and education from Minot State Teachers' College in Minot, North Dakota. She served a stint as a public school teacher, then enrolled as a nursing student at Trinity Hospital School of Nursing in Minot. Her husband was a student at the University of Minnesota Law School at the time of her appointment to the St. Barnabas faculty. Yvonne later transferred to the nursing service department as supervisor of the outpatient unit.

Beatrice Grassl

Bea was a graduate of the College of St. Teresa Program in Nursing, Winona, Minnesota. She was hired in 1955 to replace Phyllis Burke as the clinical instructor on 2 Whitney and 2 Pavilion. Three years later, she stepped up to become associate director of nursing education, replacing Ruth Schnitzen.

Marian Gruenfelder

Marian served as pediatric instructor from 1959-1961. She left St. Barnabas when her husband took a position outside of Minneapolis.

Jean Gustafson (Singh)

A native of Granite Falls, Minnesota, Jean was a 1953 graduate of St. Barnabas. Her first job after St. Barnabas graduation was at Colorado General Hospital in Denver. While there, she decided she would like to add a bachelor's degree to her resume, so returned to the University of Minnesota from which she earned a bachelor of science in nursing education in March of 1957. She and fellow St. Barnabas classmate, Avis Hernwall, had a travel itch, so they moved to England where both were employed for six months in private patient wings of a London hospital. Following that experience, they moved to Winchester, England, where both were employed at the Royal Hampshire Provincial Hospital. After six months in Winchester, they spent twelve weeks touring Scandinavian countries and the European continent. Returning home, Jean became an instructor in communicable disease and tuberculosis nursing at Minneapolis General Hospital. From Minneapolis General, she was recruited to return to St. Barnabas as the administrative assistant in the school of nursing, a position she held until the summer of 1964. She married a man from India and the couple later moved to Florida.

Maxine Gustafson

Maxine was the Teaching Dietitian in the school 1958-1959.

Ethel Haga

Miss Haga came to St. Barnabas as head dietitian in 1948. During the late 1940s and early 1950s she also carried the responsibilities of teaching dietitian, a position that at that time consisted mainly of supervising nursing students through the six weeks of diet kitchen experience to which each was assigned. Although she was a native of St. Paul, she earned her bachelor of science degree at Iowa State College in Ames, Iowa. She served a dietetic internship at Michael Reese Hospital in Chicago. She also had postgraduate study at the University of Minnesota. Miss Haga remained on the St. Barnabas staff for years, becoming one of its long-term employees. As her administrative responsibilities in the dietary department grew, she relinquished teaching students to a dietitian hired to fill the role of teaching dietitian.

Ethel Harper

Ethel joined the hospital staff in mid 1962 as a surgical nurse, but was soon transferred over to the faculty where she served as a med-surg instructor. She and her husband, a University of Minnesota faculty member, were both Canadian immigrants. At the time she joined the St. Barnabas faculty, the two were trying to adopt a child, and when a baby boy became available, she resigned to become a full-time mother to the little one.

Ruby Hass

Ruby joined the St. Barnabas faculty in November 1959 as a med-surg instructor. Her sister, Ruth, was already on staff at St. Barnabas as pediatric supervisor. The sisters were born and raised in Iowa and both were graduates of the State University of Iowa School of Nursing. Ruby remained at St. Barnabas for three years, then left in 1962 to pursue study for a master's degree at the University of Minnesota.

Ruth Hayden

Ruth joined the faculty as obstetrics instructor on September 19, 1960. She was from Wisconsin, a graduate of Milwaukee Lutheran High School and Milwaukee Hospital School of Nursing. She earned a baccalaureate degree from the University of Wisconsin in Madison. She spent the summer of 1959 touring Europe in a car which she and three other friends purchased for their tour. Ireland was their top favorite on the tour followed by Austria, Switzerland and Germany. Ruth stayed at St. Barnabas for one year.

Bernice Hennum

Bernice Hennum was instructor of pharmacology and therapeutics in 1948. The record is not clear on how long she was on the St. Barnabas faculty, but it appears it was not more than one or two years.

Mary Isely (Hermsmeier)

Mary taught nursing arts beginning in the fall of 1948. She was married over the Christmas holidays and finished out the school year, resigning in the spring of 1949. She was pregnant by that time and moved with her husband to Rochester. I lived in Rochester in 1952 and 1953 and one day met Mary in the grocery store. She had not been employed in nursing since leaving St. Barnabas. She had three little boys at that point who kept her too busy to think of working out of her home!

Mary Hess (Peterson)

Mary Hess came to Minneapolis from Wisconsin where she had graduated from the University of Wisconsin with a baccalaureate in nursing. She joined the St. Barnabas family as a staff nurse on maternity in 1961, then in 1962 she moved over to the school of nursing to develop and teach a new course in community health problems. She was very talented musically and sang in the madrigal singers group at Central Lutheran Church as well as the senior choir of Mount Olivet Lutheran Church. She sang for the wedding of a fellow faculty member, Berdine Schotzko in 1964. Mary met her husband, Bruce Peterson, in Minneapolis and the two were married in 1965 at Mount Olivet Lutheran Church. He was in YMCA work and ultimately the couple left the city when he took charge of a YMCA out of state.

Muriel Hoeflich

A graduate of the University of Minnesota School of Nursing, Muriel Hoeflich taught pediatric nursing at St. Barnabas for one year, 1949-1950. She was married to a doctor who was completing his residency at the University of Minnesota Hospitals. When she left in 1950, the couple was expecting their first child.

Mildred Holm

Millie Holm joined the staff at St. Barnabas in 1948 as supervisor-instructor in obstetric nursing. She held the dual position for a few years, but as her administrative responsibilities increased, she relinquished formal teaching to a person hired just to be an instructor in obstetric nursing. Millie continued on for several years as obstetric supervisor. She was a graduate of Northwestern Hospital School of Nursing and is remembered for her dignified demeanor. Those who got to know her well knew she had a wonderful sense of humor which lightened up every discussion in which she participated.

Virginia Howland

Virginia Howland was listed as the dietetics instructor in the 1948 bulletin issued by the school of nursing. Apparently when she resigned, her teaching responsibilities were taken over by the new chief dietitian, Ethel Haga.

Flora Hungerford

Flora Hungerford, appointed a med-surg instructor in 1968, had the distinction of possessing two baccalaureate degrees from different colleges. She held a bachelor of science degree in biology from Westmar College in LeMars, Iowa. She was also a graduate of Methodist-Kahler School of Nursing in Rochester, Minnesota. She served for a time as the health service staff nurse and counselor at Westmar College. She also worked as a staff nurse at Rochester Methodist Hospital. Feeling the need for more education, she enrolled at Case Western Reserve University in Cleveland, Ohio, from which she earned a bachelor of science degree in nursing. Coming back to Minnesota, she worked as a staff nurse in special care at Bethesda Hospital in St. Paul and later as an instructor in the Bethesda Hospital School of Practical Nursing.

Edna Jesse (Ware)

The record isn't clear, but apparently Edna Jesse served the dual role of pediatric supervisor-instructor from 1948-1950. She married between the time of her appointment to the position and her resignation in 1950. She was a 1942 graduate of St. Barnabas Hospital School of Nursing.

Helen Ann Johnson

Helen was a clinical instructor on 2 Whitney and 2 Pavilion in the late 1940s or early 1950s. When she resigned in July of 1952, it was to await the birth of her second child.

Mary Jones

Mary was appointed to the St. Barnabas faculty as a clinical instructor on 4A on January 13, 1964. She also helped to develop and later taught a new course entitled "Patient Care Management." She graduated from high school in Chesterfield, Illinois, and attended Blackburn College in Carlinville, Illinois, and Washington University in St. Louis, Missouri, from which she earned a bachelor of science degree in nursing education. She received her basic nursing from Barnes Hospital School of Nursing in St. Louis. She was married with four children at the time of her appointment to the St. Barnabas faculty. Her husband was a representative of American Hospital Supply Company. The family moved to Minnesota in September of 1961. Prior to that move, they lived in Oklahoma City where she had served as a clinical instructor in a practical nursing program. She also had experience as a supervisor-head nurse on a hospital psychiatric unit. She left the St. Barnabas faculty in 1965 to earn a master's degree in psychiatric nursing at the University of Minnesota. In 1967, she returned to St. Barnabas and served as a liaison between nursing service and nursing education. She taught inservice education programs for nursing service and helped the nursing school faculty with curriculum and faculty development. When the new combined facility opened, she was supervisor of the psychiatric unit. When Metropolitan Medical Center was formed in 1970, she was one of five assistant directors of nursing service in the new organization.

Barbara Jorenby

When she was appointed clinical instructor on 5B, December 2, 1963, Barbara Jorenby had already been a part of the St. Barnabas family for two years, since she had been a staff nurse on pediatrics beginning in 1961. She graduated from Viroqua High School in Viroqua, Wisconsin, and took her nursing education at St. Olaf College, from which she earned her bachelor of science in nursing. St. Barnabas was her first employer after graduation from St. Olaf. Her husband, Robert, was a student at Northwest Electronics Institute at the time of her appointment to the faculty.

Betty Coffman Knight

Betty was appointed a med-surg instructor about 1946. She was a St. Barnabas graduate, class of 1940.

Mabel Lagos

Mabel came to the St. Barnabas faculty as a teaching dietitian in 1959. She was a Fairmont native, receiving her basic education there and in Minneapolis. She graduated from the University of Minnesota with a bachelor of science degree in foods, nutrition and institutional management. She served her dietetic internship at the University of Minnesota Hospitals. Before she joined the faculty at St. Barnabas, she was employed at the University of Minnesota Hospitals, the Visiting Nurse Association of Minneapolis and the Nicollet Clinic. Following her 1962 resignation, she returned to the Nicollet Clinic.

Julia Larson

Julia was another person who served in the dual role of supervisor-instructor. Her field was pediatric nursing. From 1950-1954 she served in pediatrics at St. Barnabas. For a brief period during that time, she had an instructor also assigned to pediatric nursing, but it appears that she served in the dual capacity for the rest of her tenure. When she left in 1954, she went to Boston University to study for a master's degree.

Betty Lou Lia (Hogberg)

Betty Lou joined the St. Barnabas faculty in 1961 as a maternity nursing instructor. She was a graduate of the University of Minnesota School of Nursing and held a baccalaureate degree in nursing education from the university. She was married in 1963 to Rudy Hogberg, a widower with three small children, whose wife had been killed in a car accident. After her marriage, she resigned in order to have more time to spend with her new family. Later, she and Rudy had an additional little girl.

Linda Lowry

Linda was appointed a med-surg instructor at St. Barnabas in 1966. She was a graduate of St. Olaf College with a bachelor of science degree in nursing. Her experience before she came to St. Barnabas was as a staff nurse at Fairview Hospital.

Hazelle Lundell

One of the most loved of all faculty members in the history of the school was Hazelle Lundell. She was a graduate of St. John's Hospital School of Nursing in Red Wing, Minnesota. Prior to coming to St. Barnabas, she worked at Northwestern Hospital in Minneapolis, St. John's in Red Wing, Children's Memorial Hospital in Chicago and St. Cloud Hospital. She came to St. Barnabas in 1946 and worked for ten years on 2 Whitney and 2 Pavilion. In 1956, she was transferred to the school as an assistant instructor in nursing arts. Though she never earned an academic degree, she did take a number of courses to enhance her natural teaching abilities. In 1958, she was promoted to instructor in fundamentals of nursing, a position she held for the remaining years of the school. Further biographical information about Hazelle is in Chapters 14 and 16.

Marie Meader

Marie came to St. Barnabas as the nursing arts instructor in 1952. She served approximately four years in this position. She was already married when appointed to the faculty and during her tenure, she had a child. When the little girl was about two years old, Marie resigned in order to have more time to devote to her.

Betty Meehan

Betty Meehan was appointed maternity nursing instructor in 1963. She came to St. Barnabas with a degree in elementary education and previous teaching experience in public schools. She was a graduate of St. Cloud Hospital School of Nursing and held a bachelor of science in nursing administration from the University of Minnesota. She had worked in the delivery room at St. Cloud Hospital, was maternity supervisor at St. Cloud, had taught maternity nursing at St. Alexius Hospital in Bismarck, North Dakota, had been a med-surg instructor at Swedish and assistant director at Northwestern Hospital prior to coming to St. Barnabas. Mr. Meehan was with the Minneapolis Police Department.

Pat Melcher

Another Wisconsinite, Pat was appointed med-surg instructor in 1966. She received her basic nursing education at Columbia Hospital School of Nursing in Milwaukee and her bachelor of science in nursing from the University of Wisconsin in Madison. She had worked as both a staff nurse and a head nurse at the University of Wisconsin Hospitals before she moved to Minnesota.

Geraldine Sullivan Nehotte

Gerry came to St. Barnabas in 1965 as a part-time instructor in maternity nursing. She was a graduate of the College of St. Teresa in Winona with a bachelor of science in nursing. Before her marriage, she had been a med-surg instructor at Abbott Hospital and had participated with St. Barnabas faculty in the Central Teaching Program. She was married in 1955 to Bob Nehotte, an accountant. By the time of her appointment to the St. Barnabas faculty, she had become the mother of six children. She did some part-time work at Eitel Hospital between her Abbott experience and appointment at St. Barnabas.

Katherine Ness

A member of the St. Barnabas class of 1946, Katie went on to the University of Minnesota after she received her RN, graduating from the University with a bachelor of science in nursing education. She returned to St. Barnabas as a med-surg clinical instructor. In 1952, she was promoted to associate director of the nursing school, a position she held for approximately three years. She returned to university studies, earning her master's degree, after which she was employed by St. Olaf College, teaching in their nursing program. She remained with St. Olaf until she retired. As of this writing, she was still living in the Minneapolis area.

Barbara Neubauer

Apparently Barbara came to St. Barnabas in 1950 as replacement for Margaret Elvin in the position of nursing arts instructor. Little is known about her. She resigned in 1952 because of relocation due to her husband's job.

Linda Olson

Still another Wisconsinite was Linda Olson from Ridgeland, Wisconsin. She graduated from high school in Barron, Wisconsin, and earned a bachelor of science in nursing from the University of Wisconsin in Madison. She worked as a staff nurse at the University of Wisconsin Hospitals before moving to Minneapolis. She was hired by St. Barnabas as a staff nurse on 3B, but transferred over to the nursing school in 1965 as a med-surg instructor. Her husband was a student in the College of Veterinary Medicine at the University of Minnesota when Linda was appointed to the faculty at St. Barnabas.

Naomi Otterstad

A native of Appleton, Minnesota, Naomi joined the St. Barnabas faculty in 1966. She was a graduate of St. Olaf College, with a bachelor of science in nursing. Prior to her appointment at St. Barnabas, she had been a staff nurse and a head nurse on the rehabilitation unit at Fairview Hospital. Her husband, Marc, was a student at Luther Seminary at the time of her appointment to the St. Barnabas faculty.

Margaret Parren (Baach)

From Benton Harbor, Michigan, Margaret Parren, served as instructor of nursing of children from 1961 to 1963. She had a bachelor's degree in nursing education before joining the St. Barnabas faculty. When she resigned in 1963, it was to enroll at the University of Minnesota, where she earned a master of education in nursing education. Following receipt of her master's degree, she joined the staff of the Minnesota Board of Nursing, serving as associate executive secretary of the board for more than twenty years before her retirement. While at the board, she met Bill Baach, an accountant, and the two were married in the new chapel at Macalester College. As of this writing, they were living, retired, in a townhouse in Edina.

Mary Peck

Mary came on board as a med-surg instructor in 1967. She had a bachelor of science degree in nursing from the University of Wisconsin. Prior to moving to Minnesota, she was a staff nurse at the University of Wisconsin Hospital and was an instructor at General Hospital School of Nursing in Madison, Wisconsin.

Carol R. Pederson

Hired originally to serve as clinical instructor in operating room nursing, Carol served in that capacity from 1958 to 1963. In 1963, she moved out of the operating room to become a med-surg clinical instructor. Her basic nursing education was from Abbott Hospital School of Nursing with a bachelor of science in nursing education from the University of Minnesota. Her experiences, all in operating room nursing, were as a staff nurse at Cottage Hospital, Santa Barbara, California, instructor at Hennepin County General Hospital in Minneapolis and instructor at the College of St. Catherine, St. Joseph Hospital facility, in St. Paul.

Doris Peters

A Canadian by birth, Doris Peters joined the St. Barnabas faculty in 1968 as a med-surg instructor. She got her basic nursing education at Vancouver General Hospital School of Nursing in Vancouver, British Columbia. She went down to Seattle, to earn her bachelor of science in nursing from the University of Washington in Seattle. She also held a diploma in public health from the University of Western Ontario in London, Ontario. She served as a public health nurse in British Columbia and a staff nurse in emergency room nursing in London, Ontario. She also served in a staff nursing position in Renton, Washington and a nurse at the Visiting Nurse Service in Seattle before moving to Minnesota and St. Barnabas.

Donna Peterson

Donna was appointed an instructor in maternity nursing in 1968. She received her basic nursing education at Ancker Hospital School of Nursing in St. Paul. She held a bachelor of science in nursing education from the University of Minnesota. Her prior experiences included head nurse in maternity at Ancker and staff nurse in the delivery room at North Memorial

Hospital in Robbinsdale. She also served in the Army Nurse Corps before she came to St. Barnabas.

Alys Platzer

Alys joined the St. Barnabas faculty in July of 1963, replacing Margaret Parren. Alys was from Young America, Minnesota. She took her basic nursing at St. Mary's Hospital School of Nursing in Minneapolis and earned a bachelor of science from Wayne State University in Detroit, Michigan. She did postgraduate work in pediatric nursing at Children's Hospital in Detroit and worked at that hospital as a staff nurse and instructor. She then went on to Catholic University in Washington DC, where she earned a master's degree in education. She spent ten years, from 1953 to 1963, teaching in the nursing program at the College of St. Catherine in St. Paul and supervising students on med-surg units at St. Joseph Hospital in St. Paul, before joining the St. Barnabas faculty.

Alice Ramlo

Alice served as a clinical instructor on 4A for three years, 1959 to 1962.

Lillian Ramsey

In 1962, Alice Ramlo's replacement on 4A was Lillian Ramsey. She was an Ohio native who took her basic nursing at Deaconess Hospital School of Nursing in Cincinnati, Ohio, and her baccalaureate degree at the University of Cincinnati. Like so many of the younger faculty members, she had a student husband. He was working on his PhD in economics at the University of Minnesota when Lillian joined the faculty. She was one of the trio of faculty members who had babies in late 1963 and early 1964.

Ferne Saari (Hansen)

Ferne Saari became a clinical instructor in med-surg nursing in 1953. She was a graduate of the Hamline-Asbury nursing program with a bachelor's degree in nursing. She married during the time she was at St. Barnabas. She served on the faculty for more than five years.

Lulu Saunders

Lulu Saunders had graduated from St. Barnabas only one year prior to being named an instructor in the nursing school in 1920. Board of Nursing records indicate she earned the grand sum of fifty dollars per month plus room and board. She was the first instructor to be identified by name in Board of Nursing records. Apparently she stayed at St. Barnabas for two or three years. The 1923 report to the Board of Nursing indicates another instructor in the position. She moved to Rochester and served for many years on the faculty of Kahler Hospital School of Nursing where she was highly respected and well liked by those who knew her.

Jeanne Scanlon

Jeanne Scanlon was one of a handful of faculty from the east coast of the United States, who wore a distinctive little organdy cap. She joined the St. Barnabas faculty as a med-surg clinical instructor during the 1950s. She held a baccalaureate degree in nursing from one of the eastern schools, possibly Cornell. Athletics were important to Jeanne, even to scheduling a winter vacation in Switzerland so she could get in some heavy duty skiing. Unfortunately, she was ill with a respiratory infection during her entire vacation, so wasn't able to take advantage of the Swiss slopes.

Ruth Schnitzen

A native of Ohio, Ruth Schnitzen worked part-time beginning in February 1955. In May she was appointed associate director of education. She was born and raised in Wooster, Ohio, and earned a baccalaureate degree from the College of Wooster. She then went on to Western Reserve University in Cleveland, where she received both her nursing education and a master's degree. She remained at St. Barnabas for three years, until 1958.

Berdine Schotzko

For several years prior to coming to St. Barnabas, Berdine Schotzko was a Franciscan nun. She graduated from the College of Teresa with a bachelor of science in nursing. Following this, she was assigned to St. Mary's Hospital in Rochester as head nurse on an orthopedic unit. She had not taken her final vows in the Franciscan order and in 1962 she decided to leave the convent where she had spent the previous nine years of her life.

She came to St. Barnabas as the clinical instructor on 5B. She and Mary Hess, another young member of the faculty, became fast friends and Mary helped her through the adjustment to living on her own after so many years in the convent. For example, Berdine was not accustomed to living in an apartment on her own, keeping house there, cooking for herself and even learning to remember to lock the door when she left and to carry her key with her. Her wardrobe was the envy of all the faculty. Because she was starting from scratch, she could buy complete matched ensembles while other faculty members were shopping to find outfits which would coordinate with the rest of their existing wardrobe. A beautiful print dress with purple flowers in the pattern and matching purple suede pumps comes to mind as one good looking outfit she got. Another difference in her wardrobe as compared to other faculty members was that everything she wore was new, while other faculty members tended to use their new outfits for Sunday best and to wear older outfits for work.

Berdine was born and raised on a sheep farm near Sleepy Eye, Minnesota, and longed to return to the farm life style and to be near her large family of several siblings and her parents. In 1963, she married a farmer from Sleepy Eye who had been a school mate years before. Mary Hess sang for her wedding in a southeast Minneapolis Catholic Church. Several nuns from Rochester made the trip to Minneapolis for the wedding—St. Barnabas's own Sound of Music happy ending.

Jeanne Schultz

Jeanne migrated to Minnesota from her hometown of Detroit, Michigan. She attended Michigan Lutheran Seminary in Saginaw, Michigan, followed by Bethany Lutheran College in Mankato, Minnesota. Later, she enrolled at Mankato State College from which she earned a bachelor of science in nursing. She married a physicist, employed by Univac, and the couple had a four-year-old son at the time of Jeanne's appointment to the St. Barnabas faculty in 1965. At St. Barnabas, she taught patient care management.

Winifred Schweppe

Miss Schweppe was employed during the 1940s and served until 1950 in the dual role of supervisor-instructor in operating room nursing.

Ruth Stryker

Ruth joined the St. Barnabas family in 1956 as supervisor-instructor in pediatrics. During her tenure in that position, she helped to plan the pediatric unit in the new hospital. She was from St. Paul and a graduate of the University of Minnesota School of Nursing and the University School of Public Health from which she earned her bacherlor's degree. After participating in the move from the old hospital to the new one across the street, in 1959 Ruth joined the nursing service staff, leaving faculty responsibilities to Marian Gruenfelder, new to St. Barnabas that year. In nursing service, Ruth made her mark first by developing a refresher course for inactive nurses. At that time the St. Barnabas Nurses Alumnae voted to provide a scholarship each year to a student in the nursing school. In return, alumnae were asked what the hospital might do for them and an overwhelming number requested a refresher course to allow them to return to nursing practice after years at home raising children. Ruth also began a writing career during her years in nursing service. Her uncle, James Gray, was a well-known and respected author in the Twin Cities and Ruth apparently followed in his footsteps. She had several articles published in nursing journals and in 1964, she was given the Mary Roberts Writers Award for one of her articles. Later, she authored a textbook entitled, *Back to Nursing*. After ten years at St. Barnabas, she resigned in 1966 to become director of nursing education for the American Rehabilitation Foundation. Her responsibilities there included rehabilitation programs particularly for nursing home staffs. Ruth was married during those years to a widower who had a teen-age son, so she added motherhood to her impressive list of accomplishments.

Shirley Thordson (Mertz)

In 1950, Shirley came to St. Barnabas replacing Winifred Schweppe in the operating suite. She served first as a staff nurse and clinical instructor and later as head nurse, and after the move to the new hospital in 1958, she became supervisor of the operating room. She was a graduate of Hamline Asbury School of Nursing and had worked on surgical stations and operating rooms at Asbury, at Swedish and at a rural hospital before coming to St. Barnabas. She married during her many years at St. Barnabas.

Gayle Tweten

Gayle joined the St. Barnabas faculty in 1968 as a med-surg instructor. She held a bachelor's degree in nursing from the University of North Dakota. Prior to her appointment at St. Barnabas, she served as a staff nurse in intensive care and coronary care at Fairview Hospital.

Marian Steffy Ulrich

Marian was a graduate of St. Barnabas, class of 1963, who went back to Macalester College to complete her bachelor of science degree in nursing. She joined the St. Barnabas faculty on January 4, 1965, as clinical instructor on 4B. During the time she was working on her degree at Macalester, she worked for the college in their health service as well as the health service at Hamline University. She also worked part-time at Midway Hospital in St. Paul. Her husband, Dale Ulrich, taught German at Sibley High School in West St. Paul and at the time of Marian's appointment to the St. Barnabas faculty, he was taking graduate work at the University of Minnesota.

Delores Jean Wegner

Delores was a Nebraskan, graduate of Nebraska Methodist Hospital School of Nursing in Omaha and of the University of Nebraska. She came to St. Barnabas in 1962 applying for a staff position in nursing service. But when her academic credentials were reviewed by personnel, she was referred to the nursing school and hired as a clinical instructor on 5A. In 1964, she obtained a position with the International Council of Nurses and was assigned to work in Sierra Leone in West Africa.

Carol Wendt

Carol came to St. Barnabas from North Carolina. She had her bachelor of science degree from Duke University School of Nursing in Durham, North Carolina, and several credits toward a master's degree, also from Duke. Her prior experiences when she joined the St. Barnabas faculty included float and charge nurse of the out patient department at Duke Medical Center and supervisor of the emergency room at Duke Medical Center. She was appointed community health instructor at St. Barnabas in 1967.

Betty Wendtland

Betty Wendtland came to St. Barnabas in the late 1940s or early 1950s. She served as clinical instructor in maternity nursing.

Margaret Younglove

Margaret was a graduate of Asbury Hospital School of Nursing and was listed on the Minnesota Board Report of 1923 as the instructor at St. Barnabas.

Jean Zastrow

Jean was already somewhat familiar with St. Barnabas faculty members through her involvement with the Central Teaching Program when in 1966 she joined the St. Barnabas faculty. She had served on the faculty at Northwestern Hospital School of Nursing and participated in the Central Teaching Program. She received her bachelor of science in nursing from Hamline-Asbury School of Nursing. Her husband, Ken, was a salesman in the Minneapolis area. The couple had two sons, both teenagers at the time of Jean's appointment to the St. Barnabas faculty.

Reviewing the faculty list from A to Z, one can see that over the years St. Barnabas was served by nurses from many parts of the country. They came to the faculty with a variety of prior experiences and were in all age groups, the younger age group predominating, but balanced also by those with more experience. There never were any men on the faculty except those who taught preclinical classes at the University, Macalester and the Video Nursing Education program. And there were few minorities, Mary Chapus, a Nisei, being the only one who comes to mind. There probably were other instructors whose names have been lost over time. We salute the unnamed faculty, this list of seventy-eight and the twelve administrative heads who served the school.

There were other members of the school staff who reported to the School Director and whose services were as vital to the operation of the school as the services given by the instructional staff. These included the office staff, the librarians, the housemothers and the residence receptionists. Following are the names of those school staff members who played such vital roles in the development and operation of the school. As with the instructor list, there are undoubtedly others who toiled in the school, but whose names have been lost over time.

LIBRARY

Mary Clark

Mary was the librarian during the early 1950s. She may have been the first librarian employed by the school. Little information about her was available.

Silvija Kupchs

Silvija was the librarian who served longest through the history of the school. She came in 1954 and served until the school closed in 1973. Further biographical information about Silvija can be found in Chapter 21.

Eunice Michelson

Eunice was hired as an assistant to Silvija. Silvija and her husband, Paul, took five months off in the 1960s to tour Europe. Eunice filled in for Silvija during that period and acted as her assistant before and after that leave of absence. Her husband worked for the postal service in Minneapolis.

HOUSEMOTHERS AND RESIDENCE RECEPTIONISTS

Mrs. Gertrude Noyes

Mrs. Noyes is the first housemother for whom records could be found. She came to St. Barnabas as the housemother at Wellesmere in 1942. When Knickerbacker Residence was opened for upper class students in 1943, Mrs. Noyes moved to Knickerbacker. Mrs. Noyes retired in 1948. She moved from Minnesota and died July 10, 1959.

Mrs. Grace Wittig

Mrs. Wittig joined the St. Barnabas family in 1943 as the housemother at Wellesmere, which had just been designated the residence for first year students. She was originally from Eau Claire, Wisconsin. She moved to

Minneapolis in 1920 and prior to coming to St. Barnabas, for a number of years she had owned and operated an apartment house in Minneapolis. The mother of two sons and grandmother of four children, she resigned in 1953 to join her son's firm, Arrowhead Airways in Hibbing.

Mrs. Helen Cribbe Dick

Mrs. Dick was a St. Barnabas graduate, class of 1917. She replaced Mrs. Noyes at Knickerbacker. Since she was a nurse, she also served as student health director. The dual arrangement proved unworkable and in 1953, she moved to the position of full time health director for both employees and students.

Mrs. Ruth Gallup

Mrs. Gallup replaced Mrs. Dick in 1953 and when Knickerbacker was closed and Whitney Residence opened, she moved to Whitney, where she served until 1962.

Mrs. Helen Jahrow

Mrs. Jahrow replaced Mrs. Wittig at Wellesmere and served only two years. No other information about Mrs. Jahrow was available.

Mrs. Daisy Lau

Mrs. Lau came to St. Barnabas in 1954 replacing Mrs. Jahrow at Wellesmere. She was a native of Minneapolis, graduate of North High and of the University of Minnesota. She had served as a housemother at Abbott Hospital School of Nursing for ten years before coming to St. Barnabas. When Whitney Residence opened in 1960, she also moved to Whitney and shared house director responsibilities until 1962 with Mrs. Gallup. From 1962 until her retirement at the end of the school year in 1963, she was the sole house director, assisted by receptionists serving at the front desk around the clock. Mrs. Lau had two daughters, two granddaughters and two grandsons.

Mrs. Helen Bachman

Mrs. Bachman joined the St. Barnabas staff in 1963. Like Mrs. Lau, she had previous experience with house director responsibilities, though her charges were not students, but young women employed in downtown businesses. She had been superintendent of the Clara Doerr Girls Club for the eight and one half years preceding her appointment at St. Barnabas. Her childhood home was in Cannon Falls, Minnesota. Later she moved to Marshalltown, Iowa, where she graduated from Marshalltown High School and attended Central Iowa Business College. She had three sons and eight lively grandchildren. Mrs. Bachman remained at St. Barnabas until the school closed in 1973. Like Mrs. Lau, she was assisted by residence receptionists at the front desk round the clock.

Mabel Christensen and **Myrtle Foss** were the first two residence receptionists to be hired when the new system was inaugurated in 1962. Both women were married and had grown children of their own. They became very popular with the students at Whitney. In 1963, a bookstore was opened on the fifth floor of the residence. Mrs. Christensen was appointed to manage the store, which was open on a part-time basis. Textbooks used in the school were stocked there and in addition, there was a limited supply of personal care items, some gift items and candy. One item stocked in 1963 and 1964 was an eight-inch doll dressed in the blue and white checked uniform of the school. Proceeds from the bookstore went into the student activity fund. In 1966, Mrs. Christensen moved to the school office, where she served as a clerk-typist. She also was the advisor for the student newspaper, *Chat from Checks*.

Elizabeth Bingaman, Betty Boyd, Irene Butter and **Edna Castleman** served as residence receptionists following Mrs. Foss and Mrs. Christiansen. Edna and Irene had been employees at St. Andrews. When that hospital closed in 1963, they transferred to these positions in the nursing school at St. Barnabas.

School offices were in different locations through the years. In the 1940s, the school office was on the first floor of the Martin building, to the right as one entered the building. Later, that space was needed to expand the library and the offices were moved up one floor to an area labeled, the Zebra Area, so named because the walls at the west end of the area were painted with horizontal stripes. On the north side of the hall was an office for the associate director of the school, another one adjacent to it for the clerical staff and a third office on that side of the hall was for the director of nursing. Across the hall were offices for nursing arts instructors and a faculty locker and break room.

Carolyn Berg was Miss Merrell's secretary when she first took the director's position at the hospital in 1950. Carrie switched to nursing service about 1952, where she remained until she resigned to be married in 1962. She was replaced in the school office by **Rosemary Church**. Rosemary also left to be married, about 1955 or 1956.

Kay Christiansen came in the 1950s, working first as a clerk-typist, then switching to become the school's first registrar. **Elma Ann Krier (Lyon)** came on board replacing Kay, also originally as a clerk-typist, then moving into the position of registrar after Kay left. Elma Ann was divorced, with a young son when she first came to the school. Later she married and as Elma Ann Lyon, she remained for the rest of the years the school existed and on into Metropolitan Medical Center years. Though students were no longer being accepted at Metropolitan Medical Center, there was still need for a registrar to handle the records of all the graduates of the school who needed transcripts either for other schools they attended, or more often for state boards that were granting them licenses by interstate endorsement. As of this writing, Elma Ann was working regularly at the historical library established after St. Barnabas and Swedish closed their schools.

Other clerk-typists who worked in the school office were **Betty Lindsey**, who served in the late 1950s and early 1960s. She left in 1962 to spend more time with her young children. **Delores Metz** replaced her. Delores later married and stayed on as Mrs. Campbell. **Lenore Olson** came in 1967 and a **Mrs. Stenberg** after that.

As for the school offices themselves, in the late 1950s, the offices were moved from the Zebra Area to the other end of the hall on the same floor of the Martin building. When Whitney Residence was opened in 1960, the school offices were moved to the remodeled Whitney building. They took over the area of the first floor which had been occupied by X-ray during the days Whitney served as a hospital. The old front entrance of the Whitney building became a lounge and the horseshoe drive was eliminated in favor of a yard in front of the building, enclosed by a serpentine brick wall to provide more privacy and security for the school. The main entrance to the school was on the east side of the building in a new annex which housed two classrooms and the hall which extended from the entrance into the Whitney building. The receptionists' desk was on the south side of the hall where the laboratory had been when the building was still a hospital.

Eleanor Weston wrote the following in her annual report for the school just prior to the turn of the twentieth century. She was speaking of the students in the school, but her words might have been used to describe the faculty and school staff who also labored diligently over the seventy nine years the school existed. Miss Weston said, "The work done by our nurses during the year has been very satisfactory, in that they have been earnest and diligent in performing their duties. Even the most arduous and disagreeable tasks have been done with such cheerfulness that we are led to believe that they are inspired by a higher motive than simply that of duty."

Chapter 18

Nursing Service: At the Center of It All

The primary reason for establishing a hospital is to provide care for the sick and injured. Without those requiring care, there would have been no need to establish St. Barnabas Hospital way back in 1870. Recognizing the patient was the reason for being, the nursing service department was at the very center of the hospital with all other services radiating out from nursing. In the foregoing chapters of this history, we have seen that in the beginning there were no nurses. But nursing—or nurturing—was being done by the willing volunteers Mr. Knickerbacker convinced to help in his endeavor. Nursing at that time included everything that was done for the patient—personal care, food preparation, tidying up the area and laundry.

The first services to spin off from nursing were housekeeping and dietary. Volunteers tended to be the ladies of Gethsemane who had time to give service. Having time to give service probably meant they were wealthy enough to have servants at home to do the more menial and repetitive tasks to keep a household going. It is easy to see how the lady volunteers might have volunteered the services of their servants as well, bringing in food cooked at home and taking soiled linens home to be laundered by household staff. Remember, in the early days there were likely not more than four to six patients at a time requiring care, so providing food and laundry for these would have been no different than having four to six house guests, a situation fairly common among the wealthy in those days.

Over time, as the number of patients increased at the hospital, it became more practical to hire people to prepare food on site and to do laundry on site as well as to do daily cleaning. Technology was also developing as the number of people seeking care increased, with the result that separate bodies of specialized knowledge were evolving in all aspects of hospital work. For example, doctors probably observed that certain foods were more easily tolerated by certain patients, so evolved the need for special diets. The field of nutrition was expanding and there were people who were studying such things as the effects of vitamins, minerals and fiber on the digestive system. So gradually the food preparation department became the dietary department, requiring the services not only of cooks and food servers, but dietitians who understood the construction of well balanced diets for all patients, considering their special needs because of the illnesses that brought them to the hospital.

Similar scenarios could be developed for each of the departments that spun off as the rudimentary nursing of the Cottage Hospital gave way to the modern scientific practice of nursing. Examples of spin off departments were: dietary, housekeeping, pharmacy, medical records, anesthesia, physical therapy, rehabilitation, mental health and social services. There are many services available in the modern hospital which had roots in the days when everything was done for the patient by the care giver at his bedside.

As science and technology moved into the practice of medicine, doctors identified the need for diagnostic services such as laboratory and X-ray and it became necessary to add facilities and equipment to allow this work to be done. In the development of medical practice, the practice of safe, antiseptic surgery became the treatment of choice for patients with certain ailments and so operating rooms and the required equipment were added to hospitals too. And the care which nurses were providing to patients having diagnostic studies or preparing for or recovering from surgery had to be tailored to the needs of those individuals.

Ultimately, the department employing the largest number of employees was the nursing service department. The era of the volunteer care-giver gave way to the era of service being provided primarily by student nurses, learning on the job and working under the supervision of physicians and a small number of graduate nurses, who were in short supply in nineteenth and early twentieth century Minneapolis. This dependence on students to provide nursing service was demonstrated in the 1930s when effects of the Board of Nurse Examiners requirement that no new students be admitted to the School of Nursing for a period of one year went into effect. The decrease in the number of students available to give care was so deeply felt that on August 29, 1938, a special meeting of the Board of Trustees was called to discuss the problem. Minutes from that meeting state, "Miss Aird made a report in connection with the nursing situation at the hospital. She explained to the board why the hospital was not able to avail itself of the services of as many student nurses at this time as was anticipated a year ago. She strongly recommended the continuing of the nurse's training school, although it would be a period of three years before the school would function properly so that the hospital would receive the maximum benefit from it through the services of student nurses."

The nursing school made the changes recommended by the Board of Nurse Examiners and after their one year on probation, the school was restored to normal operations, but it took a while before sufficient numbers of students were available again to provide nursing service as before. This all came at the time the hospital was expanding its capacity with the construction of the Whitney building. For the first time, the hospital was forced to hire RNs and graduate nurses (those who had completed nursing programs, but had not written or passed licensure examinations.) The minutes of that special meeting of the Board of Trustees in 1938 included action by the board to pay an extra fifteen dollars per month to graduates who could not be accommodated in the nurses' residences maintained by the hospital. This was done to provide an incentive for graduates to come to work at St. Barnabas. The number of students graduated in 1938 was only nine, compared to the fifteen to thirty class sizes of the previous eighteen years. In 1939, they graduated only six, illustrating the difference that school probationary period made in the nursing service department.

Not long after that 1938 meeting, the country was off to war and staff shortages in hospitals were again a problem. This time the shortages extended into all departments of the hospital, with many men answering the call of the draft board and other men volunteering to serve in the armed forces. After the passage of the Bolton Act, which established the Cadet Nurse Corps in 1943, class sizes in the nursing school doubled the levels of 1940 admissions. This increase in the number of students helped to meet needs in the nursing service department, although at the same time there were more students, there were also fewer graduates available on the home front, since many made their contribution to the war effort by enlisting in the Army and Navy Nurse Corps.

One way staff shortages were met was by the employment of practical nurses and a new category of ancillary workers called Nurses' Aides. Practical nurses had been around for several years, many being trained in apprenticeship type programs for positions in specific settings such as mental hospitals and tuberculosis hospitals. Hiring large numbers of them in general hospitals was new in the 1940s. After the end of World War II, practical nurse training programs that provided instruction and a range of clinical experiences according to approved curricula, came into being and the majority of graduates of these programs went on to write licensure examinations to become Licensed Practical Nurses. Nurse aides received on the job training after they were hired by a hospital. Some girls with potential interest in becoming nurses, went on to training programs to become RNs and LPNs as a result of their employment originally as aides.

Thora McCauley Kron, 1940 graduate of St. Barnabas, wrote a treatise on "Team Nursing" which became the guide for nursing services at St. Barnabas in the late 1940s and through most of the 1950s. Thora was the evening supervisor at St. Barnabas for a number of years. She also served for a time on the faculty of the nursing school. So she had a good grasp of the situation on the clinical stations during the years of staff shortages and the employment of these two categories of workers new to St. Barnabas. The plan she outlined called for the division of shift staff into teams. Each team was headed by an RN, or sometimes by a senior student nurse, who had working with her practical nurses, nurse aides and student nurses. The team would be responsible for care of a block of patients. The blocks were usually determined geographically according to patient room numbers. For example, Team A might be responsible for the care of all the patients in rooms 200-210. The objective of the team was to distribute work assignments equitably and to provide a higher level of care for the patients than could be provided by the same caregivers working independently.

At Teachers' College, Columbia University, the same concept was being studied. Their thesis was that a higher quality of care could be given using a nursing team than was usual with the same team members working independently of each other. The report of their study, authored by Eleanor C. Lambertson, was published in 1953. Miss Lambertson later went on to doctoral studies and became an expert in nursing curriculum development. She came to St. Barnabas in 1963, for a very short time, to review preparations the nursing school faculty had made for a National League for Nursing accreditation visit about to be made to St. Barnabas.

The problem with the team nursing approach as it was practiced at St. Barnabas, was that it was often not possible to meet the objectives of the whole system. For one thing, patients were given room assignments on the basis of rooms which were available at the time they were admitted to the hospital. So rooms in one area might house patients requiring a whole lot more care than patients in rooms in another area of the same nursing station. Head nurses tried to be aware of this and to consider such inequities, but it wasn't always possible to equally distribute the load among teams. Another objective, difficult to meet, was providing supervision to the lesser-trained members of the team. The team leader, theoretically, was to provide supervision for the whole team, but often she was the only one on the team qualified to pass medications and to do treatments, which left her little time for supervision of other team members. Working in her favor was the fact that members of a team usually got to know each other well and they became familiar with the quality of care given by fellow team mates, so they would work together to maximize the skills of all and to compensate for the weaknesses of some. In general, St. Barnabas received few complaints about the quality of care it provided and most employers in the know looked with favor on a prospective nursing employee who had worked at St. Barnabas or had graduated from its nursing school.

In the years after World War II, nursing leaders throughout the country were looking at and discussing ways of providing for improvement of quality and delivery of nursing services to an ever expanding population. The Minnesota Nurses Association, the Minnesota League for Nursing, the Minnesota Licensed Practical Nurse Association and the Minnesota Hospital Association brought leaders in from all over the country to present workshops and seminars on improvement of patient care. Nurses from St. Barnabas were encouraged to participate in such offerings and often they were part of the planning committees for these programs. After the split of the nursing department in 1961, leaders in the nursing service department, under the capable guidance of its director, Virginia Schmidt, were freer to develop and institute new programs to improve the quality of care being offered by the department. Examples of new programs they developed at that time included pediatric pre-surgical admission orientation in 1961, a new approach to in-service education in 1964, addition of a teen-adult wing in 1964, the nursing care coordinator plan in 1965, the opening of special care areas which included intensive care as well as coronary care, 1966, and a cardiac arrest program in 1966.

When in 1970, St. Barnabas merged with Swedish Hospital to form Metropolitan Medical Center, Martha Yucel, then director of nursing service at St. Barnabas, became director of nursing service in the new corporation. Mrs. Yucel had replaced Virginia Schmidt in 1967 when Virginia resigned to be married. At Metropolitan Medical Center, Martha had a staff of five assistant directors, four of whom moved with her from St. Barnabas. The four were Ruth Darnell, Ruth Hass, Mary Jones and Anita Lillquist. Ruth Weise, who directed the nursing school at the time of the merger, was appointed director of nursing education at Metropolitan Medical Center. Both St. Barnabas and Swedish closed their nursing schools with the merger into a new corporation, but there was still a job to be done in providing in-service and continuing education for the large number of nurses employed at MMC. The fact that so many of the nursing leaders from St. Barnabas moved into the new, larger corporation, speaks well for their professional performance and the leadership they provided at St. Barnabas.

Nearly fifty biographical vignettes of nursing service personnel have been included in Chapters 14, 17, 20 and 21 of this book. In addition, eighty people from nursing service were included on the list of long term employees found in the appendix. Especially in the early years, there were several individuals for whom St. Barnabas was nearly a lifetime employer. And even at the end, when the merger with Swedish came, there were several who had been St. Barnabas staff members for years. Following are vignettes of additional nursing leaders not cited previously.

Virginia Schmidt

Virginia was the first director of nursing service appointed when the school and service were split in 1961. She was a native Minnesotan and a graduate of St. Cloud Hospital School of Nursing. She received her baccalaureate degree in nursing administration from the University of Minnesota. She had been serving as Miss Merrell's assistant director of nursing service. Her prior experiences had included service at Minneapolis General Hospital, at Peninsula Hospital in Burlingame, California and at Menorah Medical Center in Kansas City, Missouri. She remained in the director slot for six years, resigning when she married in 1967.

Marjorie Person

Marj was the classic "bootstrapper," rising from staff nurse to the director level on the basis, primarily, of her innate ability, friendly disposition and willingness to put in a full measure of work for every hour she was paid. She graduated from Bethesda Hospital School of Nursing in St. Paul. That was in the days when Bethesda offered a program of preparation for nurses who would write licensure examinations to become Registered Nurses. The hospital had an affiliation for basic sciences with Gustavus Adolphus College in those days. Later, that school was closed and a new program in practical nursing opened in its place. Marj was a graduate of the old school which prepared nurses to become RNs. She married immediately after graduation and went to fulltime responsibilities as a housewife and mother. She and her husband raised a family of three children. Eight years after nursing school graduation, she joined the staff at Fairview Hospital in Minneapolis where she worked for two years. Next came an appointment to St. Andrew's Hospital as night supervisor. She served there for six years, then went on days becoming the assistant superintendent of nurses first, and finally the director of nurses. It was Marj Person who oversaw the move to St. Barnabas when the St. Andrew's division was closed. An article describing the final days of patients and staff at St. Andrew's, authored by Marj Person, appears in Chapter 8. After that hospital closed, she transferred to St. Barnabas, first as maternity supervisor and later a combined position as supervisor of both maternity and pediatrics.

Martha Yucel

Martha was a graduate from a nursing program in the south. She held a number of supervisory and nursing administration positions in Tuscaloosa and Huntsville, Alabama, before moving to Minnesota. She came to the Twin Cities in 1960 as a result of a transfer for her husband, Edgar K. Yucel. He had been appointed supervising engineer at Remington Rand Univac. The couple had a four-year-old son. In 1960, she joined the nursing service staff at St. Barnabas as medical-surgical nursing supervisor. Later she resigned to enroll at the College of Saint Catherine in St. Paul from which she earned a bachelor of science in nursing. She also went on to earn a master's degree in nursing education from the University of Minnesota. She returned to St. Barnabas after receiving her master's degree and in 1967, she succeeded Virginia Schmidt as director of nursing service. When Metropolitan Medical Center was established in 1970, she moved from the directorship at St. Barnabas to that of director of nursing for Metropolitan Medical Center. In addition to her family responsibilities and job related responsibilities, she was active in the Minnesota Nurses' Association, serving first on the board of Third District MNA and later as president of the state level of that organization.

Ruth Darnell

Ruth was another "bootstrapper." She was a 1953 graduate of St. Barnabas School of Nursing. She was married either before graduation or shortly thereafter and juggled home responsibilities with nursing responsibilities. She worked off and on at St. Barnabas from 1953 on up through the days of the merger with Swedish. She was a staff nurse, then an assistant head nurse, a supervisor and finally an assistant director of nursing.

Marjorie Devereaux

"Devie," as she came to be called at St. Barnabas, spent nearly her entire nursing career at St. Barnabas, though she was a graduate of Kahler

School of Nursing in Rochester. She was already married when, in 1949, she joined St. Barnabas as a staff nurse. By 1951, she had risen to the position of head nurse on 4 Martin. Along the way she took a number of courses at the University of Minnesota, never earning a degree as such, though she did earn nearly forty credits for her various courses. From her position as head nurse, she went on to become a supervisor, then was appointed to a new position, one which she organized, as assistant supervisor of ancillary personnel. In preparation for that job, she took a course in on-the-job training methods. It was she who oriented, trained and then supervised nurse aides and orderlies. She was highly respected by both those whom she supervised and by her nurse colleagues as well. Ultimately, she became administrative assistant in nursing service.

Mary DeVinney

Mary came to St. Barnabas in 1948 from out-state Minnesota. She was a graduate of the nursing program at Little Falls, Minnesota. She worked as a staff nurse at St. Francis Hospital in Breckenridge, then later took a course in operating room nursing and was appointed operating room supervisor at St. Francis. From Breckenridge, she moved to Chicago were she was an operating room staff nurse at Mercy Hospital. When she came to St. Barnabas in 1948, she worked first as a part-time nurse, particularly on the 3 PM to 11 PM shift. She was married by that time and had small children at home. She continued working staff evenings and ultimately became assistant evening supervisor. Nursing students of the era remembered her for her friendliness and helpfulness toward them.

Beverly Gacek Hilt

Bev was another St. Barnabas graduate, class of 1952. After graduation she joined the United States Air Force Reserve and was trained to become a flight nurse. She lived for a time in Miami, Florida, where she had positions as an office nurse and a hospital staff nurse. Returning to Minneapolis, she worked for eleven years as a staff nurse at St. Barnabas, then was promoted to become a supervisor.

Margaret Jam

Margaret Jam came to St. Barnabas in 1952 with an appointment as the head nurse in pediatrics. She remained in that position for nearly seven years, resigning on May 1, 1959, to accept a position with the Bloodmobile. She was a native of Montana where she had most of her nursing education at Sacred Heart Hospital in Havre, Montana, finishing the last six months of her training at Sisters' Hospital in Santa Monica, California. After graduation, she worked for a time on the obstetric unit at Sisters' Hospital. She joined the Army Nurse Corps in 1945 and was stationed at Camp Crowder, Missouri, and at Brooks Army Hospital in San Antonio, Texas. After discharge, she worked for a time as a special duty nurse in Minot, North Dakota, before moving to Minneapolis and St. Barnabas.

Jean Mulder

Jean came to St. Barnabas in 1967, with an original appointment in the dual position of medical-special care area supervisor. Later she became supervisor on obstetrics. She graduated from Lutheran Hospital in Sioux City, Iowa, though she began her nurses training at Methodist-Kahler Hospital School of Nursing in Rochester, Minnesota. After graduation, she worked for three years at Lutheran Hospital and three years at a hospital in Sioux Center, Iowa. Just prior to coming to Minneapolis and St. Barnabas, she worked in the hospital at Worthington, Minnesota, as med-surg head nurse and relief supervisor.

Helen Krieg

Helen was a 1936 graduate of St. Barnabas. She worked as a staff nurse at St. Barnabas after graduation and during World War II, she served in the Army Nurse Corps. After her discharge from the army, she returned to Minneapolis and employment at St. Barnabas where she was head nurse on 3 Whitney for several years. Along the way she took some classes in ward administration at the University of Minnesota. When the move to the new hospital came in 1958, she became the supervisor of the central supply room. Her longtime assistant on 3 Whitney, Irene Peper, St. Barnabas class of 1949, became the head nurse with the 3 Whitney staff as they moved to the new hospital.

Betty Reynolds

Betty was a 1958 graduate of St. Barnabas. Following graduation, she took two years at the University of Minnesota, studying nursing education. She worked as an evening charge nurse on 4A and as a staff nurse in the emergency room. Ultimately, she became the evening house supervisor.

Irene Sobotka

Irene came to St. Barnabas in October 1955 with an appointment as associate director of nursing service under Dorothy Merrell. A native of Chicago, she received her basic nursing education at Roseland Community Hospital School of Nursing in Chicago. For advanced education in nursing, she turned to the University of Minnesota where she earned a bachelor of science in nursing education and a master's degree in nursing administration. While at the University, she was elected to Sigma Theta Tau, the national honorary society for nursing. She was active in the Minnesota Nurses Association. She remained at St. Barnabas for six years, being replaced in 1961 by Virginia Schmidt.

Betsy Sperbeck

Betsy was a St. Barnabas graduate, class of 1952. After graduation, she stayed on at St. Barnabas, working in central service and the emergency room. After the move to the 1958 hospital, she became health service director for the hospital. Betsy was a native Minnesotan, born and raised in Winona.

Diane Schweizer

Diane received her bachelor of science in nursing from Gustavus Adolphus College. Later she also earned a master of science from the University of Colorado. Returning to Minnesota, she served for two years as a nurse clinician at Bethesda Hospital in St. Paul before joining the staff at St. Barnabas in 1968 as a supervisor on the fourth floor.

Betty Waldron

Betty was one of the long-term employees at St. Barnabas. She was a graduate of Eitel Hospital School of Nursing in Minneapolis. She spent three years as the assistant night supervisor at Eitel and another two years doing private duty nursing. Along the way she was married and had children. When she came to St. Barnabas in 1949, it was as a single mother, for her marriage had ended. She worked first as a staff nurse and later as a supervisor on evenings and nights. She remained at St. Barnabas until retirement.

Hannah Walseth

The first associate director of nursing service hired after Dorothy Merrell became director of nursing, was Hannah Walseth, who remained at St. Barnabas for approximately five years. She grew up in southwestern Minnesota and was a graduate of the University of Minnesota School of Nursing. During her first months at St. Barnabas, she lived in a private room at Knickerbacker Residence. Later, she moved to a south Minneapolis house which she shared with Katherine Ness and Dorothy Merrell. The three ladies remained lifelong friends, even after Dorothy's move to California.

As was said of the faculty in Chapter 17, members of the nursing staff, particularly the supervisory staff of nursing service, represented all age groups and variations in background. It may be significant that a greater number of St. Barnabas graduates went on to supervisory positions in nursing service than to faculty positions in the nursing school. Perhaps it reflects well on the good basic preparation they had from the nursing school and the long tradition of quality care for patients at St. Barnabas.

Chapter 19

Establishment of Supporting Departments

With the opening of the Martin building in 1894 and the increase in bed capacity to 75 patients, the increased workload for administration and nursing had to be relieved. And so began the development of supporting departments in the hospital. "Supporting" meant personnel of these departments did not have regular close contact with patients, but the services they provided were necessary to the operation of the organization. Often these services were beyond the scope of nursing. Other services were those that enabled the hospital to function more effectively and efficiently. Most likely dietary, housekeeping and engineering came first. By 1907, laundry had split off from housekeeping, adding another department.

An interview conducted with Amanda Evenson indicated that when she came on staff in housekeeping in 1907, there were only fifteen women working in the entire hospital (excluding nursing) and these fifteen were in housekeeping, dietary and the laundry. Later, maintenance would split off from engineering and two kinds of chiefs were named in engineering, the operating engineer and the maintenance engineer. A booklet describing the hospital, dated 1916, listed a dietitian on staff, so we assume dietary existed as a department by that time and likely much earlier than that. By 1963, 132 different job categories stood behind patient care at St. Barnabas. To illustrate this fact and to commemorate Hospital Week, in May of 1963, employees representing the 132 jobs were positioned on the lawn outside of the hospital and a photo was taken which appeared the next day in the Star Tribune. A copy of that picture is included in this book.

A breakdown of budget figures in 1953 revealed the following percentages of budget for each department in the hospital: Dietary, 8%, General Office (included Medical Records, Personnel and Purchasing) 9.6%, Operating Room, 4.9%, Anesthesia, 2.4%, Delivery Room, 1.7%, Pharmacy, 4.7%, Nursing Service, 32.8%, Nursing School, 4.1%, Laboratory, 6.3%, X-ray, 4.5%, Housekeeping, 5%, Laundry, 2.4%, Maintenance, 3.2%, Electro-encephalography Lab, .32% and Photo Lab, .5%. In addition, 7.1% of the budget went to heating, lighting and power for the hospital and 2.8% to depreciation. The same article which included these data compared a number of factors from 1941 to 1942 and 1951 to 1952. During this ten year period, the number of patients admitted doubled, babies born doubled, surgical procedures doubled, but the average patient stay decreased from eight days in the 1940s to 5.6 days in 1951-1952. The increase in X-ray and laboratory examinations was really dramatic—in 1941-1942 there were 25,930 laboratory examinations. This figure increased to 102,733 in the following ten years. X-ray examinations increased from 3,340 in 1941-1942 to 11,363 in 1951-1952. Medical advances made during World War II accounted for most of the differences since the physical facilities at St. Barnabas were the same for both time periods.

The supportive service departments which came into being during the years St. Barnabas Hospital existed included the following:

ADMITTING AND INFORMATION DESK

Clara A. Johnson began in admitting in 1945 and continued to head that department until her retirement in 1968. **Violet Julius** also served in the department as did **Marge Elias**. Marge's relationship with St. Barnabas was first as a volunteer, then as a part-time employee in admitting and information desk. Later she switched to full-time and a position as a ward clerk on one of the clinical units.

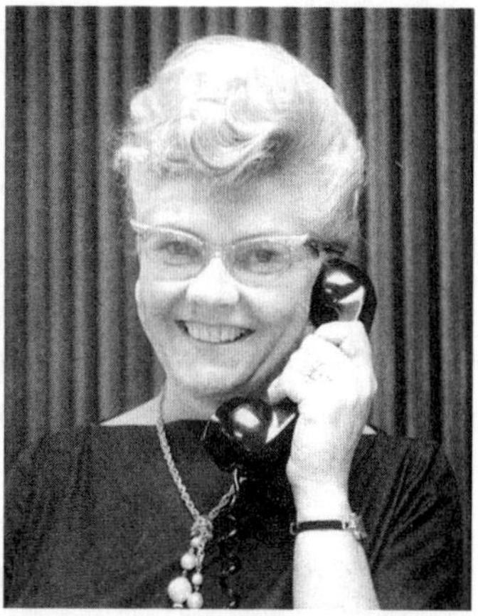

Vi Julius

BUSINESS OFFICE

There were offices pictured in a 1916 booklet about the hospital. They were labeled the "Front Office" and the "Cashier's Office." The front office likely was the office of administration. The administrator probably did all the hiring, firing, buying and general problem solving. Likely all transactions involving money were handled from the cashier's office. Following World War II, a business office was established. In 1949

Marvyl Apelt was named supervisor of the business office and credit manager. Part of her work as credit manager would be picked up by a new social services department when Marvyl retired in 1967. There was a position in and before 1930 and on into the 1940s that was labeled "superintendent". The position appeared to be the second in command after the administrator or director of the hospital and it seems likely that this person carried on the functions later picked up by the business office.

CENTRAL SUPPLY

The forerunner of central supply was known as "central service" and was housed in a very small room in the Whitney building, next to an equally small pharmacy. The RN in charge of central service served double duty as the emergency room nurse. The emergency room was a small examining room just across the hall from central service. Whether or not there was a central service before the Whitney building was built is not known. The RN in charge of central service in the 1940s was St. Barnabas graduate **Mae Carlson**, class of 1928. She was assisted by **Josephine Holmberg Pletscher**, St. Barnabas class of 1946 and **June Golden** and **Shirley**

Dolvin, both 1949 St. Barnabas graduates. When Mae retired, Shirley was chosen to be in charge of central service and emergency room. She moved in 1958 to the new hospital as head nurse in the emergency room. **Mildred Carstens (Johnson)**, class of 1951 also worked in central service for a few months following her graduation. In the 1958 building, central supply and the emergency room were split from one another and, in fact, were situated in completely different areas, not even on the same floor. While Shirley was assigned to the emergency room in the new hospital, **Helen Krieg**, St. Barnabas class of 1936, who had been head nurse on 3 Whitney was in charge of central supply. **Irene Peper**, St. Barnabas class of 1949, who had been Helen's assistant head nurse on 3 Whitney, served for a time in charge of central supply after Helen retired, but missed having regular patient contact and moved up to take charge of 5A with the staff which had moved from 3 Whitney. **Sylvia Chadwick**, also a St Barnabas graduate, class of 1926, also worked in central supply in the 1958 building. When St. Barnabas and Swedish merged in 1970, the chief in central supply was a man, **Angelo DeVito**.

COMMUNITY RELATIONS

The Community Relations office came into being in 1957 with the appointment of **Jean Houle**. Previous to Jean's hiring, community relations had been handled in the personnel office. Jean had an outgoing, friendly manner plus many business contacts in the community from previous positions she held. She adapted all of her previously acquired skills to develop a sound program so when she moved to another company in 1962, she passed a well organized program to her successor, **Bette McTaggert**. By1970, when Metropolitan Medical Center had replaced St. Barnabas and Swedish hospitals, community relations was handled by two people, **Karen Erickson** and **Jane Schulzenberg**.

CONTROLLER

Francis P. Brodin was the first controller at St. Barnabas. He joined the hospital staff in 1950 and remained until 1956 when he was replaced by **William E. Wells Jr.** Mr. Wells remained on the staff through the rest of the days of St. Barnabas and beyond into Metropolitan Medical Center days.

DENTAL SERVICES

It is unclear how long this department existed. It was pictured in the 1916 booklet about the hospital. Perhaps as more dentists opened offices of their own, there was no longer a need for this service to be offered in the hospital.

DIETARY

In a report written in 1902 by John I. Black, President of the Board of Trustees, reference is made to improvements made that year in the kitchen, which, it appears, was on the top floor of the new Martin building. There was an elevator in the center of the Martin building which would have made it possible to distribute food cooked on the top floor to patients on the lower floors. When the Corridor building was added to the Martin building, the kitchen was moved over to the corridor wing. Apparently by that time it was evident that the odors of food cooking were irritating to some patients. Later, when the Pavilion building was erected, dietary moved to the ground floor there, taking it completely away from patient care areas. In the 1958 building dietary and the employee cafeteria were in the basement of the building.

No reference is made to the person in charge of the kitchen in the early years. The 1916 booklet lists Margaret Holden as the dietitian, though there is no indication how long she held this position and whether or not the position was held by someone else at an earlier date. She may well have been the first dietitian on the staff at St. Barnabas. It seems possible that before there was a dietitian, the department may have been run by someone who was just a good cook. **Elvera Spotts** was the head dietitian during the 1940's. She resigned in 1947, though later she returned as a faculty member in the school of nursing. She was replaced by **Ethel Haga**, who was not only a dietitian, but was in charge of both patient and employee food service. Miss Haga stayed on to become one of the long-term employees of the hospital.

Over the years there were several other dietitians on the staff assisting Miss Haga. One such person was **Betty Griffin**. After working at St. Barnabas for a time, she was appointed the dietitian at St. Andrew's and was in charge of food service there. **Robert Abrahamson** was listed as the food service manager at MMC in 1970.

ENGINEERS

Charlie Engstrom joined the St. Barnabas staff in 1911 as assistant operating engineer, indicating there was already someone else in the operating engineer spot at that time. This department probably went back to the opening of the Martin building in 1894 though there is no record indicating how many employees there were nor who they were. Charlie became the operating engineer after a while and stayed on at St. Barnabas for 50 years and 10 months before his 1961 retirement. The function of the operating engineer was to keep the boilers for heat and hot water running. Later, another category, maintenance engineer, was created for the person hired to service and repair the boilers. **George Klahr** occupied that position in 1954, though there is no indication of how many Maintenance Engineers there were before George. It is possible that position was created about 1928 which was the year **Elmer Parker** was named chief engineer. Elmer hired on in 1926 as the night engineer, but was promoted to the chief spot two years later. He held that position until his retirement in 1953. By 1958, maintenance, engineering, laundry and housekeeping came under the administrative umbrella of one position, the director of general services. **Don Tallman** was hired to fill that position beginning in 1958. He stayed at St. Barnabas for four years. During that time, possibly with the move to the new hospital, the position name was changed to supervisor of buildings and grounds. **H. P. (Bill) Haugen** was hired with that title in 1962 and stayed for five years before moving on to a similar position in the White Bear Lake school system. In 1970, **Don MacRae** was listed in the position. It is likely he came on board in 1967 when Bill Haugen resigned.

HOUSEKEEPING

Records indicate there was a housekeeping department as early as 1902 and probably even before that. It is possible it came with the opening of the Martin building. There is no record of the names of the early heads of this department, though reference was made to the position in early reports. **Mae Curry**, who joined the staff in 1949 as executive housekeeper, is the earliest housekeeper listed. There is no date for Mae's resignation, but it appears her replacement was **James A. Cook** who came on board as executive housekeeper in 1958. James Cook was replaced one year later by **Donn Cook**. When Donn Cook resigned in 1963, the job of executive housekeeper went to **Alice Jonquist**, who had begun employment at St. Barnabas as a floor maid in 1941. Alice died in 1967 and there is no record of the name of her replacement. **Victor Froehlke** is listed as executive housekeeper in 1970, so it is possible he joined the staff to replace Alice.

Over the years from the Martin building to the 1958 hospital, the work of both engineers and housekeeping expanded as more beds were added with each building project and each of the new buildings came with new equipment up-to-date for the time. Use and care of the new equipment required new skills of the persons employed in these departments.

LAUNDRY

There was a laundry at St. Barnabas as early as 1907 and likely even before that. It is known that Amanda Evenson, a long-term employee in housekeeping, reported there were women working in the laundry at the time she was employed in 1907. The earliest laundry employee we can identify by name was **Axel Mattson**, who joined the staff in 1923 and remained until his retirement in 1953. Axel's job in the laundry was not specified in the information left about him, but it is possible he was the man in charge of the operation. In 1956, **Alaric W. Dupont** was hired to supervise installation of new equipment in the laundry and he stayed on then as head of the department until 1962. His replacement was **Frances Goodman** who served for five years. His responsibility included supervision of the laundry at Swedish as well as St. Barnabas. He resigned in 1967 to accept a similar position at the University of Minnesota Hospitals. **Roger Hanson** replaced Mr. Goodman and was with the hospital through the merger into Metropolitan Medical Center.

MEDICAL ARTIST

Robert C. Benassi was hired in 1954 to be the medical artist for the hospital. His office was at Smith House on the southwest corner of Seventh Street and Ninth Avenue South. The position lasted only a short time. Perhaps there was not sufficient call for his services to make the position economically viable.

MEDICAL LIBRARY

The Medical Library was created in 1942 and named for George S. Grimes, a long time member of the board of trustees. The library was located adjacent to the doctors' staff room and its operation was supervised by the librarian hired for Staples Memorial Library in the school of nursing.

MEDICAL PHOTO LAB

This facility was opened in 1950 under the direction of **Less Hier**. After Mr. Hier resigned, the facility was closed. It had been housed at Smith House.

MEDICAL RECORDS

Justine Hansen was in charge of the medical record department from 1937 to 1958. It is likely she was the first to head this department. It is not known who took her place in charge of medical records, but it may have been **Sue Peska**. Sue was medical record librarian prior to her 1966 resignation to have a baby. **Sandra Helgeson** was listed as the department head in 1970.

OCCUPATIONAL THERAPY

This department was new with the building of the joint facility with Swedish Hospital. **Kathy McFarland** is listed in charge in 1970. She may have been in the position from the time the department opened.

PATIENT ACCOUNTS AND PAYROLL

There were two new positions listed in a report issued for Metropolitan Medical Center in 1986. **Kris Fallon** was in charge of payroll at that point. The name of the person responsible for patient accounts was not listed.

PERSONNEL

Dorothy Touhey is the first personnel director listed in information available at this writing. She came in 1953, staying only two or three years before being replaced by **Lowell M. Vandervort** 1954 or 1955. Mr. Vandervort's title was director of personnel and community relations. Community relations was split off from personnel in 1957 with the hiring of Jean Houle to work fulltime on just community relations. During Mr. Vandervort's tenure, the personnel office was on 3 Corridor. By 1958, with the opening of the new hospital, personnel was moved to larger quarters on the tunnel level of the new building. **Fred Manthey** was director of the department at that time, a position he handled capably for several years. **Bruce Storrustan** is also listed in the department during the years before the merger to become Metropolitan Medical Center, but it isn't clear what his position was. In 1970 at MMC, **John Dunlap** was listed as personnel director.

PHARMACY

In the Whitney building, the pharmacy was located on the first floor, down the hall from the switchboard and admitting, next to central service. That may have been the first location from which a registered pharmacist operated. **Polly McIntire** (her surname is uncertain at this writing) held the position in the 1940s. She worked only day hours and when she was off duty, medicines and intravenous fluids were dispensed by the nurse/supervisor on duty. Polly was replaced about 1949 by **Joe Markovic**, who handled the department alone at first. **Russell Strom** came next, first as assistant pharmacist and later, in 1965, he became the chief pharmacist. Both Joe and Russ were avid bowlers and regulars on the St. Barnabas teams. Working with Joe and Russ was **Marly Ervasti**, who was on the pharmacy staff from 1956 to 1966. Also joining the staff in 1956 was **John Dearman**. John served for only two years, then left in 1958 to become the pharmacist at St. Andrew's, a position he held until St. Andrew's closed in 1963. At that time, he returned to St. Barnabas, apparently as chief pharmacist until Russ Strom assumed that position in 1965. John's move in 1965 took him to sunny California. From 1957 until 1963, **Gary Folsom** was on staff as an assistant pharmacist. He met and married a St. Barnabas graduate during those years, Deanna Carter, class of 1958. When the Folsoms left Minneapolis in 1963, they moved to Parkers Prairie where Gary was employed as the chief pharmacist in the brand new community hospital there. **Robert Paulson** came on as assistant pharmacist at some time during those years, possibly 1965. Both he and Marly Ervasti were in an Army Reserve unit stationed at Fort Snelling. In 1970, both Russ and Bob resigned and opened a pharmacy of their own in the new St. Barnabas office building across Eighth Street from the hospital. **Robert Nordin** was chief pharmacist and **Louis Balster** an assistant when Metropolitan Medical Center came into being.

PURCHASING

Margaret Muntifer was the first purchasing agent for whom information could be found. She worked at St. Barnabas from 1948 to 1958. The name of the next person to fill this position is unavailable, but records do indicate that **Richard Carlstrom** was hired as purchasing agent in 1963.

RESEARCH

Chapter 22 describes the research programs carried out at St. Barnabas. Until 1970, there apparently was no central department for research, rather each team planning to work on a given project would be given permission and space to do it. But it appears there was no central coordination of the projects for the first twenty or more years. In 1970, a department was created at Metropolitan Medical Center, under the direction of **Dr. Henry Bates**.

SOCIAL SERVICE

Marvyl Apelt in the business office had been carrying on some social service activities for years before a separate department was established, though that was not her primary responsibility and her professional background did not include formal education in social work. As the hospital increased in size, it was no longer feasible to ask the business office staff to carry this extra responsibility. So in 1967, a social service department was created and **Susan Erickson** and **Fern Loomis** were hired to staff it. **Joni Holtz** is listed as responsible for social service at MMC in 1986.

SWITCHBOARD

In the Whitney building, the switchboard was in the same area near the front entrance as admitting and the information desk. Several employees who ultimately moved to other responsibilities, started at the switchboard. It must have been a difficult and frustrating job because the switchboard was right out in the open, with a sliding glass window facing the main hall. The poor operator was interrupted frequently by visitors, doctors, hospital staff and anyone else looking for something or someone. **Vivian Provo** became an operator in 1955 and in 1958 moved to new surroundings, a private area in the basement level of the new hospital. Gone were the frequent interruptions of earlier years. Along with the new location came a change in title as the switchboard became the communications center.

WASHBURN CLINIC

Not really a department of the hospital at all, but rather a tenant activity of the hospital, was Washburn Clinic, which, beginning in February 1951, was located on 3 Martin. The Clinic was a child guidance clinic which was operated by the Department of Psychiatry of the University of Minnesota Medical School. Washburn Clinic was named for Cadwallader

Washburn, who had played a role in the early days of St. Barnabas. The clinic remained at St. Barnabas for only a few years. The reason for moving it is not known. Perhaps they needed more space or space more accessible to the clientele they served. Or Perhaps St. Barnabas needed that space for its own purposes. The nursing school offices and staples library occupied that area after the clinic was gone and before the move to the remodeled Whitney Residence.

THE VOICE OF ST. BARNABAS

Another service which was not really a department of the hospital, but was closely identified with it, was the paper, the *Voice of St. Barnabas*. Its creator was **Muriel Riddiford**, who edited the paper from the first issue in 1952 until 1962. It came out four to six times per year, depending mainly on how much news was available and when Mrs. Riddiford, who did this as a volunteer activity all those years, had the time available to give to it. After Jean Houle was hired in community relations, Mrs. Riddiford worked with her on the *Voice*, but she retained editorship herself.

Mrs. Riddiford had a staff of volunteer reporters from every department and every clinical area in the hospital who contributed the news items Mrs. Riddiford edited and published. Prior to each issue, there would be a meeting of all volunteer reporters and Mrs. Riddiford would discuss the focus of the next issue and give a deadline for submission of news.

After Mrs. Riddiford's retirement, the paper continued to be published along the same lines she had established. With the merger into Metropolitan Medical Center, both the name and the focus of the paper changed. *Scope* replaced The *Voice of St. Barnabas* and later the focus changed again and with it came another name change to *Dimensions Of Metropolitan Medical Center*. For old-time employees accustomed to their *Voice* during its eighteen years of existence, the new papers never quite measured up to the original. I was one of the aforementioned volunteer reporters. I relied heavily upon all three papers for documentation of information about the hospital that I have included in this book. But I relied especially on the *Voice of St. Barnabas*.

Chapter 20

Greatest Resource St. Barnabas Had–Its Employees

A retirement plan was established for St. Barnabas employees beginning 1 July 1963. It was a non-contributory plan with funds being supplied entirely from the hospital. It covered all full-time employees and part-time employees who worked at least 24 hours per week on a regular basis. Vesting began at ten years of employment.

The other primary reward for long term employment was an employee recognition dinner. It was given annually on a day during the week of Florence Nightingale's birthday to honor employees who had worked at St. Barnabas (also St. Andrew's for the years it was a division of St. Barnabas) for ten years or more. Pins were given in recognition of ten years' service and then for each five-year interval beyond ten.

The program from the 1972 dinner identified twelve employees who were termed members of the "Diamond Club." This was the first time the term "Diamond Club" appeared on a recognition day dinner program. At that dinner, long-term Swedish employees were also recognized since the two hospitals had become divisions of Metropolitan Medical Center beginning in 1970. Perhaps the "Diamond Club" designation had been used in earlier years at Swedish. To be designated a member of the "Diamond Club", one had to have served at least twenty-five years on staff.

Topping the Diamond Club list on that 1972 program was **Florence Watts Buck**, 1928 graduate of St. Barnabas School of Nursing, who had worked at that point for thirty-two years at St. Barnabas. She retired in 1973 with thirty-three years of employment as an RN at St. Barnabas and Metropolitan Medical Center. Not only was Florence a St. Barnabas graduate, but both of her daughters also graduated from the school, Joanne Watts Torres in 1951 and Joyce Watts Dudley in 1953.

Another St. Barnabas graduate who logged thirty-eight years of employment at the hospital was **Ruth Anderson Reynolds**, class of 1923. She married soon after graduation and lived for several years in smaller communities in Minnesota, raising a family of three children. In 1938, she returned to Minneapolis and employment in maternity at St. Barnabas. She began as a staff nurse and progressed up the chain of command serving as assistant head nurse, then head nurse and finally supervisor and coordinator. She was interviewed for the "Familiar Faces" column in a 1958 issue of the *Voice*. The interviewer described her as one who obviously enjoyed her work and who was cheerful, efficient and always willing to help others.

Other St. Barnabas employees on that Diamond Club list from 1972 were **Callista Cashman**, who had twenty-five years in nursing service, **Mary Conroy**, who had twenty-six years in the laboratory, **Hazelle Lundell**, who had twenty-five years, first in nursing service, then later on the faculty of the nursing school, and **Ann Smith**, who had twenty-six years in housekeeping.

Margaret Johnson was also listed as a member of the club. More information about Margaret is included later in this chapter. Among the twelve listed were six others who had been Swedish Hospital employees. Together, the twelve members of the Diamond Club of 1972 had given 352 years of service to St. Barnabas and Swedish.

Six employees were listed as members of the Diamond Club in 1986: **Elma Ann Lyon, Irene Peper, Marion Picha, Gilma Prestemon, Karen Rasmussen** and **Doris Pearson**.

The *Voice of St. Barnabas* records that 138 St. Barnabas employees honored at the 1970 dinner had given a total of 2094 years of service to St. Barnabas and St. Andrew's. Similar calculations for other years were not published, but likely that figure was comparable for each year preceding 1970. Invitations for the annual dinner went out not only to current employees, but also to retired employees living in the Minneapolis area and their years of service up to retirement were computed with current employees to determine the total years of service.

From accounts of recognition services for other years, we find that **Charley Engstrom** topped the all time list for longevity of employment. Charley came to St. Barnabas in 1911 and was employed in engineering for fifty-one years before he retired. He was only twenty-two years old in 1911 and his principle task was the firing of the boiler which provided heat and hot water for the hospital. Ultimately, he became the operating engineer, the post he held until his retirement in December of 1961. Upon retirement, Charley moved to the Odd Fellows home in Northfield.

A co-worker with Charley in engineering was **Elmer Parker**. He came to St. Barnabas on July 28, 1926, expecting to stay on the night shift for about two weeks. But he changed his mind and became one of the very long-term employees at the hospital. He was on nights for seven years, then became chief engineer and stayed on until retirement. His intent during his youth was to become a doctor and, in fact, he attended the University of Wisconsin for one year at which time he married and dropped out of college to make a living for his family. Late in his employment, Elmer was quoted as saying "One of the things that is outstanding about St. Barnabas as a place to work is its family feeling. You couldn't find a homier place to work."

The person who served the second highest number of years was **Amanda Evenson**, who was on the staff of St. Barnabas, in housekeeping, for forty-eight years. She came to St. Barnabas in 1907 as an immigrant from Norway. She became seriously ill soon after her arrival in America and she had to be hospitalized for several weeks. During that time, she became familiar with the inner workings of a hospital and decided that is where she would like to work. She began her long years of employment at St. Barnabas on January 10, 1907, and remained on staff until her retirement in 1955. Many changes occurred in those forty-eight years and Amanda, loved by all who knew her, witnessed many of those changes.

Two men shared the honor of having served the next largest number of years, forty-three. **Ray Erickson** came to St. Barnabas as a house orderly in 1919. A few years later he transferred to the operating room, serving as an orderly there for thirty-five more years. Ray was featured in the "Familiar Faces" column of the *Voice of St. Barnabas* in June of 1954. The column opens with "St. Barnabas Hospital has a chief surgery orderly who can qualify for his first million miles pushing a stretcher."

Ray had spent about one year working as an orderly in three other Minneapolis hospitals before he came to St. Barnabas. The first operating room in which he worked after coming to St. Barnabas was the one in the old Martin building. Then he moved to the new suite in the Whitney building in 1937 and in 1958 he moved to the "new" St. Barnabas operating room suite. Generations of nursing students, apprehensive about their first service in the operating room, soon felt at home because Ray was there to lend a hand in orienting them to the location of almost anything they could be asked for during their operating room experience. Soon after the move to the new hospital in 1958, Ray transferred to central supply where he covered evening and night shifts. The *Voice* records, "His industry and attention to detail remained at the same high level" (in Central Supply compared to Operating Room). Ray retired for health reasons in 1963.

The other forty-three year man was **Axel Albertson**, painter in maintenance. He came to St. Barnabas the same year as Charley Engstrom (1911), but retired eight years before Charley did. By coincidence, Axel died 28 February 1963, just about the time that Ray Erickson, the other forty-three year man, retired. Axel was another of our Norwegian immigrants, coming to this country at age twenty after having served a stint with the merchant marine on a German ship. During those years at sea, he learned the painter trade. For his first ten years in the states, he worked as a painter in Chicago. He came to Minneapolis in 1911 and began his long years of employment at St. Barnabas. Like Amanda Evenson, Axel saw many changes during his forty-three years here. Axel and Mrs. Albertson raised a sizable family, four daughters and two sons, at their south Minneapolis home.

Isaac Aaker, chef in dietary, came to St. Barnabas in 1923 and served in dietary for forty years before his retirement in June of 1963. During all those forty years on the job, Isaac took almost no time off for illness. Isaac's wife was employed at General Mills, though the *Voice* does not indicate whether she also had a long history there as Isaac had at St. Barnabas. The couple had one son, Gordon, and two grandchildren with whom they enjoyed regular visits. Isaac retired from dietary to his yard and his flower garden, the two prime hobbies of his life.

Isaac's counterpart at St. Andrew's was **Eva Beihoffer**, who began her employment at St. Andrew's in 1932. She had the distinction of being the first cook hired at St. Andrew's. Eva was also featured in the "Familiar Faces column of the *Voice of St. Barnabas* (March-April 1955). The article describes her very large family in these terms:

> Eva has reared four of her own children, and has been a mother to nine others. Most of the nine foster children were between the ages of 12 and 14 when Eva began caring for them. The first two, Mary and Ann, were taken in when Eva bought a home and found that no provision had been made by the former owner, their father, for the girls. The next child, Bruce, is a nephew of her husband. Jerry was a little boy whose family refused to care for him. Esther was next, a girl from Eva's hometown of New Auburn, Minnesota.
>
> The Beihoffer daughters, Velva and Mary, brought Myrtle home with them from work when they found she had no home. Edith was an orphaned girl whose marriage had been unfortunate. She brought her infant son, Dick, to Eva, and both were made welcome.
>
> Buzz Beihoffer, the oldest son, as hospitable as the rest of the family, brought to Eva a friend who needed a home. He was the last of the family to arrive.
>
> All these young people lived with Eva until they were married or entered the service. However, the habit of home cooking was hard to break and Eva continued to cook for the many relatives and friends constantly coming to her home.

Certainly Eva would have qualified as a "Big Heart Award" winner. What greater way to demonstrate Christian values than the way chosen by Eva.

Axel Mattson came to St. Barnabas the same year as Isaac Aaker, 1923. He retired earlier than Isaac, so had fewer years on the job, but was still well over thirty years at retirement. Axel worked for all those years in laundry.

Another of the long-timers at St. Barnabas was **Justine Hanson**. She came to St. Barnabas and medical records in 1921, remaining on staff for thirty-four years. She came from teaching school in North Dakota and worked a variety of jobs at the hospital, serving at the admissions desk, on the switchboard, at the information desk, in the business office and in purchasing. When the Whitney building was opened in 1937, she moved to medical records where she remained until retirement. She was a great favorite with the medical staff, all of whom she got to know well over her long years of service. She became an active member of the American Association of Medical Record Librarians in 1940 and became well known for her contributions to that organization. Not only was she a favorite with the medical staff, but she always had time for students and alumnae of the nursing school. She was made an honorary member of the St. Barnabas Nurses Alumnae in 1946. The women's board also honored her with a vote of appreciation for the many services she rendered to them.

Justine was known to many in the hospital as "Hans." She was remembered for her dry sense of humor. Hans looked forward to having time in retirement for her favorite pastime, reading, but she died soon after she retired.

Clara A. Johnson, admitting, came to St. Barnabas in 1928 and stayed for thirty-eight years. Initially, she was a part-time employee hired to cover during the summer vacation period. But that vacation extended into thirty-eight years. Like Justine Hanson, she filled a variety of different positions at first, starting as an elevator operator, moving to the switchboard and finally, in 1945, to admitting. Ultimately, she became the chief admitting clerk.

During her long tenure at St. Barnabas, people were often confused by the amount of work it appeared she did in two totally different fields. It seems there was another Clara Johnson, also a long-timer on staff at the same time. She was **Clara O. Johnson**, head nurse on 2 Whitney. Clara O. was known by some of her friends as "the Duchess" because of her aristocratic bearing. In 1955, she was featured in the "Familiar Faces" column of the *Voice of St. Barnabas*. Let's look to see what the interviewer had to say about her:

> Who is she—this person with sparkling eyes and a gay, ready wit, who directs her floor with an easy manner and smooth efficiency? It's Clara Johnson, head nurse on 2 Whitney of course! Daughter of a Lutheran minister, Miss Johnson was born in Chicago. After graduating from St. Olaf College with a degree in music, she took nurses' training at LaCrosse Lutheran Hospital in Wisconsin.
>
> For three years, she was in charge of surgery at the E.E.N.T. Infirmary in Chicago, and later came to Minneapolis as assistant head nurse at Northwestern Hospital. In 1939, Miss Johnson joined the St. Barnabas Hospital nursing staff, becoming head nurse on 2 Whitney, which ever since, has remained under her excellent supervision.

It is interesting to note that in the history of the Whitney building, only one other head nurse served on 2 Whitney, and she served only the first two years that building was in use as a hospital. Clara served almost the entire twenty-one years the Whitney building served as a home for clinical services of the hospital.

Friendliness, efficiency and empathy were character traits which Clara possessed. Both her staff and her patients were comfortable knowing Clara was in charge She had many outside interests. As one would expect, with her degree in music she was an accomplished musician and often served as organist for hospital chapel services. She also played bridge on a regular basis with others of the supervisory staff of nursing service. She almost always traveled to some distant place for her vacations and usually came back with a deep tan, the envy of many. In her quiet times she liked to knit or read a good book.

Clara worked at St. Barnabas for at least twenty-seven years before she retired—all of those as a head nurse. Again, that is a record few could equal.

At least five others served thirty years or more on the staff at St. Barnabas. **Hazel Johnson** came in 1922 and stayed at least thirty-three years. **Albert Erickson**, maintenance, came in 1918 and stayed thirty-seven years. **Jack Leffingwell**, X-ray, was on staff from 1923 to 1955. A biographical sketch of Jack is included in Chapter 7.

Another who would be remembered by older St. Barnabas graduates was **Alpha Elf**. Alpha came in 1934 and worked most of the next thirty years in the Wellesmere linen room where students turned in soiled uniforms and cotton personal laundry and picked up the same after they had been laundered and ironed. Students who sent cotton pajamas to the laundry through the Wellesmere linen room would hear Alpha say, as she checked off the items they were to pick up, "Oh yes, you have two pairs of Peeyays, too." Dear Alpha was a kindly Scandinavian lady who just never learned to pronounce her Js!!

Still another person who was on staff for more than thirty years served before anyone living today would remember. **Harriette Hartry** came to St. Barnabas in 1899 and remained on staff for thirty-one years. She served in the beginning as the superintendent of nurses, then in 1907 was made the superintendent of the hospital, a post she capably filled until 1930. She must have been quite a lady.

Serving as director of nurses during most of Miss Hartry's tenure as hospital superintendent was **M. Dorothy Rhodes**. Miss Rhodes was a 1906 graduate of St. Barnabas School of Nursing. She assumed the top position in the nursing department in 1916 and remained in that job until 1938, covering a period of some difficulty in nursing service and the nursing school. Details of that are covered in Chapter 14. She, too, must have been quite a lady. There were still many nurses around St. Barnabas during the early years I was on the school faculty who remembered Miss Rhodes and spoke of her frequently.

Helen Parker Hayden was a 1936 graduate of the nursing school. Helen had worked in X-ray during her days as a student nurse and upon graduation and after she received her RN, she joined the X-ray department where she worked for more than thirty years until retirement. More about Helen's contributions to St. Barnabas will be found in Chapter 7.

Co-workers in the post-anesthesia recovery room from its opening in the early 1950s were RNs **Inga Peterson** and **Margaret Johnson**. Inga came to St. Barnabas in 1941 and worked for several years on 5 Pavilion before moving to PAR. She served for more than twenty-five years at St. Barnabas. Margaret came in 1944 and served for twenty-seven years. She was one of the Diamond Club members listed on the 1972 program for the recognition dinner. Apparently Inga retired before that year for she would also have been a member of the Diamond Club, but was not listed on that program.

Irene Nelson, a Canadian, found her way down to Minnesota in 1939 and stayed on to work the rest of her professional career in the United States. She worked first at St. Mary's in Rochester, then moved up to Minneapolis and the University of Minnesota Hospital. In 1942, she came to St. Barnabas. She began her years at St. Barnabas working as a staff nurse on 2 Whitney. After a number of years, she moved to 2 Pavilion where she was named head nurse. When the hospital was moved in 1958 to the "new" St. Barnabas, she moved with her staff to 4B. In 1964, after twenty two years at St. Barnabas, she resigned and was replaced as head nurse by **Gilma Prestemon**, who had been her assistant for a number of years on 2 Pavilion and later on 4B. Gilma was a 1951 graduate of St. Barnabas who stayed on after graduation and worked her entire nursing career at St. Barnabas. She progressed from staff nurse to assistant head nurse to head nurse and later became a supervisor on neurology after St. Barnabas and Swedish combined to form Metropolitan Medical Center. Gilma was well liked by all who knew her. She was intelligent and thoughtful, though her quiet manner belied the wisdom she possessed. She died in 2001. In my opinion she was one of the best nurses St. Barnabas school of nursing ever produced.

Coming to the United States from Canada with Irene Nelson was **Joyce English**. Though Joyce never qualified for recognition as a long-time employee of the hospital, she is mentioned because in the combination of years she worked at St. Barnabas along with the years she served in her next position, she was a long-time presence at St. Barnabas. Joyce served for several years as the head nurse on fourth Martin, then left the employ of St. Barnabas to go to work for Drs. Carl Rice and Jacob Strickler, who in the early 1950s established a research program at St. Barnabas in cooperation with Baxter Laboratories. Their aim was to develop more nutritious parenteral fluids. Joyce coordinated the program, making rounds with the two doctors and keeping notes of her daily observationsof their patients who were on intravenous fluids. She worked in close cooperation with Jeanne Jensen, Medical Technologist in charge of the research lab which the two doctors maintained on 3 Corridor. Joyce had a great sense of humor, but at the same time she was most knowledgeable of the craft of nursing. She was generally well liked and respected throughout the hospital.

One of Joyce English's closest friends at the hospital was **Marian Holt**. Marian had been married to a physician, but after his early death, she came to work at St. Barnabas in 1946 as the first ward clerk employed by the hospital. She was assigned to maternity. One of her prime responsibilities was getting the information required to have an official birth certificate prepared for every newborn. She interviewed each new mother and from the information supplied, she submitted the application for birth certificate to the State of Minnesota, which then issued the birth certificate for the baby. Ultimately, there was enough demand for her services that she specialized in the birth certificate work. She was identified at times as a member of the medical records staff and at other times as a member of the maternity staff, but her responsibility remained the same, getting and recording the information needed to develop an accurate birth certificate for each newborn. Ironically, though she spent more than twenty years working with new mothers and being concerned with newborns, she had no children herself. After Dr. Holt's death, Marian made a home for her bachelor brother in a big Victorian house across the street from Pioneer Hall at the University of Minnesota and just a stone's throw from the University Hospital. She and Joyce English seemed a most unlikely pair of friends, but they enjoyed years of playing pranks on each other every day.

A twenty-year member of the housekeeping staff was **Ethelyn Hagstrom**. She began her employment at St. Barnabas on a part-time basis in 1947. Later, she moved to a full- time position as the maid assigned to 5 Pavilion. After the move to the new hospital in 1958, Ethelyn served as a float. Her quiet, friendly manner allowed her to fit in readily wherever she was assigned to work, whether for a day or a week or even longer. Ethelyn was a member of one of the St. Barnabas bowling teams which also afforded her another opportunity to get to know fellow employees she did not see every day on the job. A colleague of Ethelyn's in the housekeeping department was **Rachel Flemming**. She came to St. Barnabas in 1941 and was assigned to be the station maid on 2 Pavilion. She remained with that staff when they moved in 1958 to 4B in the new building. Rachel was featured in the "Familiar Faces" column of the *Voice* in 1965. She was asked by the interviewer what she considered to be one of the improvements of the new building as compared to Pavilion. She replied that would have to be the windows in the new building which could be washed on both outside and inside from the safety and comfort of the inside of the building. The interviewer for that column stated, "Rachel is well known for her excellent work performance and her kindness shown to patients." It was a hallmark of St. Barnabas Hospital that members of all departments understood they were there to be a part of serving sick people.

Still another long-time member of the housekeeping staff was **Rose Ennis**. Her employment at St. Barnabas was broken by an interval of four years away from the hospital. She first came to St. Barnabas in 1928 and worked for ten years, then resigned and later came back in December of 1942. One of Rose's cherished values was punctuality. She was proud of the fact that in all of her years at St. Barnabas (at least twenty four), she was never late for work even once. Rose had a sister who worked in dietary at Swedish for thirty years, many of them the same years Rose was across the street at St. Barnabas. Another sister worked down the street about three blocks as a nurse aide at Minneapolis General for twenty-three years. Rose's twin sister also worked in the hospital arena, at Veterans' Hospital in south Minneapolis. You might say working in health care settings was popular in that family.

Still another long-time member of the housekeeping department was **Alice Jonquist**, who worked her way on up through the ranks to become chief of her department in 1963, and serving until her death in 1967. This in spite of the fact that Alice walked with a limp, a residual effect from a childhood bout of polio. As was true of the three department members just described, Alice was also featured in the "Familiar Faces" column of the *Voice*. The interviewer said, "Everyone knows Alice—one of the most popular folks in the St. Barnabas family."

What a compliment and what a legacy to leave for those remembering her in the future. Alice was particularly proud when a patient or visitor would comment about the outstanding cleanliness of the hospital. Though she was by nature a quiet person, she conducted the business of her department with efficiency and good grace, earning the cooperation of her department members, never demanding their performance. Alice worked at St. Barnabas for twenty-six years beginning in 1941.

Working for the housekeeping department, but not in the hospital proper, was **Emily Nelson** who retired in 1963 after twenty years of service as the maid on first floor at Wellesmere, then later on the second floor of the Whitney Residence. Students whose rooms were cleaned by Emily over her twenty years at St. Barnabas remember her kindness toward them.

An eighteen-year employee of the business office was credit manager and supervisor, **Marvyl Apeltt**. She joined the St. Barnabas family in 1948 and like so many other St. Barnabas employees made the big move across the street to the new building in 1958. Marvyl's skills weren't limited to the business office. In the days before a social service department, it was Marvyl who worked with patients needing help in paying their hospital bills. Prior to her service at St. Barnabas, she had taught school for seven years and worked for a number of years for a group of jewelry stores in downtown Minneapolis. She brought a wealth of different experiences to her job which enhanced her performance in supervising credit accounts for the hospital. Fishing and camping on lakes on Minnesota's northern border were favorite hobbies of Marvyl and her husband.

Two employees from the nursing service department retired in the spring of 1963, one having served fifteen years on the staff, and the other, fourteen years. **Helen Pfleuger** came to St. Barnabas as a staff nurse anesthetist in 1948 and had become chief anesthetist at the time of her retirement. Fellow employee, Ebba Martinson, in writing for the *Voice* about Helen's retirement said one of Helen's character traits was orderliness, that she wanted a place for everything and she always kept everything in its place. Accordingly, the going away gift to her from her colleagues in anesthesia was a purse with many different compartments in it.

Helen was very active in the Minnesota Association of Nurse Anesthetists during her tenure at St. Barnabas.

Another nursing service employee, known well to students who rotated through night duty as a part of their training, was **Kristian Thingstad**, night orderly. Whenever nurses on night duty needed an extra hand, Kris was there to provide it for them. He came to St. Barnabas in 1949, retiring in 1963. He was Norwegian born and fit in well with the Scandinavian climate of Minneapolis in the 1940s and 1950s. The person who wrote for the *Voice* about Kris's retirement paid tribute to him with these words: "If there is any truth in the saying 'The devil finds mischief for idle hands to do,' the devil must have found Kris very unproductive! Every move Kris made was 'on the double.'"

Kris was born and reared with his seventeen brothers and sisters on a farm near Hamar, Norway—seventy miles north of Oslo. After retirement, he went back to Norway for a lengthy visit with all his family there.

Juliet White, nurse aide, worked for twenty years on 2 Whitney from her arrival in April of 1943 until just two weeks before her death in April of 1963. Known as "Whitey" to co-workers and patients, alike, she was seen as helpful and dependable in all that she did. She was loved and highly respected by her co-workers and patients on 2 Whitney.

Another twenty-year employee was **Sofie Christensen** who was a nurse aide in pediatrics. Writing about Sofie for "Familiar Faces" was her co-worker, later head nurse, Carmen Kjellsvig, who wrote that Sofie received her training in a Danish hospital, working there as a nurse aide in the emergency ward. Sofie and her husband emigrated to the United States in 1939. They couldn't speak a word of English when they arrived, so Sofie enrolled in English as a second language course at Vocational High School. She joined the St. Barnabas family in 1951 and credited working there with helping her to improve her language skills. .

Eunice Roesler was a ward clerk at St. Barnabas, beginning on 2 and 3 Whitney in 1947 and moving to 5A when the new building opened in 1958. In 1960, she retired, but continued to work part-time as needed. One of her great interests was music, particularly playing the organ. She had a Wurlitzer organ in her home, and sometimes shared her talents by playing the organ for Sunday morning chapel services at the hospital. She was a deacon in her Presbyterian Church and a member of Eastern Star. Five years after her retirement Eunice told someone she wasn't yet a senior citizen because she didn't have time for that!

A review of all of these biographical vignettes of those who served St. Barnabas for so many years shows there was no one particular department which had an edge on employees with longevity of employment. In addition to those described in this chapter, there were several nursing supervisors who served at St. Barnabas for many years. Their biographical sketches are included in Chapter 18. In the Appendix will be found a list of all those who received awards at the annual recognition dinners.

What motivated so many to come to St. Barnabas and remain on staff for 20-30-40 years and some for even more than that? There was a perception then that success in life involved getting a good job early in life and keeping it. Loyalty to one's employer was a cherished value. And often one chose a dwelling place near to the job. That convenience of being near to the place of employment was also cherished and many preferred not to upset the arrangement by taking another job. Once ownership of an automobile became the expected norm, basically, after World War II, all of that changed and we became a more mobile society. As more and more people owned automobiles and roads leading into the city were improved, it became possible, even expected, that one could live in the suburbs or a rural area and still commute to a job downtown. Those more distant dwelling places then became centers of circles in which were located different opportunities for employment in many different directions. Gradually, the once cherished value of loyalty to one employer eroded as the expectation of getting a job and keeping it for a lifetime changed to an expectation of having four, five, six or more jobs, each a better opportunity than the one which preceded it. Truly the greatest resources St. Barnabas had in the first 50-75 years of its existence was its employees. Their loyalty and pride in being a part of St. Barnabas nurtured the hospital as it grew and expanded.

Chapter 21

Displaced Persons on Staff

Following World War II, when the Soviet Union moved into the Baltic states of Latvia, Lithuania and Estonia, large numbers of the citizens of these countries moved west to escape life under Soviet domination. At the same time, there were citizens of the Soviet Union who also chose to leave, or were forced to leave, who turned to the west for new lives. Most moved through Germany and stayed there for a time before moving on to the United States under sponsorship of various individuals and/or organizations. Once in the United States, many found it difficult to get established in professions that they had practiced in their homelands because they could not produce documentation of their professional credentials and could not speak the English language. Ordinarily a prospective emigrant would secure such documentation before leaving the homeland, but in the late 1940s and early 1950s many chose not to try to get such documentation fearing reprisals should the government authorities know of their intentions to leave.

Two people whose journey finally brought them to St. Barnabas were Jacob and Sophie Karaby, who came to the United States in 1950, from Odessa in the Ukraine, USSR. In Odessa it had been Dr. Jacob Karaby and his nurse wife, Sophie, but when they arrived in the United State in January of 1950, they lacked the documentation to prove their professional backgrounds. They also lacked English language skills needed to practice in American hospitals. They lived their first two years in Rochester, where Jacob was employed at Rochester State Hospital. In April 1952 they moved to Minneapolis and Jacob found work as an orderly at St. Barnabas. Sophie also joined the St. Barnabas family as a dishwasher in the lab. On May 11, 1955, both became United States citizens. "The rest of the story" is unknown with regard to Jacob and Sophie Karaby, but in many cases, with development of English language skills, more schooling in the United States and obtaining United States citizenship, these displaced persons were able to move up the ladder to successful lives more comparable to the professions they had in their home countries.

A couple who started the hard way in the United States, but later were able to follow the professions they had known earlier, was Bela and Margit Gallo, who came in the early 1950s from Latvia. Margit worked for a time as an LPN on 2 Whitney. Ultimately, Bela was able to secure his MD in Minnesota and the family moved to Silver Bay, a new taconite community on the north shore of Lake Superior. Their daughter, Cookie, was born there. She had two brothers a bit older than she, though the places of their births are not known to me. After a time practicing at Silver Bay, Dr. Gallo moved his family to Ironwood, Michigan, where he established a very successful medical practice. My husband and I visited the Gallos in Ironwood in 1960. In 1990, we chanced to run into their son, who was then a docent at Taliesin, the home and museum of Frank Lloyd Wright in Spring Green, Wisconsin. Bela and Margit had died by that time, but they had lived and practiced as Dr. and Mrs. Bela Gallo of Ironwood, Michigan, from the time we saw them in 1960 to the end of their lives.

Another displaced person, or "DP" as they were called by some, was Emilija Liesha. She and her husband came to the United States from Estonia in the early 1950s. Like Margit Gallo, Emilija worked on 2 Whitney, but she was a nurse aide rather than a nurse. She was several years older than Margit Gallo and lacked the English language skills Margit had. Like many others, the Lieshas fled Estonia and were unable, or afraid, to carry with them their professional and educational documents from Estonia.

Still another displaced person who joined the St. Barnabas family in the 1950s and stayed on to become a long-term employee was Silvija Kupschs. The following is quoted from an article written by Elma Ann Krier for the May-June 1952 issue of the *Voice of St. Barnabas*.

> September 10, 1954, was a lucky day for St. Barnabas…it was the day that Mrs. Silvija Kupchs began her employment as librarian. Since that time she has been in charge of the school library, the medical library and ward libraries and has done the technical work for the laboratory and administrative libraries.
>
> Mrs. Kupchs was born and raised in Latvia. She received her degree in Romance languages and education from the University of Riga and taught French, Latvian, voice and penmanship in the French Liceum. Later, she was in charge of the French College Library in Germany. In 1949, Silvija and her mother found their way to the United States and settled in New York.
>
> From there they went to Grand Rapids, Michigan, where she met and married a fellow Latvian, Paul Kupchs. From Michigan, they moved to California, but within a year returned to the Midwest and settled in Minneapolis.

In her spare time, Silvija was secretary of a Latvian academic group. She also enjoyed music, cooking, sewing and, of course, reading. Their house was on the east side of the river, but the Kupchs still called Minneapolis their home. Paul was a chemist for a St. Paul firm. His mother lived with them during their Twin City years and acted as their housekeeper. A humorous incident involving this lady and the author of this book took place about 1962. Silvija had a day off and something came up at the nursing school for which a quick answer from Silvija was needed, so I called her home. Her mother-in-law answered the phone. She spoke no English and I, of course, no Latvian, but I was able to deduce that Silvija was not there. As the lady talked, though I couldn't understand a word of it, I interjected "Ja" every once in a while. The next day Silvija reported to me that someone had called the previous day and her mother-in-law thought it may have been a call from the nursing school. Silvija said, "She didn't know who called, but it was someone who spoke Latvian."

Coffee room discussions with Silvija during the years she served in the hospital libraries was most interesting. The struggle she and her mother endured to escape from Latvia and to survive until they reached the United States brought the gravity of the Cold War home to faculty members who participated in these discussions.

Silvija lived on after retirement until 2001. Paul, who outlived her, arranged to have her cremated. With the help of their long-time friend, Ruth Weise, he sent her ashes back home to Latvia for interment.

Chapter 22

Research Programs

St. Barnabas was the first private hospital in the Twin Cities to establish a research program. It all began in the late 1940s with Drs. Rice and Strickler who, with support from Baxter Laboratories, conducted research on the nutritional value of parenteral fluids. Registered nurses and nursing students of that era found themselves adding a number of sterile ingredients to bottles of intravenous fluids sent up from pharmacy. The substances most frequently added were absolute alcohol (for pain management as well as for the nutritional value it added to fluids) and vitamins. The research program established by Rice and Strickler included a full-time medical technologist (Jeanne Jensen) who worked from a laboratory located on the third floor of the Corridor building and a full-time registered nurse (Joyce English) who kept tabs on all the patients who received the fluids with added nutrients. Joyce met the patients when they first came to the doctors' office and were scheduled for surgery. She made rounds every day with the doctors, visiting each patient and documenting effects of the fluids they were getting. She saw each patient again in the office when they came back for post-operative follow-up care. Financial support for the program came from Baxter Laboratories which had a detail man on their staff who regularly visited the two doctors, Jeanne and Joyce and other St. Barnabas staff members who might be involved with the research being done.

The next research project at the hospital came with the establishment, under the direction of Dr. John Wild, of a program for detection of breast cancer. The piece of equipment developed by Dr. Wild's team was called an "echograph." It worked on a similar principle to the ultra sound diagnostic equipment in use today. Dr. Wild's team was housed at first on 3 Corridor and later across the street at Smith House. That program was terminated in 1960.

The most extensive of the early research programs was one offered in association with the University of Minnesota. Dr. Laurence O. Pilgeram, a university faculty member, directed this program on detection, prevention and treatment of arteriosclerosis. Dr. Pilgeram's team included five full-time biochemists and two part-time graduate students in biochemistry. The project began with the hiring of Dr. Pilgeram in 1957 and ended with his resignation in 1965 to take another position in the field.

Recognizing the value of the research programs, in 1956 the Board of Trustees incorporated the St. Barnabas Hospital Research Foundation. The foundation provided a good deal of the support for Dr. Pilgeram's work. The auxiliary also made substantial contributions to the research programs from fund-raisers which they sponsored. In 1966, the St. Barnabas Foundation merged with Swedish to become The Swedish and St. Barnabas Hospitals Foundation. The new foundation had a fifteen-member board which included representatives from the boards of trustees, the research staff, administration of the two hospitals and medical staff from both hospitals. Over the years, the foundation received grants from many sources including private individuals, The Onan Family Foundation, which gave a $50,000 grant to the St. Barnabas Foundation in 1963 and the Louis W. and Maud Hill Family Foundation which contributed $50,000 to the joint foundation in 1967.

The St. Barnabas Hospital Research Foundation and later The Swedish and St. Barnabas Hospitals Foundation provided support for a number of different research programs. Among those they supported were a study of cancer of the colon, headed by Drs. Lloyd Sherman and R. J. Tenner; a study of rheumatoid arthritis done under the direction of Dr. Paul Bilka; a project studying tumor control with an antigen compound prepared from the patient's own tumor. Drs. Donald Amatuzio, Lyle Hay and Henry Bates headed this 1967 project. Dr. Bates later was named head of the research department established at Metropolitan Medical Center. Two projects, each a one-year project, were funded by the American Cancer Society. One of those was a study of the role of viruses in human leukemia and cancer immunology. The other project funded by the American Cancer Society was a tumor clinic in which cancerous tumors of both in-patients and outpatients were studied. The cancer society provided just one year of funding for this project, but plans adopted by the project included follow-up studies of all cancer patients who participated.

After the merger of Swedish and St. Barnabas to become Metropolitan Medical Center, a research department was established with Dr. Henry Bates as its director. In *Dimensions Of Metropolitan Medical Center*, November 1976 issue, Dr. Bates said, "If you're going to engage in biological research, you must have remarkable patience. Advances are made in ten to twenty year increments, and you must be willing to accept the failures, which far outnumber the successes."

An example of a diagnostic tool used commonly today which was developed at St. Barnabas is the cardiac stress test. It was developed in 1963 under the direction of Dr. Arthur C. Kerkhof. The original objective was to develop a screening tool for prospective deer hunters. The results of the test gave the hunter an evaluation of his fitness to withstand the rigors of deer hunting. From that original, limited objective came broader use in diagnosing heart disease in all kinds of patients.

Chapter 23

St. Barnabas Bowlers

Membership on a St. Barnabas bowling team provided an off duty activity for several St. Barnabas employees over a period of many years. Membership on the teams was open to any employee and it often happened that a department head or supervisor would be playing on a team with the most junior member of another department. In the beginning, there were both men's and women's teams. As time went on, the sexes were mixed on several teams. In 1959, a bowling league for six Minneapolis hospitals was established. The six hospitals who participated in the league were: Swedish, Mt. Sinai, Abbott, Eitel, Lutheran Deaconess and St. Barnabas. Their bowling season ran from mid September to mid-April.

There were two teams from St. Barnabas playing in the hospital league, St. Barnabas 1 and St. Barnabas 2. In addition, the hospital had a league of its own which included seven teams with names such as the Bumble Bees, the Stingers, the Hornets, the Wasps, the Queens, the Workers, the Saint Bees, the Drones and the Honey Bees. During the 1950s and 1960s, St. Andrews also had bowling teams and there were weekly competitions between the two hospitals. The St. Barnabas League played all of its games at Hiawatha Lanes in South Minneapolis. The *Voice of St. Barnabas* included the latest on activities of all the teams in a regular column called "Pin Patter."

Chapter 24

And So It Ended

On March 24, 1970, a Centennial Advisory Committee met in the administrative conference room at St. Barnabas. Members of the committee, chosen by administration and the Board of Trustees, were Dr. C. Fred Quest, president of the Board of Trustees, Dr. Joseph P. Spano, representing the medical staff, Mrs. H. M Baskerville of the auxiliary, Mr. Robert Taylor and Mr. Lowell Kruse of hospital administration, and Mrs. Karen Erickson, community relations director at St. Barnabas. I also served on the committee as an alumnae member and former director of the nursing school. At that time I was the Executive Director of the Minnesota League for Nursing.

Each member of the committee was asked to recruit members from the group he/she represented to serve on a subcommittee which would develop ideas to be presented regarding programs to be included in the celebration of the 100th anniversary of the hospital. Dates for the celebration had been selected as, March 4, 1971 through St. Barnabas Day, June 11, 1971.

No record was available to me concerning meetings or suggestions of any of the subcommittees except nursing. Being a pack rate by nature, I had filed the minutes of the one meeting held by the nursing subcommittee and somehow, in spite of eight interstate moves and one international move we made after my husband took a position with the federal government in 1975, the minutes of that meeting survived to the present day. According to those minutes, members of the nursing subcommittee met on April 16. Members of the subcommittee were Silvija Kupchs, Hazelle Lundell, Joyce Massahos, Fran Bly, John Travers, Gilma Prestemon, Anita Goldbarg and Jan Grill. They all agreed upon three criteria as guides for selecting activities for the celebration. First, that events planned should have some value to the community as well as to the hospital. By community they meant either the community as a whole, or just the nursing community in the Twin Cities. Second, that some written materials be produced in recognition of the occasion to preserve a written record of the celebration. Third, that the celebration be planned to inspire pride among students, faculty, staff and alumnae of St. Barnabas.

The subcommittee on that day came up with ten suggestions for possible activities. During the days following the meeting, five more were suggested to me. Each member of the subcommittee accepted individual responsibility for working on a specific program if the suggestion for that activity were to be selected for the celebration. Suggestions made for nursing included a multi-media presentation showing the history of the hospital and the school, a doll display showing changes in the student uniform over the years, a two day conference to be entitled, "Charting the Future" and preparation of a written history of the hospital and the school. The present book, in more formal and amplified form than envisioned, is fulfillment of that suggestion since I agreed to work on that history.

After its initial meeting in March of 1970, there were no further meetings of the Centennial Anniversary Committee. Instead, each member of the committee received a letter, co-signed by Dr. Quest, president of the St. Barnabas Board of Trustees, and Myron C. Carlson, president of the Board of Trustees of Swedish Hospital. The letter, which follows, was dated, July 28, 1970, 6:00 P.M.

> Because of your importance to the success of our hospitals, we wanted to inform you as quickly as possible that the boards of trustees of The Swedish Hospital and St. Barnabas Hospital, have approved the plan of consolidation of our two organizations at their meeting just ended.
>
> Final consolidation is subject to the approval of the two hospital corporations. All of us are convinced that we have taken a significant step toward advancing the cause of health care in this area. We know that, with your continued support and guidance, the new Metropolitan Medical Center will become one of the finest private complexes in the nation.

The move toward merger of the two hospitals began four years earlier when on Sunday, July 10, 1966, ground was broken for construction of a joint facility, built on what had been Ninth Avenue South, the street which ran north and south between the two hospitals. The building was a three-story building, with connections on each level to the existing buildings of both hospitals. It housed services which had not been available previously at either hospital, though they were services which existed in some of the other hospitals in the Twin Cities. Those services included a fifty bed psychiatric unit and mental health center; a rehabilitation unit expanding the physical medicine departments available at the two hospitals; a thirty bed long-term care unit; a medical library; and teaching clinics for outpatient diagnostic and treatment services.

Actually, joint planning and sharing between the two hospitals began even earlier than the 1966 joint facility. An article which appeared in the Summer 1964 issue of the *Voice of St. Barnabas* outlined several ways the two hospitals were already sharing services and facilities. For example there was an interconnecting steam line between the two hospitals that provided constant heat, should anything happen to the heating system of either hospital. There was a joint intern-resident teaching program, established in 1959 in an effort to provide better advanced training for medical school graduates stationed at the two hospitals. This program was the first of its kind in Minneapolis. Operation of both hospital laundries under the management of just one joint manager. At that point, the arrangement did not include joint purchase of linens, but this was being discussed for the future. The radiology departments of both hospitals were jointly purchasing a radioactive tracer isotope used to determine blood volume. This material "wears out" quickly and since a minimum amount had to be purchased, joint purchase of it by both hospitals saved money. The Swedish Hospital radiology department had a machine for cobalt treatments and St. Barnabas Hospital patients could be sent across the street for therapy there. The physical medicine department at St. Barnabas Hospital had equipment for doing electromyograms, a test performed to determine injury to nerves in muscles. For this test, Swedish Hospital patients were being sent across the street to St. Barnabas. St. Barnabas had thermal blankets and a circle electric bed which was available when needed in either hospital.

The overriding factor driving both hospitals to share in the ways outlined was the bottom line figure. With health care costs increasing all over the United States, comprehensive health planning was called for by government action. Using expensive health care dollars to the greatest, while also the most efficient extent possible was the objective of CHP.

When Metropolitan Medical Center was formed by the merger of St. Barnabas and Swedish, the boards of the two hospitals felt they had found the way to utilize corporate funds more effectively and efficiently. In the Special Consolidation Issue of the *Voice*, Frank Walter, president of the new corporation said, "Let us recognize that we have a unique opportunity to serve the health needs of our community in ways previously beyond our separate capabilities. We face many difficult decisions in the months ahead, but let us accept and relish the challenge."

That special consolidation issue of the *Voice* described the new organization in these terms: "The new Metropolitan Medical Center is an impressive combination of resources and personnel—with an equally impressive potential for future development. Collectively we have over nine hundred beds, assets of nearly $25 million, an annual budget of $20 million, and over 2,300 employees, forming one of the twenty largest private hospital complexes in the country. As a major health resource, we have a special obligation to be responsive to the needs of our community and to plan in a way that helps to meet those needs."

The board of directors of MMC had thirty-six members, eighteen from the St. Barnabas board and eighteen from the Swedish board. The two boards did have different distributions of personnel serving among their members. St. Barnabas leaned more heavily toward representation from the churches who had been the originators of the old hospital, while Swedish, not having a church affiliation, leaned toward more representation from their medical staff.

The chairman of the new board was Myron C. Carlson from the old Swedish board and the vice chairman was Dr. C. Fred Quest from the St. Barnabas board.

In a sense, this new beginning for Metropolitan Medical Center was an ending too. The earlier close identification of the Episcopal churches of the city with St. Barnabas was changed. The same could be said for Swedish and their original objective of providing a hospital associated with the culture and traditions of Swedish immigrants in Minneapolis.

For eighteen years the consolidation of the two quite different organizations worked. Red ink on the bottom line, however, was a continuing problem.

In 1988, the corporation of two disparate groups was enlarged to three with the addition to the corporation of Mount Sinai Hospital. There was the hope the new, larger corporation could assure a future for all three groups, but this new corporation lasted only three years. The Metropolitan-Mount Sinai Medical Center closed its doors forever on June 30, 1991. The buildings they occupied were purchased by Hennepin County Medical Center and renamed the Hennepin County Medical Center-Medical Specialty Center.

With so many hopes for success, what happened? *Minnesota Medicine*, December 1991 issue, in its cover story entitled "Heritage Lives On After the Doors Close," tried to explore the reasons why. One opinion cited was that of Dr. Paul Olson, MD, who almost literally grew up at St. Barnabas, where his father, Dr. Philip Olson, had been a radiologist in the 1960s. He said, "The seeds of destruction were probably sown back in 1970 when MMC was the premier hospital in the cities." He felt MMC's failure to secure high-reimbursement specialty services meant inevitable disaster down the road. He cited Abbott-Northwestern's heart institute as an example of planning for a positive future. Perhaps the naïve belief in providing for the sick among the poor and needy of the community, which had been the St. Barnabas philosophy from the beginning, was an outdated concept. Dr. Olson's reference to "high-reimbursement" was aimed at Medicare and

Medicaid reimbursement to hospitals, which often did not cover the costs to the hospital of caring for elderly patients. In hospitals which treated a greater number of younger patients as well and admitted substantial numbers of patients for complicated diagnostic and treatment facilities unique to that institution, the inequity of government reimbursement could be offset by charges made for other services. But at MMC the proportion of elderly among the patients admitted was too high to allow this in the absence of specialty services such as those to which Dr. Olson referred.

Another doctor who voiced an answer to the question of why was Dr. Charles R. Meyer of Consultants in Internal Medicine in Minneapolis, speculated, "MMC was already oversized within two years after the building program was completed in 1970. We continued to struggle with a plant that was out of proportion to what was needed and a patient population which was declining."

Continuing on in the aforementioned article, Dr. Olson was quoted as saying that during the years after the final merger, staff physicians knew the hospital would close. "We weren't led to believe that, but we felt that. We were living with that for five years. The last few managers probably realized it was doomed to close, but they were limited in what they could do."

Dr. Olson stated doctors were saddened by the decision to close. "I grew up at MMC. My father was a radiologist at St. Barnabas. Some of the best physicians in town were at this hospital—it had a fine medical staff. The nursing staff was outstanding...We saved a lot of lives, got a lot of things done here. It was a wonderful place. It was like old-time medicine at its best. I thought of it as my home."

You, the reader, decide what happened. Did St. Barnabas just lose focus when the necessity for mergers came to the fore? What would Bishop Knickerbacker have done?

The story of St. Barnabas would not be complete without providing special mention of the last four administrators of the hospital, all of whom came with educational preparation in hospital administration, something which had not been available to administrators in earlier years.

Nellie Gorgas

Miss Gorgas came to St. Barnabas at a time the challenges were as great as any of the subsequent administrators would be asked to face. The staffing

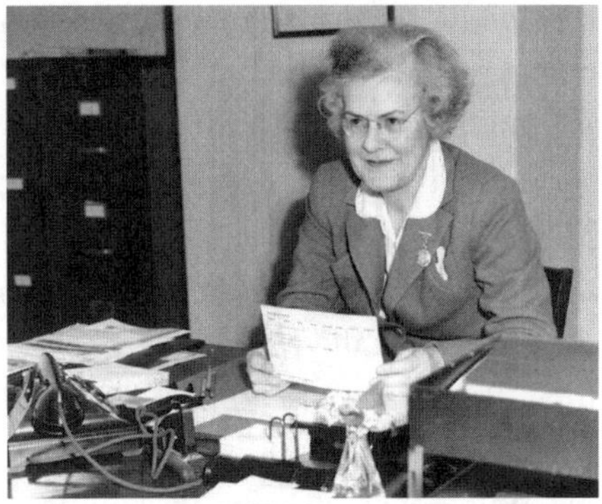
Nellie Gorgas

shortages described in connection with the one-year probation placed on the training school by the Board of Nurse Examiners were a reality, followed by even greater shortages caused by the exodus of staff people who served in World War II. In spite of it all, she did a remarkable job in keeping things going in the hospital. Her management style was different than that of the men who would be her successors. All of the men were married and had home and family responsibilities. Miss Gorgas was not married and she lived in a room at the Curtis Hotel, so she had almost no household chores to think about. The hospital was her world and her life. She could be found at the hospital all hours of the day and night. Her management style was a more folksy, personal style than those who followed her. She knew most of the employees by name and something about them, including even the student nurses. She was a warm, intelligent and dedicated lady, highly respected by her employees and by her colleagues in Twin City hospital circles. Had she been younger and in better health, she may well have made the transition from old-style to modern hospital management to a greater extent than she was able to do.

Dr. Karl S. Klicka

One of the first challenges Dr. Klicka faced on coming to St. Barnabas, was negotiating, along with Dorothy Merrell, director of nursing, for the establishment of a new preclinical affiliation for the nursing school. The school was in the early days of a cooperative teaching program for student nurses from Abbott, Northwestern and Eitel Hospitals, called the Central Teaching Program. The program has been described in Chapter 15 of this book. All four schools had been using the University of Minnesota for instruction of student nurses during their first six months in nursing school. The university had informed all four that they would no longer be able to provide instructional services to them. Macalester College in St. Paul agreed to provide the needed instruction for two semesters in the freshman year to replace the two quarters at the university. The new arrangement provided challenges which had not existed before. St. Barnabas students attending the university could walk to and from classes, or take a streetcar, since that service was available right outside the hospital door on Seventh Street. But Macalester College was far too great a distance to walk, so arrangements had to be made to bus students there. Bussing entailed a degree of liability for the hospital in the event the bus should be involved in an accident enroute to St. Paul It sounds simple when we think of it now, but these were mighty challenges for a new administrator trying to become oriented to a new position, a new community and new people. Dr. Klicka and Miss Merrell worked well together, making the transition easier. At the same time he was facing challenges in the nursing department, he was modernizing business office and administration operations. A controller, Frances P. Brodin, was hired. A personnel director, Dorothy Touhey, was also hired. These two and others were to provide more individual expertise to their departments than was available previously. Operations which had been crowded together in small offices near the front entrance of the hospital were spread out, utilizing rooms at one end of the third floor of the Corridor building.

Dr. Klicka remained at St. Barnabas only three years at which time he was offered the position of assistant administrator at Presbyterian Hospital in Chicago, one of the most prestigious hospitals in the Upper Midwest. He was replaced on June 1, 1954, by Robert W. Bachmeyer.

Robert W. Bachmeyer

Mr. Bachmeyer came to St. Barnabas from the Chicago area. He had grown up on hospital administration principles. His father was in hospital administration before him and he had authored the text which would become the Bible of hospital administrators all over the country. One of Mr. Bachmeyer's first challenges was management of two hospitals in different parts of the city, since St. Andrew's Hospital in Southeast Minneapolis had become a division of the St. Barnabas Corporation. Acquisition of St. Andrew's added eighty beds to those available for treatment of St. Barnabas patients. This was viewed as a less costly way to add beds, than the alternative of building a new building. And it did provide continuity for patients from southeast Minneapolis who were accustomed to using the hospital in their own neighborhood. Ultimately, the need to build new facilities to replace the aging Martin and Corridor buildings, became urgent and Mr. Bachmeyer's next challenge was the planning and building of the 1958 hospital. With new and larger facilities came the need for new staff as well, adding to his challenges.

In 1963, the decision was made to close the St. Andrew's Division. The cost saving envisioned with the purchase of that hospital in 1953 did not become reality. The physical plant at St. Andrew's was aging and the convenience of having all the hospital facilities under one roof outweighed the altruistic objective of providing a neighborhood hospital for the people of southeast Minneapolis.

In July of 1963, Mr. Bachmeyer resigned in order to become director of a large hospital complex in Youngstown, Ohio.

Frank S. Walter

Frank Walter came to St. Barnabas from Philadelphia, Pennsylvania, where he had been administrator at Methodist Hospital for the eight years between 1955 and 1963. He was a graduate of the University of Oregon and held a master's degree in business administration from the University of Chicago. Like Robert Bachmeyer, he had grown up speaking hospitaleze since his father, Frank J. Walter, was also a hospital administrator, serving Good Samaritan Hospital in Portland, Oregon, at the time of the younger Frank's appointment to St. Barnabas. Mr. Walter's challenges included the guidance of the nursing school in the establishment in 1964 of the Video Nursing Education program, the first program of its kind anywhere in the United States. A description of that program and the events leading up to it can be found in Chapter 15. The cooperative efforts with Swedish Hospital, leading to the building of the joint facility in 1966 and later to the formation of Metropolitan Medical Center in 1970 were major challenges for Mr. Walter. With the formation of MMC, he was appointed president of the new organization.

Chapter 25

Epilogue

In the spring of 2004, word began appearing in Minneapolis publications regarding a new use for part of the old St. Barnabas Hospital complex. *Skyway News* first ran an article on November 3, 2003, describing projects aimed at redevelopment for new purposes of several old sites in the city. One of the projects, labeled "Elliot Park site," involved one of the buildings of the old St. Barnabas, specifically, the Pavilion building. The Central Community Housing Trust was interested in remodeling the building to make it a facility for housing and training homeless youth to enter the job market.

But establishing ownership of the building was a question to be answered before anything could be done. Apparently when Metropolitan-Mount Sinai Medical Center was taken over by Hennepin County Medical Center, the two remaining buildings on the north side of Seventh Street were not included in the deal. The Whitney building was in use for a time as a facility for housing families of patients being treated for kidney disease at the medical center, but the Pavilion had stood empty for several years. An article appearing in the Star Tribune on August 20, 2004, quoted a spokesman for Allina Corporation, owners of the MMC property, as saying, "We weren't even certain it was ours." The question came because although Allina had acquired the buildings of MMC, the Episcopal Diocese retained ownership of the land north of Seventh Street on which the buildings stood.

The *Star Tribune* article went into some detail concerning the process of establishing ownership of the property. Ultimately, the trail led to a Mr. Nerland who was a senior vice president of investments at Smith Barney in St. Paul. Mr. Nerland was a trustee of the Minnesota Episcopal Diocese and he was able to unravel the mystery surrounding ownership of the property. Allina Corporation was willing to donate the vacant building and with Mr. Nerland's help, the Episcopal Diocese agreed to donate the land for the project. Mr. Nerland had earlier been involved in raising funds to convert dilapidated structures in the city into "safe, supervised housing for kids headed for self-sufficiency and a better life." Mr. Nerland was quoted saying, "The diocese thought this was a great project because it's not too big. After all, there's only about 30,000 Episcopalians in Minnesota…It's going to serve an underserved population. On any given night there's 1,000 homeless youth on the street. And only seventy overnight shelter beds and 221 transitional housing beds in the Twin Cities. The teens at St. Barnabas Apartments will have to apply to live there, and focus on improving their lot."

The article goes on to describe the new facility. There will be thirty-nine efficiency apartments in the five-story building. Youth who are selected for the program will live in the apartments, paying 30% of whatever they earn once they become employed. Federal government funds will subsidize the remaining cost of maintaining the apartments. The organization which will staff and supervise the facility is called YouthLink, a social service agency. They work with homeless youth in rehabilitation and job training to encourage them to become productive, self-sufficient young adults. The new facility will also include thirteen apartments for indigent working adults. The adults will pay $500 per month for their apartments.

The *Star Tribune* article goes on:

> The units are being developed for about $140,000 apiece, modest by today's costs. There are no Jacuzzis or video game lounges. But there will be an intake area, counselors, supervised study halls and more. Each kid will work to a customized education and work plan aimed at completing high school and gaining full-time employment…Most of the 1,000 homeless youth, ages 16 to 20, who are on the street in the Twin Cities have fled their homes because of unmet basic needs, sexual abuse, violence or drug and alcohol abuse. Many of these kids, according to police and social workers, resort to prostitution or drug dealing. Most sleep where they can because they can't afford rent or have no rental history or permanent employment.

St. Barnabas Apartments will open its doors approximately 1 April 2005. We think the Reverend Dr. Knickerbacker would highly approve. Not only is the name he chose for the hospital to be applied to the apartment building (Barnabas, the Son of Encouragement continues to encourage), but the facility will be serving the very kind of young people for whom he felt such concern when Cottage Hospital was opened so many years ago. What a fitting rebirth for the institution he founded.

Appendix A

St. Barnabas Milestones

1871	Cottage Hospital, twelve beds in rented house, the first hospital in Minneapolis.
1874	Move to Sixth Street location.
1883	Hospital is incorporated as St. Barnabas Hospital.
1884	St. Barnabas Medical Staff organized for the first time (had been volunteer doctors previously).
1894	First nursing student admitted to new School of Nursing; Martin building is opened.
1897	First graduation, School of Nursing.
1901	St. Barnabas Alumnae formed. First nursing school alumnae in the city.
1906	Wellesmere Nurses Residence built—first nurses' home in Minneapolis.
1910	Pavilion Building added to the hospital.
1911	St. Andrew's Hospital is founded.
1920	Contributions sent from St. Barnabas Alumnae to memorial fund for nurses who died in action in WWI.
1921-26	Alumnae adopted a war orphan from France, Francois Pichon.
1926	Twenty-fifth anniversary of the Alumnae was observed.
1937	Whitney Building was built, the first air conditioned hospital in the United States.

1938	St. Barnabas received a flag from the Red Cross for having the most alumnae as Red Cross nurses. Predated establishment of nursing for the armed services, all service nurses were recruited by the Red Cross.
1940s	First research programs begun. St. Barnabas was the first private hospital in the Twin Cities to establish medical research programs.
1942	Entire graduating class of nurses volunteered for service in the Army Nurse Corps. Cadet Nursing Program established at St. Barnabas.
1943	Old Asbury Hospital purchased; becomes Knickerbacker Residence for students.
1948	The Central Teaching Program established. Program originally included nursing schools at Abbott, Eitel, Northwestern and St. Barnabas Hospitals.
1949	University affiliation for sciences and social sciences terminated and new program established at Macalester College in St. Paul. Eitel closed its school that year leaving just three schools in the Central Teaching Program.
1950	Radiologic Technician training program established.
1952	St. Barnabas Bowl award for medical staff established.
1953	St. Andrews Hospital purchased—became a division of the St. Barnabas corporation. The St. Andrews Division closed in 1963.
1958	New $5,500,000 hospital was opened and dedicated.
1958	St. Barnabas Auxiliary was formed by the merger of the old Women's Board, Junior Board and Medical Staff Auxiliary.
1959	Whitney Building was rededicated as nursing school facility.
1960	Alumnae Scholarship Program was established.
1961	Volunteen or Candystriper program was established for the summer months.

1962	Macalester terminated its program with the Central Teaching Program. Video Nursing Education Program was established with KTCA-TV, the first program of its kind in the United States. Participants in the VNE program included all three of the CTP schools plus Mounds-Midway School of Nursing in St. Paul and St. Mary's Junior College in Minneapolis.
1966	For the first time in the history of the nursing school, men were admitted as students.
1967	Joint facility with Swedish Hospital was built on ninth Avenue South, the street separating the two hospitals.
1970	St. Barnabas merged with Swedish Hospital. The new corporation was known as Metropolitan Medical Center. It existed from 1970 to 1988.
1973	Last graduation, school of nursing
1988	Mt. Sinai joined MMC to form a new corporation that existed until 1991 at which time the entire MMC facility was purchased by the city and became a part of the Hennepin County Medical Center.

Appendix B

Articles of Incorporation

ARTICLE I

Name

The name of the corporation shall be Saint Barnabas Hospital.

Purpose

Its general purpose shall be, in the name of Jesus Christ and through His Church, to relieve the sick, wounded and disabled, irrespective of sex, nationality, color, or religious creed, by providing a place for the care of such persons, with medical attendance, nursing, food and clothing.

Location

It is and shall be located in the City of Minneapolis, County of Hennepin, and State of Minnesota.

ARTICLE II

The Bishop, Bishop Coadjutor and Bishop Suffragan, if any, of the Protestant Episcopal Church of the Diocese which includes or may hereafter include Hennepin County and the City of Minneapolis, and all Rectors of Churches of the same religious body within said county, shall be ex-officio members of said corporation. Each Protestant Episcopal parish within the City of Minneapolis, or within Hennepin County, shall be entitled to one member of said corporation and an additional member for every 300, or major fraction thereof, of communicants of such parish. In determining the right of representation, the report of such parish to the last Diocesan Council shall be conclusive as to the number of communicants of such parish. Such members shall be elected annually and be certified to the Secretary of the corporation by the Rector, Clerk of the Vestry, or other officer of such parish, and such person so certified shall remain a member thereof until such time as his successor has been certified to the Secretary of this corporation in like manner.

Nothing herein contained shall be construed to deprive of his or her membership in this corporation, as provided in the original and amended Articles of Incorporation, but no life memberships shall be hereafter created.

ARTICLE III

Stock

Said corporation shall have no capital stock.

ARTICLE IV

Officers

Section 1. The officers of the corporation shall be a President, Vice President, Secretary and Treasurer.

Board of Trustees

Section 2. There shall be a board of management of the business affairs of said corporation, consisting of:

(1) Not less than ten nor more than eighteen regular Trustees to be elected for terms of three years, except that in the first instance one or more of such regular Trustees may be elected for a term of one or two years each, so that, as nearly as possible, one third of the regular elective members of the Board of Trustees shall have their term of office as Trustees expiring with each annual meeting of the corporation. The number of regular elective members of the Board of Trustees to be elected each year (within the limits as to the total number of such elective members above stated) shall

be determined by resolution adopted by the members of the corporation at their annual meeting each year, and except and until changed at an annual meeting the last prior determination so made by the members of the corporation at a preceding annual meeting shall continue in full force and effect.

(2) So long as this corporation shall supervise or conduct the operation of the hospital activities of The Sheltering Arms, a Minnesota corporation, not to exceed six additional Trustees, to serve for a term of one year each, shall be elected from the members of the Men's Advisory Committee of the Sheltering Arms, the number so to be elected each year to be determined by resolution of the members of this corporation at each annual meeting.

(3) The Bishop of Minnesota or the Bishop Coadjutor of Minnesota (whichever shall have jurisdiction of a majority of the Minneapolis Parishes of the Protestant Episcopal Church) shall be an ex-officio member of the Board of Trustees.

(4) The Board of Trustees shall, at the time and place of their annual meeting herinafter provided for, elect by ballot a President, Vice President, Secretary and Treasurer for the term of one year and until their successors are elected, and whose duties shall be such as usually pertain to such offices or as may be provided for in the By-Laws of the corporation. The President, Vice-President, and Treasurer shall be elected from the Board of Trustees, but the Secretary need not be a member of the Board of Trustees.

Annual Meeting

Section 3. The annual meeting of the corporation shall be held at Saint Barnabas Hospital in said city on the festival of Saint Barnabas, at the hour of seven thirty p.m., but if said festival shall fall on Sunday, such annual meeting shall be held on the day next following, at the same hour and place.

Election of Trustees

Section 4. At each annual meeting of the corporation there shall be elected by ballot four Regular Members of the Board of Trustees (other than members of the Men's Advisory Committee of the Sheltering Arms) for a term of three years. No Regular Member of the Board of Trustees who shall have served for three consecutive full terms as a Regular Member of the Board of Trustees shall be eligible for re-election for a period of one year, except and unless the Board of Trustees by resolution presented to the annual meeting requests abrogation of this rule and said request be granted by the vote of a majority of the members present and in attendance at said annual meeting, a quorum being present. Whenever and as often as and as long as this corporation shall be in charge of the operation of the Polio Hospital conducted at Minneapolis, Minnesota, by the Sheltering Arms, there shall be elected at each annual meeting of the corporation by a ballot such number of members of the board of Trustees, for a term of one year each, from the members of the Men's Advisory Committee of the Sheltering Arms, at the annual meeting, as provided in Section 2 of this Article IV. Members of the Board of Trustees need not be members of this corporation. Not less than three quarters of all members of the Board of Trustees at any time shall be communicants of the Protestant Episcopal Church.

Reports of Officers, Committees, Etc.

Section 5. At each annual meeting of the corporation the reports of the officers and committees of the board of Trustees, with reports of officers of the Hospital, shall be read, covering the work done during the year; these reports shall then be given to the Board of Trustees to be acted upon.

Provision in Case of Failure to Hold Annual Meeting

Section 6. In case of any failure to hold an annual meeting or to elect Trustees at the time herein appointed, such election may be held at any subsequent special, regular, or annual meeting of the corporation, and the term of any outgoing Trustees shall continue until their successors are elected.

Provision to Fill Vacancy

Section 7. In case of any vacancy in any of said offices, or in said Board of Trustees, by failure to accept, death, resignation, or other cause, the vacancy may be filled by said Board at any annual, special or regular meeting.

Absence of Officers Provided For

Section 8. In the absence of any officer, his place may be temporarily filled by the Board if empowered to do so by the by-laws.

Provision for By-Laws
Chaplain, Superintendent, Physicians
Powers of Officers
Power to Amend By-Laws
Right of Patients to Choose Physician

The Board of Trustees may enact and adopt by-laws, and provide therein for the management and manner of transacting the business of the corporation; for committees of the Board, prescribing their powers and duties; for the employment of or appointment of a Chaplain, who shall be a minister of the Protestant Episcopal Church; for the employment of a Superintendent, one or more hospital physicians, and such other assistants, agents, nurses and servants as the Board may deem proper, regulating their duties; also prescribing, so far as the Board may deem proper, so far as the powers, authority and duties of the officers of the corporation, and containing regulations respecting all the other matters which can conveniently be provided for by means of by-laws. And such by-laws may be altered, changed or amended at the meeting of said Board, or at any other meetings, when so provided by said by-laws. But no regulation shall be made by said Board which shall prevent paying patients, at their option and at their own cost, from being attended in the hospital by any medical practitioner in good standing in the profession whom said patients may themselves select and employ.

Trustees Authorized to Call Meetings of Corporation

Section 9. Said Board of Trustees may also call meetings of the members of said corporation for consultation and advice, or for the amendment of these Articles whenever it shall deem proper so to do.

Appendix C

Board of Trustees

June 11 was St. Barnabas Day. Several important events were scheduled for that day down through the years. The Annual meeting of the hospital corporation was always to be on St. Barnabas Day or June 12 if St. Barnabas Day fell on a Sunday. How June 11 came to be recognized as St. Barnabas Day is unknown.

1883
Original Board of Trustees, representing twelve Episcopal parishes in Minneapolis, held their first meeting on August 28, 1883.
The Honorable Isaac Atwater served as President of the Board, 1883-1888.
Fred. R. Peet, Secretary
George H. Christian, Treasurer
Thomas B. Welles
The Honorable William Lochern
The Reverend Treadwell Walden
The Reverend A. R. Graves
Richard Martin
R. W. Jordan
Charles M. Hardenbergh
William Saeger
John I. Black

Another citation lists Edward Martin and William Watts Folwell as board members, but it is unclear as to when they served.

1887
LeRoy Robertson elected Secretary of the Board

1893
John I. Black, President.
L. R. Robertson, Secretary
The Reverend H. P. Nichols
The Reverend J. J. Faude
The Reverend F. R. Millspaugh
C. M Hardenberg
The Honorable J. C. Reno
Professor William Watts Folwell
George S. Grimes
Hector Baxter
A. G. Dunlop
A. S. Lovett

Members of the board who served on the Building Committee for the Martin building:
The Honorable J. C. Reno
J. I. Black
A. G. Dunlop
C. M. Hardenberg
George S. Grimes

1901
Hospital Annual report indicates the following resignations of Board members, but it is unclear when they served on the Board.
Dr. Webb—rector at either Gethsemane or St. Mark's.
The Reverend T. P. Thurston
The Reverend T. W. MacLean
J. W. Lawrence
Henry Doerr
R. A. Macgregor
M. H. Coolidge

1902
John I. Black, President

1904
C. B. Lyons

1907
George S. Grimes, President (Served as President until 1936.)

1915
C. E. Purdy

1916
The Reverend Dr. James E. Freeman, President
Dwight M. Baldwin, Vice President
L. R. Robertson, Secretary
M.C. Williams, Treasurer
Executive Committee: George S. Grimes, A. G. Dunlop and M. C. Williams
The Reverend William P. Remington
The Reverend Stanley S. Kilbourne
Hector Baxter
O. P. Briggs
E. C. Garrigues
C. E. Purdy

Committee appointed to raise funds to clear hospital debt (1916):
The Reverend Dr. James E. Freeman
F. M. Prince
C. M. Harrington
H. C. Clarke
G. H. Christian
C. T. Jaffray
H. R. Lyon
F. B. Snyder
E. C. Cooke

A.R. Rogers

1917
The Rev. Dr. James E. Freeman, President. (served in interim during absence of Mr. Grimes
Dwight Baldwin, Vice President
L. R. Robertson, Secretary (secretary for 33 years beginning in 1887)
M. C. Williams, Treasurer
Hector Baxter
O. P Briggs,
Stanley Kilbourne
C. E. Purdy
E. C. Garrigues
A.G. Dunlop

1922
Charles M. Case

1925
George S. Grimes, President
C. E. Purdy, Secretary (served as secretary 1920-1931)
Hector Baxter
Dwight Baldwin,
Charles M. Case
Mr. Danforth
Mr. Fenn
The Reverend Mr. A. E. Knickerbocker
Dr. Osgood
Mr. Rundell

1936
Charles M. Case, President

1937
Charles M. Case, President (replaced June 1937 by Charles Bolles Rogers)

E. A. Rundell, Vice President
J. Fred Quest, Treasurer
Stelle S. Smith, Secretary
Dwight M. Baldwin
George S. Grimes
C. M. Hardenbergh
The Right Reverend Stephen E. Keeler
The Reverend A. E. Knickerbocker
Robert B. McFerran
The Reverend Austin Pardue
Charles E. Purdy

1938
Charles Bolles Rogers, President (served until September 1944)

1944
Charles B. Sweatt, President (served last three months of 1944)
David E. Bronson, Vice President
Clarence M. Hardenburgh, Secretary
Walter G. Hudson, Treasurer
Charles M. Case
John C. Cornelius
James M. Dain
Jule M. Hannaford
The Right Reverend Stephen E. Keeler, Ex-Officio
C. Palmer Jaffray
Arthur P. Kemp
Sumner T. McKnight
Harold H. Tearse
David R. West
Edwin White
Valentine Wuertele

1946
Charles B. Sweatt, President
David E. Bronson, Vice President

C. M. Hardenbergh, Secretary
Walter G. Hudson, Treasurer
Board Members:
John C. Cornelius
James M. Dain
Jule M Hannaford
The Reverend John S. Higgins
C. Palmer Jaffray
Arthur P. Kemp
J. Fred Quest
Sumner T. McKnight
David R. West
Edwin White
Valentine Wuertele
Ex-officio: The Right Reverend Stephen E. Keeler

1948
Charles Bolles Rogers, President (1946-1951)
David Bronson, Vice President
C. M. Hardenbergh, Secretary
Walter G. Hudson, Treasurer
James M. Dain,
Donald W. Green
John W. Gregg
Jule M. Hannaford
The Reverend John S. Higgins
C. Palmer Jaffray
Arthur P. Kemp
Sumner T. McKnight
Neil Messick
J. Fred Quest
Edwin White
Paul Wishart
Valentine Wurtele
The Right Reverend Stephen E. Keeler, Ex-Officio

1949
Charles Bolles Rogers, President
Valentine Wuertele, Vice President
C. M. Hardenburgh, Secretary
Walter G. Hudson, Treasurer

1958
Valentine Wuertele, President (1952-1959)
Newell P. Weed, First Vice President
John W. Gregg, Second Vice President
Clinton Morrison, Secretary
Donald W. Green, Treasurer
David E. Bronson
The Reverend Harlan Coykendall
Robert DeHaven
Arthur D. Hyde
Raymond O. Mithun
Gerry E. Morse
C. F. Quest
Samuel H. Rogers
John S. Pillsbury, Jr.
Mrs. Lucian S. Strong
Sheffield West
Mrs. H. B. Stoker, Ex-Officio
The Right Reverend Hamilton H. Kellogg, Ex-Officio

1959
David Bronson, President
Samuel H. Rogers, First Vice President
John W. Gregg, Second Vice President
Charles W. Mooers, Treasurer
Donald W. Green
Gerry E. Morse
The Reverend Harlan Coykendall
Robert DeHaven
Arthur D. Hyde

Raymond O. Mithun
John S. Pillsbury, Jr.
Mrs. Lucian S. Strong
Newell P. Weed
Sheffield West
Valentine Wuertele
Louis N. Zelle
The Right Reverend Hamilton H. Kellogg, Ex-Officio
Mrs. Richard McNutt, Ex-Officio

1960
David Bronson, President
Samuel H. Rogers, First Vice President
John W. Gregg, Second Vice President
Clinton Morrison, Secretary
Donald W. Green, Treasurer
Gerry E. Morse
Robert DeHaven
The Reverend Harlan Coykendall
Arthur D. Hyde
Raymond O. Mithun
John S. Pillsbury Jr.
C. F. Quest
Mrs. Lucian Strong
Newell P. Weed
Sheffield West
Louis N. Zelle
The Right Reverend H. H. Kellogg, Ex-Officio
Mrs. Richard McNutt, Ex-Officio
Robert W. Bachmeyer, Ex-Officio

1961
Samuel H. Rogers. President
John W. Gregg, Vice President
Clinton Morrison, Secretary,
Donald W. Green, Treasurer

Dr. W. B. Reynolds
Raymond O. Mithun
John S. Pillsbury Jr.
Newell P. Weed
Louis N. Zelle
Valentine Wuertele

1962
Samuel H. Rogers, President
Sheffield West, First Vice President
C. F. Quest, Second Vice President
Clinton Morrison, Secretary (1953-1962)
Charles W. Mooers, Treasurer
The Reverend Russell Ewald
Maurice Adelsheim Jr.
David E. Bronson
Robert DeHaven
C. Edward Howard
Georrge D. McConnell
Raymond O. Mithun
Gerry E. Morse
John S. Pillsbury Jr.
Dr. Wm. G. Reynolds
Newell P. Weed
Wheelock Whitney Jr.
Louis N. Zelle
The Right Reverend Hamilton H. Kellogg, Ex-Officio
Dr. Donald G. Bohn, Ex-Officio
Mrs. E. Williams Burke, Ex-Officio

1963
Samuel H. Rogers, President (1961-1965)
C. F. Quest, First Vice President
Sheffield West, Second Vice President
Maurice Adelsheim Jr., Secretary
Charles W. Mooers, Treasurer:

Welles B. Eastman
John S. Pillsbury Jr.
Dr. W. B. Reynolds
Robert DeHaven
C. E. Howard
The Reverend Russell V. Ewald
G. D. McConnell
Louis N. Zelle
Wheelock Whitney Jr.
Gerry E. Morse
David E. Bronson
Raymond O. Mithun
Theodore Burton
Newell P. Weed, Advisor
John W. Gregg, Advisor
Valentine Wuertele, Advisor
Mrs. Lucian S. Strong
The Reverend Harlan Coykendall
Mrs. R. L. Thorfinnson, Ex-Officio
The Right Reverend Hamilton H. Kellogg, Ex-Officio
Dr. Archie M. Smith, Ex-Officio

1964
Raymond O. Mithun, President
C. F. Quest, Vice President
Maurice Adelsheim, Jr., Secretary
Charles W. Mooers, Treasurer
David E. Bronson (Served on the board for 30 years)
Theodore P. Burton
Robert DeHaven
Welles B. Eastman
The Reverend Russell Ewald
C. Edward Howard
George D. McConnell
Gerry E. Morse
John S. Pillsbury Jr.

Dr. Wm. B. Reynolds
Wheelock Whitney Jr.
Louis N. Zelle
Newell P. Weed
Valentine Wuertele
The Rev. Harlan Coykendall
John W. Gregg
Mrs. Lucian Strong
The Right Reverend Hamilton H. Kellogg, Ex-Officio
Mrs. Philip Olson, Ex-Officio
John W. Gregg, Advisor
Valentine Wuertele, Advisor
Mrs. Lucian Strong, Advisor
The Reverend Harlan Coykendall, Advisor

1965
Raymond O. Mithun, President
C. F. Quest, First Vice President
Sheffield West, Second Vice President
Maurice Adelsheim Jr., Secretary
Charles W. Mooers, Treasurer
David E. Bronson
Theodore P. Burton
Robert DeHaven
Welles B. Eastman
C. Edward Howard
The Reverend Bernard W. Hummel
George D. McConnell
Gerry E. Morse
John S. Pillsbury Jr.
Dr. Wm. B. Reynolds
Samuel H. Rogers
Wheelock Whitney Jr.
Louis N. Zelle
The Reverend Harlan Coykendall, Advisor
John W. Gregg, Advisor

Mrs. Lucian S. Strong, Advisor
Newell P. Weed, Advisor
Valentine Wuertele, Advisor
The Right Reverend Hamilton H. Kellogg, Ex-Officio
Dr. Archie M. Smith, Ex-Officio
Mrs. Philip A. Olsen, Ex-Officio

1966
Raymond O. Mithun, President
C. F. Quest, First Vice President
Horace Hitch

1967
Raymond O. Mithun
C. F. Quest, First Vice President
George D. McConnell, Second Vice President
Maurice Adelsheim, Secretary
Charles W. Mooers, Treasurer
Theodore P. Burton
Robert Cosgrove
Welles B. Eastman
Grover Forster
Horace Hitch
D. Edward Howard
The Reverend Bernard W. Hummel
The Right Reverend Hamilton H. Kellogg
Gerry E. Morse
Dr. Wm. B. Reynolds
Robert Watson
Sheffield West
Wheelock Whitney Jr.
David E. Bronson, Advisor
John W. Gregg, Advisor
Samuel H. Rogers, Advisor
Valentine Wuertele
Dr. Richard Frey, Ex-Officio

Mrs. Ben E. Mostrom, Ex-Officio

1970
George D. McConnell, President
C. F. Quest, Vice President
Maurice Adelsheim Jr., Secretary
Charle W. Mooers, Treasurer
Theodore P. Burton
Robert C. Cosgrove
Grover W. Forster
Frank D. Kiewel
Raymond O. Mithun
Gerry E. Morse
Dr. Wm. B. Reynolds
Dr. Jacob Strickler
Robert D. Watson
Welles Eastman
Horace Hitch
The Right Reverend Hamilton H. Kellogg
Walter Davies Jr.
Bruce C. Winslow
Dr. Richard Frey
David E. Bronson, Advisor
John W. Gregg, Advisor
Valentine Wuertele, Advisor
Mrs. Harry Murphy, Ex-Officio

1971
C. F. Quest, President
Horace Hitch, Vice President
Maurice Adelsheim; Jr., Secretary
Walter Davies Jr., Treasurer
Robert DeHaven (Also served 1958-1965)
George Fox
Walter Saunders

Appendix D

Administration Directors and Teams

1871-1883
The Rev. David Knickerbacker

1883-1884
The Rev. Mr. Cummings, rector of Gethsemane

1884-1890
Mrs. Alice A. Pew. First appointed matron, then became acting superintendent of the hospital. (It appears she held both jobs concurrently for a time.)

1890-1907
Unknown

1907-1930
Harriett S. Hartry appointed superintendent of the hospital on August 16, 1907. (She had served as superintendent of nurses since December 2, 1899.)

1930-1937
Uncertain, but it appears it may have been S. W. Rice.

1937
S. W. Rice (Whitney Building dedicated.)

1937-1948
Nellie Gorgas (Active in hospital administration circles in the upper midwest.)
Martha Lockman served as superintendent under Miss Gorgas until 1948.

1948-1949
George Barthel. Served as superintendent for a short period under Miss Gorgas and took over the reins when she became ill and was forced to resign.

1949-spring of 1954
Dr. Kenneth Klicka

1954-1963
Robert W. Bachmeyer

1963-1970
Frank S. Walter

Appendix E

Officers, Women's Board, Auxiliary & Later the Combined Auxiliary

"On May 23, 1893, a board of directors consisting of women, three from each parish of 300 communicants or more and two from each having a less number, were elected. It is expected they will be of great benefit and usefulness in the future management of the Hospital."

1893
St. Mark's Parish: Mrs. James W. Lawrence, Mrs. R. S. Burhyte and Miss Kate Welles.
Gethsemane Parish: Mrs. A. M. Smith, Mrs. F. F. Davis and Mrs. W. A. Edwards
St. Paul's Parish: Mrs. A. W. Paris, Mrs. M. H. Coolidge, Mrs. Harris
Holy Trinity Parish: Miss H. Rollett, Mrs. J. C. Cockburn, Mrs. P. M. Thompson
All Saint Parish: Mrs. J. A. Adams, Mrs. M. Han
St. Luke's Parish: Mrs. F. H. Hall, Mrs. C. G. Williams
Grace Parish: Mrs. Thomas Cox. Mrs. C. E. Hixon
St. Andrew's Parish: Mrs. W. M. Wilkinson, Mrs. Bockman

1894
WOMEN'S BOARD
Mrs. J. W. Lawrence, President
Miss Rollet, Secretary-Treasurer

1916
WOMEN'S AUXILIARY
Miss C. J. Welles, President
Mrs. R. M. Peters, Vice President
Mrs. John Plum, Secretary
Mrs. H. M. Lyon, Treasurer
Mrs. A. L. Aylmer
Mrs. W. R. Appleby
Miss J. M. Adancourt
Mrs. C. H. Bigelow
Mrs. R. B. Ballard
Mrs. L. R. Boswell
Mrs. S. S. Cargill
Mrs. N. H. Chase
Mrs. J. H. Daunt
Mrs. S. L. Fraser
Mrs. H. W. Gibson
Mrs. W. W. Hawes
Mrs. L. V. Haddox
Mrs. John Hickerson
Mrs. J. S. Kilbourne
Mrs. Lewis Kedney
Mrs. F. P. Lothman
Mrs. H. C. Maugham
Mrs. F. E. Mix
Mrs. W. R. Murray
Mrs. W. L. Nesbitt
Mrs. S. W. Patton
Mrs. E. S. Stebbins
Miss V. Stebbins
Mrs. G. Stevens
Mrs. C. F. Stremel
Mrs C. H. Simons
Mrs. J. W. Taylor
Mrs. Leon Warner
Mrs. Frank Wilkinson

JUNIOR AUXILIARY
Miss Helen Wheeler, President
Mrs. Orren Safford, Secretary-Treasurer
Miss Marjorie Boardman
Miss Katherine Dwinnell
Miss Katherine Eastman
Mrs. Elsie D. Freeman
Mrs. Lawrence McCoy
Miss Dorothy Record
Mrs. Wilbur Shaw
Mrs. Thomas Skiles

1933
ST. BARNABAS STAFF AUXILIARY (newly organized)
Mrs. W. B. Holt, First President
Mrs. G. S. Cabot, First Vice President
Mrs. A. J. Hammond, First Treasurer
Mrs. G. P. Schmidt, First Secretary

1944
WOMEN'S AUXILIARY
Mrs. Norman Johnson, President
Mrs. Robert Meech, Vice-President
Mrs. Paul Wishart, Secretary
Mrs. Record Bauman, Treasurer
Mrs. Sewall D. Andrews Jr.
Mrs. Floyd W. Bennison
Mrs. Donald W. Green
Mrs. Charles L. Harris
Mrs. John M. Harrison
Mrs. Lynn Johnson
Mrs. R. T. LaVake
Mrs. Addison Lewis
Mrs. C. A. Lyman
Mrs. Stanley M. Lyman

Mrs. Robert F. Pack
Mrs. L. S. Strong
Mrs. C. B. Sweatt
Mrs. Harold H. Tearse
Mrs. Amos L. Warner
Mrs. F. B. Wells
Mrs. D. R. West
Mrs. Alfred Wilson

1946
WOMEN'S BOARD
Mrs. Robert Meech, President
Mrs. John M. Harrison, Vice President
Mrs. Charles L. Harris, Secretary
Mrs. Record Bauman, Treasurer

STAFF AUXILIARY
Mrs. Hanford L. Russell, President
Mrs. Harold H. Sutcliffe, Vice President
Mrs. J. H. Plum, Secretary
Mrs. Edgar Chapman, Treasurer

1948
WOMEN'S BOARD
Mrs. Sewall Andrew, President
Mrs. John Harrison, Vice President
Mrs. Harold H. Tearse, Secretary
Mrs. F. B. Wells, Treasurer

STAFF AUXILIARY
Mrs. Harold H. Sutcliffe, Acting President
Mrs. J. H. Plum, Secretary
Mrs. Edgar Chapman, Treasurer

1949
WOMEN'S BOARD

Mrs. Lucian Strong, President
Mrs. Paul Wishart, Vice President
Mrs. David Bronson, Secretary
Mrs. B. A. Buckmaster, Treasurer

STAFF AUXILIARY
Mrs. Harold Sutcliffe, President
Mrs. W. S. Langley, Vice President
Mrs. John Plum, Secretary
Mrs. Edgar Chapman, Treasurer

1952
WOMEN'S BOARD
Mrs. Theodore Noll
Mrs. M. W. Goldsworthy
Mrs. John Lowe
Mrs. J. E. Tappan Jr.
Mrs. Helen C. Dick, Nurses' Alumnae Representative

1953
WOMEN'S BOARD
Mrs. Paige Lehman, President

AUXILIARY
Mrs. Harold Sutcliffe, President

JUNIOR WOMEN'S BOARD
Mrs. Wheelock Whitney, President

STAFF AUXILIARY
Mrs. Archie Smith, President

1954
WOMEN'S BOARD
Mrs. Paige Lehman, President
Mrs. W. T. Noll, Secretary

Mrs. C. L. Hodgman, Treasurer
Mrs. Ben Greer, Assistant Treasurer
Mrs. Carl Anderson
Mrs. C. Lewis Barthalomew
Mrs. William Curran
Mrs. R. L. Dunton
Mrs. C. R. Fike
Mrs. Jack Hilley
Mrs. John W. Hunt
Mrs. E. H. Lindemann
Mrs. Archie M. Smith
Mrs. J. Boyd Spencer
Mrs. Ralph C. Turnquist
Mrs. Robert Wilson

ASSOCIATE BOARD
Mrs. David Bronson, President

JUNIOR WOMEN'S BOARD
Mrs. Arthur Ostrander, President
Mrs. Nat Robbins Jr., Vice President
Mrs. David Bull, Treasurer

STAFF AUXILIARY
Mrs. Harry Johnson, President

1955
WOMEN'S BOARD
Mrs. Elmer Salzman, President
Mrs. Samuel Rogers, Vice President
Mrs. Totten Heffelfinger, Second Vice President
Mrs. George Hagen, Corresponding Secretary

1957
WOMEN'S BOARD
Mrs. Samuel Rogers, President

1958
COMBINED AUXILIARY (After 1958, there was only the Combined Auxiliary)
Mrs. Harry B. Stoker, President

1959
Mrs. Richard McNutt, President
Mrs. Arthur Lyman, Vice President
Mrs. David Cochran, Corresponding Secretary
Mrs. Robert Onan, Recording Secretary
Mrs. Arthur Kerkhof, Treasurer

1960-61 (Elections moved to spring)
Mrs. John E. Andrus, Recording Secretary
Mrs. Brace Bennitt, Jr., Corresponding Secretary
Mrs. Arthur Kerkhof, Treasurer

1961-62
Mrs. Howard Whitney, President
Mrs. Geoge Olmsted, Vice President
Mrs. D. Philip Seifert, Corresponding Secretary
Mrs. Philip A. Olson, Recording Secretary
Mrs. Jakob Strickler, Treasurer
Mrs. Robert Onan, Director at Large

1962-63
Mrs. E. William Burke, President
Mrs. Paul Pederson, Senior Vice President
Mrs. Newell Weed, Vice President
Mrs. John Cummings, Corresponding Secretary
Mrs. John MacDonald, Treasurer
Mrs. William Price, Assistant Treasurer
Mrs. Philip Olson, Director at Large

1963-64
Mrs. Paul Pederson, President

Mrs. Ross Thorfinson, Senior Vice President
Mrs. John Kellogg, Vice President
Mrs. Robert Hays, Recording Secretary
Mrs. Donald Forman, Corresponding Secretary
Mrs. John McDonald, Treasurer
Mrs. William Price, Assistant Treasurer
Mrs. Page Lehman, Director at Large

1964-65
Mrs. Ross Thorfinson, President
Mrs. Ramona Miller, Puppet Chairman

1965-66
Mrs. Philip Olson, President
Mrs. Eugene Kulesh, Executive Vice President
Mrs. John Kellogg, Vice President, Coffee and Gift Shops
Mrs. Philip McNairy, Vice President, Community Relations
Mrs. H. N. Baskerville, Jr., Vice President, Special Projects
Mrs. B. E. Mostrom, Vice President, Volunteer Services
Mrs. J. Boyd Spencer, Recording Secretary
Mrs. Elliot Gillespie, Corresponding Secretary
Mrs. Donald Forman, Treasurer
Mrs. Brace Bennitt, Jr., Assistant Treasurer
Mrs. J. H. Strickler
Mrs. R. W. Hayes
Mrs. Ross Thorfinson, Past President
Mrs. James Hirsch, Puppet Chairman

1968-69
Mrs. Harry A. Murphy, President
Mrs. Jakob H. Strickler, Vice President, Policy
Mrs. R. L. Thorfinnson, Vice President, Gift Shop
Mrs. Philip A. Olson, Vice President, Coffee Shop
Mrs. Brace Bennitt Jr., Vice President, Community Relations
Mrs. Roberg L. Awsumb, Vice President, Special Projects
Mrs. Philip McNairy, Vice President, Volunteer Services

Mrs. F. R. Fles, Recording Secretary
Mrs. Julius Bonnelo, Corresponding Secretary
Mrs. Frank Mork, Jr., Treasurer
Mrs. Paul E. Pederson and Mrs. H. M. Baskerville, Directors at Large
Mrs. B. E. Mostrom, Past President

1969-70
Mrs. Geoge Olmsted, President
Mrs. W. F. Van Gorder, Vice President, Policy
Mrs. Edward Forbes, Vice President, Special Projects
Mrs. Robert Reed, Vice President, Volunteer Services
Mrs. Kenneth Schultz, Recording Secretary
Mrs. John Smith, Corresponding Secretary
Mrs. W. B. Bendell, Treasurer
Mrs. Ken Oelschlager, Assistant Treasurer
Mrs. W. R. Frank, Director at Large
Mrs. Harry Murphy, Past President

Appendix F

Medical Staff Roster, 1970
(Including years of service)

Internal Medicine
D. S. Amatuzio
Donald Bell, 13 years
Reuben Berman, 18 years
Henry Bloch, 12 years
Malcolm Blumenthal, 7 years
Donald Bohn, 21 years
Paul Bowlin, 11 years
John G. Bradley
John Cardle, 4 years
James Cole, 16 years
Dale H. Correa, 24 years
Willis M. Duryea Jr., 5 years
E. P. Eichhorn, 7 years
Rafael Fernandez, 4 years
William Flory, 6 years
Richard Frey, 18 years
Mark C. L. Hanson
John N. Heinz, 5 years
Edward A. Johnson, 13 years
John Johnson
Charles P. Kolars, 12 years
Russell Lindgren, 32 years
James McKenna, 9 years
Frank Martin, 16 years
John Middlebrook
J. C. Miller, 31 years
O. L. N. Nelson, 31 years
Bruce C. Nydahl, 3 years
Rolland A. Olson, 6 years
L. R. Scherer, 33 years
Ralph M. Silas, 7 years
Lowell Weber
Cabot Wohlrabe, 19 years

Cardiology
Arnold Adicoff, 4 years
David G. Jones, 16 years
Robert Schultz, 4 years

Dermatology
Charles Balogh, 17 years
Isadore Fisher, 23 years
Elmer Hill, 23 years
Carl W. Laymon, 24 years
S. L. Mandel, 17 years
Milton Orkin, 4 years
Willard C. Peterson, 6 years
Alvin Zelickson, 10 years

Neurology
James Allen
Lawrence Farber, 9 years
Richard Galbraith, 6 years
Malan Hurr, 7 years
John M. McKelvey
Harold Noran, 24 years
Lawrence Schut, 4 years
R. C. Stoltz, 18 years

Physical Medicine
Joseph Engel, 19 years
Miland Knapp, 35 years
Arthur Quiggle, 16 years

Psychiatry
William Brauer, 4 years
Donald Daggett, 12 years
C. O. Erickson, 23 years
John Haas, 3 years
Andrew Leemhuis, 21 years
Glen Lewis, 5 years
Murray Locke, 5 years
Robert Meller, 13 years
Jennings Peteler, 12 years
John C. Regan, 12 years
John Schumacher, 4 years
Jack Wallinga, 16 years

Pathology
Wayne Chadbourn, 15 years
Nathaniel Lufkin, 32 years
John Popowich, 8 years
Richard Reece, 6 years

Radiology
S. Harley Calin, 10 years
Frank Mork Jr., 8 years
Philip Olson, 16 years

Rheumatology
Paul Bilka, 20 years

Pediatrics
Stuart Arey, 28 years
David Bloom, 7 years
Robert Bugenstein, 11 years
Lawrence Erickson, 19 years
Elizabeth Jerome, 20 years
Arthur K. Larson, 15 years
Nancy Lund, 5 years
William Mulholland
Lloyd S. Nelson, 22 years
Theodore Papermaster, 22 years
Deane Petersen, 17 years
L. F. Richdorf, 30 years
John D. Tobin, 23 years
A.V. Stoesser

Obstetrics-Gynecology
Marion Grimes, 40 years
Donald M. Larson, 5 years
Roger C. Larson, 5 years
David C. Lees, 6 years
John Maunder, 16 years
Mancel T. Mitchell, 23 years
John T. Moehn, 23 years
Mitchell Pincus, 13 years
Owen F. Robbins, 23 years
S. B. Solhaug, Jr., 16 years
William A. Treat, 5 years

Terrell F. Yeager

General Practice

C. A. Aling, 37 years
Clarence Arlander, 33 years
Herbert Billman, 5 years
T. J. Bloedel, 30 years
Albert Corniea, 47 years
Kenneth Dedeker, 5 years
John Eichenlaub, 7 years
Charles Friend, 22 years
Lester Gallett
Gary Good, 12 years
Harold Kadesky
Frank J. Kucera, 49 years
Otto A. Lenz, 33 years
Abraham B. Litman, 11 years
Gerald Midrum
A. Harold Mork
Frank E. Mork, 21 years
Leonard Moyer, 9 years
Maxine Nelson, 20 years
Carl J. Olson, 21 years
Eugene Ott, 16 years
B. J. Palen, 15 years
Charles Peluso, 22 years
M. K. Plasha, 17 years
Henry Quist, 14 years
R. E. Risch, 18 years
Wayne Rydburg
Franklin Sidel, 14 years
Archie Smith, 29 years
John E. Smith, 14 years
C. A. Strunk, 17 years
Barbara Subak, 15 years
D. M. Thysell, 3 years
Lloyd Whitesell, 33 years
Matthew Yelle
Charles W. Zinn

General Surgery

James G. Anderson
Frank Ankner, 19 years
Stuart Arhelger, 13 years
Roger Becklund, 5 years
Edwin Benjamin, 33 years
Harold Benjamin, 33 years
Herman Bentz
Lyman Clay, 33 years
Daniel P. Cortez, 6 years
Harrison Farley, 9 years
Robert Hammerstrom, 14 years
William A. Hanson, 9 years
Lyle J. Hay, 12 years
Hermann W. Heupel, 4 years
David Hickok, 7 years
Carter Howell, 15 years
Daniel W. Huebert, 13 years
Angelo Johnson,15 years
Arnold Kremen, 16 years
Clarence Kusz, 9 years
Lawrence Larson, 12 years
John Linner, 13 years
Donald MacKinnon, 23 years
Elmer Martinson, 12 years
Hamlin Mattson
Daniel Moos, 24 years
E. Theodore Palm, 4 years
John Parrott, 9 years
Clifford Phibbs, 9 years
Nathan Plimpton, 24 years
Carl O. Rice, 34 years

John Rosenow, 21 years
A. M. Sborov
W. G. Schaefer, 42 years
Horace G. Scott, 22 years
Joseph Spano, 38 years
Jacob H. Strickler,22 years
O. J. Campbell, 25 years
A.A. Zierold, 33 year

Anesthesia

Florence Bouthilet, 13 years
Edward Hustad, 3 years
Mark Kim, 8 years
Donald Limbeck, 17 years
Marvin Stewart, 18 years
D. Stuart Weatherhead, 13 years

Dental Surgery

Dean Brandsness, 5 years
Ralph Christensen, 9 years
Harold Panuska, 9 years
Vernon Day Smith, 9 years

Plastic Surgery

Harry A. Johnson, 4 years
Conrad Karleen, 3 years
Lyle Kragh, 12 years
Walter Lynn

Thoracic Surgery

Paul Gannon, 4 years
Joseph Garamella, 13 years
Nathan K. Jensen, 23 years
Frank Johnson, 13 years
William D. Kelly, 4 years
Joseph Kiser, 3 years
Michael Lynch, 9 years
Charles A. Peterson
Theodore Peterson, 3 years
W. Robert Schmidt, 20 years

Orthopedic Surgery

Robert Barnett, 15 years
Wesley Burnham, 23 years
Lester Carlander, 20 years
Frederick Drill
Harry B. Hall, 28 years
John Moe, 24 years
Roland Neumann
Lumir Proshek, 4 years
Edward L. Salovich, 11 years
Elmer R. Salovich, 8 years
Robert Soiseth, 6 years
Kenath Sponsel, 20 years
A. Bruce Sundberg, 5 years
Joseph Tambornino
Wayne Thompson
Francis J. Trost, 7 years

Ophthalmology

Donald Cundy, 23 years
Bourne Jerome, 23 years
Winston Lindberg, 12 years
Sidney Nerenberg, 9 years
Mark L. Norman Jr., 15 years
Karl Sandt, 22 years
Irving Shapiro, 15 years
Howard Shaw, 19 years

Otorhinolaryngology

Benjamin Bofenkamp,21 years
John Glaeser, 6 years

Ekrem Gozum, 5 years
Kurt Pollak
Robert Richardson, 11 years
George Tangen, 8 years

Otorhinolaryngology & Ophthalmology

Clyde Cabot, 27 years
Robert Wheeler, 19 years

Neuro-Surgery

Paul S. Blake, 19 years
Harold Buchstein, 30 years
David Johnson, 15 years
C. Kent Olson, 21 years
Leonard Titrud, 24 years
Erich Wisiol,8 years

Pediatric Surgery

Tague Chisholm, 24 years
Felix McParland, 13 years
Bernard Spencer,16 years
John Waldron, 7 years

Proctology

Charles Neumeister, 9 years
Lloyd Sherman, 15 years
Robert Tenner, 24 years

Urology

Samuel Beirstein, 11 years
John P. Cooper, 13 years
Charles Donald Creevy, 3 years
George Garske
Paul Hartig, 8 years
Gerald Koos, 4 years
Bruce Linderholm
E. George Olsen
J. A. Polzak, 18 years
William Price, 17 years
Milton Reiser, 5 years
Richard Rodgers
Baxter Smith, 24 years
R. T. Soderlind
Joseph Twidwell
Edgar Webb, 26 years

Honorary Staff

Isabel Cameron, 24 years
Frank T. Cavanor, 24 years
Wallace Cole, 28 years
Henry D. Diessner, 24 years
Gilbert L. Doxey, 24 years
Herman E. Drill, 1 year
Edward T. Evans, 24 years
Hewitt Hannah
Reuben A. Johnson, 24 years
Ralph Knight, 13 years
William J. Kucera Sr., 24 years
Leonard Lang, 4 years
Stanley Maxeiner, 2 years
Harold Michelson, 24 years
Irwin H. Moore, 23 years
Reuben Rosenwald, 24 years
Adam Smith, 24 year
Karl Waldron
Kenneth W. Wilder, 24 years
Robert Wilder, 24 years
Arthur A. Wohlrabe, 24 years
R. S. Ylvisaker

Others

Dennis Kane, 5 years
Jerry Schottler, 5 years
Jane Diehl, 3 years
Ali Hakim, 3 years
John L. Howell, 3 years
C. Richard McKinley, 3 years
Gerald Mindrum, 3 years
V. George Nagobads, 3 years
Charles Ostrov, 3 years
Loran Pilling, 3 years
U. S. Anderson, 2 years
Aydin Bilgutay, 2 years
Merrill Chesler, 2 years
Roger Farber, 2 years
George Hilgerman, 2 years
Emerson Hoppes, 2 years
Henry Horecki, 2 years
Freeman Kovack, 2 years
James Lillehei, 2 years
Thomas Litman, 2 years
William Luckey, 2 years
Glen Sawyer, 2 years
John Seymour, 2 years
James Swenson, 2 years
John Bergstrom, 1 year (1970)
Michael Bromer, 1 year (1970)
John Curran, 1 year (1970)
Alan L. Goldstein, 1 year (1970)
William Goodchild, 1 year (1970)
Sergio Grossling, 1 year (1970)
Charles Lukinac, 1 year (1970)
Timothy Magee, 1 year (1970)
Charles North, 1 year (1970)
Rodney Peterson, 1 year (1970)
Thomas Rose, 1 year (1970)
Sheridan Stevens, 1 year (1970)
Richard Tudor, 1 year (1970)
Catherine West, 1 year (1970)

Appendix G

Medical Staff Officers

1884
Original Medical Staff.
(Prior to 1884, doctors served on a volunteer basis and were not organized.)
Thomas S. Roberts, Chief of Staff

Surgeons

J. E. Moore
Knute Heogh
J. C. Stewart
J. W. McDonald

Internists

Thomas S. Roberts
H. B. Bracken
J. T. Moore
C. H. Hunter

Specialists

A. W. Abbott
H. McI. Morton
M. P. Vanderhorck
J. H. Martindale
R. O. Beard

1951
Clarence E. Arlander, Chief of Staff

1953
Archie M. Smith, Chief of Staff

1954
O. L. N. Nelson, Chief of Staff
R. G. Tinkham, Vice Chief
H. F. Buchstein, Secretary-Treasurer
Archie M. Smith, Councillor

Department Heads
L. R. Scherer, Internal Medicine & Medical Specialties
L. B. Clay, General Surgery
O. F. Robbins, Obstetrics and Gynecology
Lloyd S. Nelson, Pediatrics
M. E. Knapp, Physical Medicine
L. F. Sherman, Surgical Specialties
Bourne Jerome, Ophthalmology and Otolaryngology
A. W. Naslund, Roentgenology
P. C. Engelhart, General Practice
A. H. Mork, General Practice
W. T. Walsh, General Practice
H. W. Peterson, St. Andrew's

1955
A. H. Mork, Chief of Staff
L. F. Sherman, Vice Chief
J. T. Moehn, Secretary-Treasurer
O. L. N. Nelson, Councillor

Department Heads
William T. Walsh, General Practice
Archie M. Smith, General Practice
H. A. Johnson, General Practice

Harold H. Noran, Medicine
Joseph P. Spano, General Surgery
Benjamin Bofenkamp, Surgical Specialties
M. T. Mitchell, Obstetrics and Gynology
Elizabeth Jerome, Pediatrics
N. H. Lufkin, Pathology
Sheffield West, Board of Directors
R. W. Bachmeyer, Ex-Officio
Telmer O. Peterson, Ex-Officio

1956
Lloyd F. Sherman, Chief of Staff

1957
William T. Walsh, Chief of Staff
Lloyd F. Sherman, Retiring Chief
Edgar A. Webb, Vice Chief of Staff
John T. Moehn, Secretary-Treasurer

1958
Edgar A. Webb, Chief of Staff
William T. Walsh, Retiring Chief
Charles R. Peluso. Vice Chief of Staff
Donald G. Bohn, Secretary

Chiefs of sections
Nathan C. Plimpton, Surgery
Joseph A. Resch, Medicine
Deane Peterson, Pediatrics
Mancel T. Mitchell, Obstetrics and Gynecology
Wesley H. Burnham, Surgical Specialties
Robert G. Tinkham, General Practice

1960
Mancel T. Mitchell, Chief of Staff

1961
Charles R. Peluso, Chief of Staff
Mancel T. Mitchell, Retiring Chief of Staff
Donald G. Bohn, Vice Chief of Staff
Philip A. Olson, Secretary-Treasurer

Chiefs of sections
Donald G. Bohn, General Surgery
Owen F. Robbins, Obstetrics and Gynecology
Theodore G. Papermaster, Pediatrics
Arthur G. Kerkhof, Medicine
Harold Mork, General Practice
Robert G. Tinkham and Clarence E. Arlander, Exec. Com.

1962
Donald G. Bohn, Chief of Staff
Charles R. Peluso, Retiring Chief of Staff
Philip A. Olson, Vice Chief of Staff
Archie M. Smith, Secretary-Treasurer

1963
Donald G. Bohn, Chief of Staff
Archie M. Smith, Vice Chief of Staff
Philip A. Olson, Secretary-Treasurer

Chiefs of sections
Russell Lindgren, Internal Medicine
Jacob H. Strickler, General Surgery
Elmer J. Hill, Medical Specialties
Robert Schmidt, Surgical Specialty
John B. Maunder, Obstetrics and Gynecology
Henry P. Staub, Pediatrics
Carl J. Olson, Leo Zaworski and Charles A. Aling, General Practice

1966
Richard Frey, Chief of Staff

John Smith, Vice Chief of Staff
S. H. Calin, Secretary-Treasurer
Archie M. Smith, Counselor

Chiefs of sections
Arthur K. Larson, Pediatrics
Paul Bilka, Medical Specialties
James Cole, Internal Medicine
William Price, Surgical Specialties
Joseph P. Spano, General Surgery
Mitchell Pincus, Obstetrics and Gynecology
Eugene Ott, Charles Friend, Carl J. Olson, General Practice
Wayne Chadbourn, Pathology

1967
Richard Frey, President
John E. Smith, Vice President
S. H. Calin, Secretary-Treasurer
Archie M. Smith, Counselor

Chiefs of sections
Charles Kolars, Internal Medicine
Paul Bilka, Medical Specialties
Jacob A. Strickler, General Surgery
William Price and Robert Barnett, Surgical Specialties
Mitchell Pincus, Obstetrics and Gynecology
Arthur K. Larson, Pediatrics
Maxine Nelson and Charles Friend, General Practice
Wayne Chadbourn, Pathology
Sheffield West, Frank S. Walter, Robert J. Taylor and Lyle Hay, Executive Officers
Donald G. Bohn, Stuart R. Arhelger, Elizabeth Jerome, Mancel T. Mitchell and Charles R. Peluso, Proctors

1968
John E. Smith, President

Jacob H. Strickler, Vice President
S. Hartley Calin, Secretary-Treasurer
Richard Frey, Counselor

Section officers, Executive Committee
Charles Kolars, Internal Medicine
Paul Bilka, Medical Specialties
John Parrott, General Surgery
Erich Wisiol and George Tangen, Surgical Specialties
Mitchell Pincus, Obstetrics and Gynecology
Arthur K. Larson, Pediatrics
Maxine Nelson and Charles Friend, General Practice

1970
Jacob H. Strickler, President
Charles Kolars, Vice President
Wayne Chadbourn, Secretary-Treasurer
John E. Smith, Counselor

Section officers
Barbara Subak and Henry Quist, General Practice
Lawrence Farber, Internal Medicine
Charles Balogh, Medical Specialties
Mancel T. Mitchell, Obstetrics and Gynecology
John Parrott, General Surgery
Robert Barnett and Sidney Nerenberg, Surgical Specialties
Lloyd Nelson, Pediatrics
Miland Knapp, Physical Medicine

Appendix H

St. Barnabas Bowl Winners
(Became Charles Bolles-Rogers Award in 1972)

1952 Dr. S. Marx White
1953 Dr. Henry L. Ulrich
1954 Dr. Edgar J. Huenekens
1955 Dr. Thomas A. Peppard
1956 Dr. Silas C. Anderson
1957 Dr. George E. Fahr
1958 Dr. Ralph T. Knight
1959 None
1960 None
1961 Dr. Moses Barron
1962 None
1963 Dr. Arthur Zierold
1964 Dr. Thomas J. Kinsella
1965 Dr. Thomas Lowry
1966 Dr. Orwood J. Campbell
1967 Dr. Leonard Lang
1968 Dr. Carl O. Rice
1969 Dr. Stanley Maxeiner
1970 Dr. Herman Drill
1971 Dr. Lawrence Richdorf
1972 Dr. C. Donald Creevy
1973 Dr. John W. Johnson
1974 Dr. Cecil J. Watson
1975 Dr. Ragnvald S. Ylvisaker
1976 Dr. Tague Chisholm and
Dr. Lyle French
1977 Dr. Reuben Berman
1978 Dr. Arnold Anderson
1979 Dr. Robert Priest
1980 Dr. John Moe
1981 Dr. John I. Coe
1982 Dr. Edward Horns

Appendix I

Long-Term Employees
(Year of employment and years of service)

1899
Harriette Hartry, Superintendent of Hospital and Superintendent of Nurses, 31 years

1907
Amanda Evenson, Housekeeping, 48 years

1911
Charles Engstrom, Engineering, 51 years
Axel Albertson, Painter, Maintenance, 44 years

1916
M. Dorothy Rhodes, Director of Nurses, 22 years

1918
Albert Erickson, Maintenance, 37 years

1919
Ray Erickson, Orderly, 43 years

1921
Justine Hanson, Medical Records, 34 years

1922
Hazel Johnson, Dietary, 33 years

1923
Isaac Aaker, Chef, 40 years
Jack Leffingwell, X-ray, 36 years
Axel Mattson, Laundry, 32 years
Robert Aguilar, Administration, more than 30 years

1924
Ruth Reynolds, RN, Maternity, 38 years

1926
Elmer Parker, Engineering, 27 years

1927
Clara A. Johnson, Business Office, 40 years, worked part-time after retirement from 40 years full-time

1928
Louise Kassenborg, Laundry, more than 25 years

1932
Eva Beihoffer, Dietary, St. Andrew's

1934
Alpha Elf, Wellesmere Linen Room, 30 years
Arthur Manske, Engineer, St. Andrew's
Sopha Janjigian, Housekeeping, 18 years

1935
Lilah Day, Dietary, St. Andrew's

1936
Helen Hayden, X-ray, 32 years

1937
Matilda Engstrom, Laundry, 21 years

1938
Hulda Ostlund, 28 years

1939
Florence Buck, Head Nurse 5 Pavilion, 3B, 33 years
Clara O. Johnson, Head Nurse, 2 Whitney and 4A, 27 years
Clara Peterson, Housekeeping, 25 years

1940
Andrew Wahlstrom
Nancy Torrens, Housekeeping, 12 years
Gertrude Noyes, House Mother, Wellesmere and Knickerbacker

1941
Rachel, Flemming, Housekeeping, 25 years
Alice Jonquist, Housekeeping, 25 years
Inga Peterson, RN, 5 Pavilion and Post Anesthesia Recovery, 25 years
Ruth Kiely, Nurse Anesthetist, at least 17 years

1942
Zora Donaldson, Nurse Aide, 5 Pavilion, 17 years
Mathea Christenson, Maternity, 24 years
Rose Ennis, Housekeeping, 20 years
Irene Nelson, Head Nurse, 2 Pavilion and 4B, 22 years
Gertrude Braun Sears, Nursing School, 10 years
Alice Dawson, Physical Therapy, more than 22 years

1943
Anna Backer, Dietary
Mary Burns, Dietary
Emma Chadwick, Dietary
Dorothy Day, Nurse Anesthetist, more than 20 years
Doris Johnson, LPN
Mary McMahon
Emily Nelson, Maid, Wellesmere and Whitney Residence, 20 years

Juliet White, Nurse Aide, 2 Whitney and 4A, 20 years
Elsie Swanson, Dietary, St. Andrew's, 11 years
Irene Mortensen, X-ray
Lena Youngberg, Nursing
Mae Carlson, RN, Central Service and Emergency
Anna Larson, Dietary, St. Andrew's
May O'Neil, Dietary, St. Andrew's
Bertha Schwanke, Housekeeping, St. Andrew's

1944
Margaret Johnson, LPN, Post Anesthesia Recovery, 27 years

1945
Minnie Swanson
Mary Conroy, Laboratory, 26 years
Edith McGuire
Ann Smith, Maid, Knickerbacker and Whitney Residence, 26 years
Clara Tuma, Maid, Wellesmere and Whitney Residence, 18 years

1946
Callista Cashman, Evening Supervisor, Head Nurse ICU, 25 years
Mary Curtis, LPN, 2 Pavilion and Post Anesthesia Recovery, 17 years
Dorothy Eddy, RN, Newborn and Premature Nurseries
Clara Holt, Dietary
Marian Holt, Clerk, Medical Records and Maternity
Hazelle Lundell, RN, 2 Pavilion, Nursing School Faculty, 27 years
Stella Rasmussen, Dietary, St. Andrew's
Ed Shema, Engineer, St. Andrew's
Margaret Jam, HN Pediatrics, 13 years

1947
Violet Borgen, Housekeeping, 17 years
Ella Burnikel
Ruth Dahlin
Ethel, Haga, Dietician
Ethelyn Hagstrom, Housekeeping

Ann J. Olson, Laundry
Helen Pfleuger, Nurse Anesthetist, 15 years
Dorothy Sheridan, Business Office
Kristian Thingstad, Orderly, 14 years
Mildred Holm, Maternity Supervisor and Instructor, 15 years
Carol Holle Paulson, Head Nurse Pediatrics
Dorothy Sheridan, Bookkeeper, more than 17 years

1948
Helen Krieg, Head Nurse 3 Whitney, CSR, 26 years
Hazel Leshovsky
Mary Misica, LPN, 2 Pavilion
Winnifred Phillips, Night Supervisor, St. Andrew's
Patricia Taylor, Laboratory
Adolph Wade, Painter, Maintenance
Mary DeVinney, Assistant Evening Supervisor, 20 years
Margaret Muntifer, Purchasing, 10 years

1949
Marvyl Apelt, Credit Manager, 18 years
Nora Crawford, LPN, 2 Whitney, 4A, Intensive Care, at least 15 years
Marjorie Devereaux, Nursing Administration
Isabel Kroona, Operating Room Technician
Irene Peper, Assistant Head Nurse 3 Whitney, Head Nurse 3B, 37 years
Eunice Roesler, Ward Clerk, 13 years
Margaret Walbom, Laundry
Betty Waldron, Evening Supervisor, Assistant Director Nursing. Service, 27 years

1950
Shirley Thordson Mertz, Operating Room Supervisor, 25 years
Ruth Balzer
Ruth Fink, Dietary
Nettie Garin, Laboratory, at least 11 years
Dorothy Merrell, Director of Nursing, 11 years
Alice Ostrowski

Olga Ziemelis, Housekeeping
Marcia Eckert, Night Supervisor

1951
Elsa Apinis, Nurse Aide, Operating Room
Robert Apinitis, Central Service, 15 years
Lillian Bleckert, Fourth Floor, St. Andrew's, at least 12 years
Sofie Christensen, Nurse Aide, Pediatrics, 20 years
Emma Cimbulis, Nurse Aide, 3 Whitney and 5A
Katharine Frydrych, Nurse Aide, St. Andrew's Operating Room, Central Supply Room, 20 years
Janet Hokanson, Evening Supervisor, St. Andrew's
Anna Holovka, Dietary, St. Andrew's
Betty Griffin, Dietary, St. Andrew's
Thelma Duncan, Admitting
Violet Julius, Information Desk, 15 years
Marie Knutson, Housekeeping
Herta Lapins, RN, Operating Room, 20 years
Esther Leary, Housekeeping
Robert Nilson, Laundry, 12 years
Esther Olson, Housekeeping, 14 years
Marjorie Person, Nursing Administration, St. Andrew's, 17 years
Lucinda Robinson
Florence Sullivan, Ward Clerk, 4 Martin and 5B, 20 years
Jack Sutfin, Janitor, Wellesmere and Whitney Residence, 16 years
Harriet Wick, Dietary, 20 years

1952
Melvina Anderson
Anna Danell
Minnie Ehlin
Lela Erickson
Perry Gilfillan, Chaplain, 24 years
Lavilla Hering, Fourth Floor St. Andrew's, at least 11 years
Fred Isler
Elza Kruklis, Dietary, Central Supply, 12 years

Anna Kula, Dietary
Ottelie Kvernstoen, Supervisor, Operating Room, St. Andrew's
Agnes Lighter, Dietary, at least 10 years
Mary Miller
Esther Olson
Gilma Prestemon, Assistant Head Nurse 2 Pavilion, Head Nurse 4B, 22 years
Sylvia Rosenau
Norma Seebach, Head Nurse, 4 Martin, 4B
Sylvia Senn, RN, Post Anesthesia Recovery

1952
Belle Smith, Central Service, 12 years
Don MacRae, Maintenance, 30 years

1953
Margaret Hadley, Information Desk, 15 years
Roshell Borchert, Housekeeping
Delores Carnes, Night Supervisor
Maxine Grigsby
Olena Hanezarow
Willie Hester
Doris Pearson, Business Office, 33 years
Pearl Ramin, Switchboard, St. Andrew's, 10 years
Anna Salovich, Housekeeping
Jessie Wood
Grace Bailey, RN, float
Katherine Erickson, Laboratory
Marilyn Larson Nelsen, RN, 3 Whitney, 5A, Evening Supervisor

1954
Juta Mahakar, Play Lady, Pediatrics
Mabel Miller, Operating Room
Walt Rasula, X-ray, 10 years
Mabel Sharp, Ward Clerk, 5 Pavilion, 3B, Central Supply
Russ Strom, Pharmacy at both St. Andrew's and St. Barnabas

Shirley Dolvin, RN Central Service. Emergency Room
Silvija Kupchs, Librarian, 16 years
Marian Picha, Secretary, Laboratory, 32 years
Eloise Sharrow, Coordinator, Maternity
Mildred Tupper, LPN, Newborn Nursery, 15 years
Lillian Hoover, Ward Clerk, 4A, 15 years
Daisy Lau, House Mother, Wellesmere, Whitney Residence, 10 years
Leona Bush, Housekeeping, more than 10 years
Margery Breyen, Dietary

1955
Beverly Ewert, Nurse Anesthetist, 30 years
Vivian Provo, Switchboard, 10 years
Leslie J. Krob, Administration, 11 years
Ruth Anschutz
Gertrude Berlin
George Klahr, Chief Engineer
Angeline Owens
Therisa Van Kalsbeek, St. Andrew's

1956
Myrtle Larson
Myrtle Lee, Anesthesia
Dorothy Olson, Ward Clerk, Operating Room, 15 years
William Wells, Comptroller, 12 years
Dorothy Allard, RN, Float, 30 years

1957
Lucy M. Turk, Communications, 10 years
Elma Ann Lyon, Nursing School Registrar, 25 years
Beverly Gacek Johnson, Evening Supervisor, 33 years

1958
Karen Rasmussen, Assistant Head Nurse and Coordinator, Labor and Delivery Room, 29 years
Dalton Israelson, Carpenter, 10 years

Florence Dochow, Assistant Head Nurse 5 Pavilion and 5A
Renee Klassen, Assistant Head Nurse, Coordinator, 4A, 10 years
Jane Medhus Lundgren, 14 years

1960
Stanley Berge, Housekeeping, 10 years
Mildred Crawford, Dietary, 10 years
Alice Dawson, Physical Therapy, 10 years
Sophie Dulski, Dietary, 10 years
Mabel Elkins, Dietary, 10 years
Marilyn Erickson, Ward Clerk, 5B, 10 years
Gladys Folsom, Coffee Shop, 10 years
Derald Johnson, X-ray, 10 years
Harvey Krenz, Housekeeping, 10 years
Katherine Lanigan, Dietary, 10 years
Katherine Lee, Housekeeping, 10 years
Esther Lincoln, Central Service, 10 years
Margaret Loewen, Accounting, 10 years
Marilyn Nelsen, RN, 5A, 10 years
Emma Nelson, Central Supply, 10 years
Phyllis Ness, Nurse Aide, 10 years
Barbara Newell, LPN, Special Care, 10 years
Adina Ottem, Housekeeping, 10 years
Marie Protasiewicz, Dietary, 10 years
Minnie Quast, Housekeeping, 10 years
Milton Ramm, Purchasing, 10 years
Helen Rusin, Ward Clerk, 3B, 10 years
Rosemary Tschida, 2A, 10 years
Marie Wincek, Coffee Shop, 10 years
Jean Winkels, RN, 10 years
Fern Krikku Marty, 10 Years
Yvonne Barstow Allen, 42 years

1961
Doris Gaddis Haglund, RN Pediatrics, Labor and Delivery Room, Evening Supervisor, 11 years

1962
Mary Ellen Baxter, Nursing School Faculty, 10 years
Mabel Christensen, Nursing School Receptionist, 10 years
Mabel Erickson, Laundry, 10 years
Susan Fleming, Operating Room 10 years
Ruth Nevels, Physical Therapy, 10 years

1968
Arlene Fuller, Medical-Surgical Nursing, Obstetrics and Gynecology, 22 years

1970
Rosemary Sadler Olson, LPN 2 years, then RN 9 years

1971
Mary Ann Meyers Bacha, RN, 31 years
Linda Grover Busby, RN, 31 years

Appendix J

Distinguished Early Alumnae St. Barnabas Hospital School of Nursing
(Year of graduation shown)

During its 79-year history, St. Barnabas Hospital School of Nursing produced 1,660 graduates. The following are early graduates who made substantial contributions to nursing and to their communities.

Minnie Patterson (1897)

First graduate and pioneer in Red Cross nursing in Minnesota; she was active in public health nursing and organized and served as the first director of the Visiting Nurse Association in Minneapolis. Through her efforts, along with others, the Glen Lake Sanitarium was opened for treatment of Minneapolis residents who had tuberculosis.

Ella Gibson Birum (1894)

Ella was the youngest student ever admitted and graduated from St. Barnabas Hospital School of Nursing. She was just sixteen years old when she enrolled in 1894, having already attended Wilder College. Minnie Paterson took this very young orphan girl under her wing and they became best friends as well as classmates in spite of ten years difference in their ages.

Eleanor Hamilton (1898)

She served on the first Minnesota State Board of Nurse Examiners, established in 1907. She was chief anesthetist at St. Barnabas for a number of years.

Charlotte Roberts (1898)

She was the first secretary of the local nurses' association.

Bertha Erdman (1899)

She was the first director of the University of Minnesota School of Nursing, established in 1909. Unfortunately, her tenure at the university was very short because she developed tuberculosis and had to resign.

Caroline Rankielaur (1901)

She was a charter member of the Minnesota Nurses Association, organized in 1905; She was also one of the advocates of state licensure for nurses, leading to the appointment of the Minnesota State Board of Nurse Examiners, which later became the Minnesota Board of Nursing. She also served on the board.

Anna Armitage (1906)

She was head nurse in maternity at St. Barnabas from graduation until at least 1916. Some time later, she converted to Roman Catholicism, entered a convent and became Sister Aquinas. As Sister Aquinas she served for several years as the superintendent of nurses at St. Mary's Hospital in Minneapolis. Later she served in the same capacity at St. Michael's Hospital in Grand Forks, North Dakota.

Helen Vail Stevens (1906)

She left Minneapolis soon after her graduation to become associated with the Visiting Nurse Association of Pittsburgh and Allegheny County in Pennsylvania. She served as director of that organization for 23 years. During World War I, she served as an army nurse on both the French and German fronts. She returned to Pennsylvania and public health nursing, later moving to the Visiting Nurse Service of New York City where she was a supervisor. And still later she returned to Minneapolis as educational director of the Visiting Nurse Association of Minneapolis. In 1960, she received the Award of Merit from the Public Health Nursing Service of the Pennsylvania Public Health Association. She was the first nurse ever to receive this award, given in recognition of a career dedicated to the field of public health..

M. Dorothy Rhodes (1906)

She served as director of nurses at St. Barnabas from 1916-1938, the longest period of time in the history of the hospital that one person served in that position.

Leola D. Ellis (1909)

Served for 37 years as the public health nurse for Goodhue County, Minnesota, retiring in 1958. Was recognized for outstanding work in tuberculosis case finding and follow up. Received awards in both 1952 and 1953 from the Minnesota Tuberculosis and Health Association.

Ella Mae Thompson (1915)

She was a field consultant of the National Association of Practical Nurse Educators.

Amelia Peterson Gunderson (1916)

Nurse anesthetist who worked at first at St. Barnabas, then became the personal anesthetist for Dr. Owen Wangensteen, traveling with him wherever he did surgery. President of the St. Barnabas Alumnae Association and treasurer of that organization for twenty-five years. Active member of Gethsemane Episcopal Church, every month driving to Cambridge, Minnesota, to conduct chapel and communion services there at the State School. Member of the Gethsemane Altar Guild, diocesan president of the Daughters of the King as well as president of the Gethsemane chapter of the same organization. The motto of the organization and the one by which Amelia lived was: "I am but one, but I am one. I cannot do everything, but I can do something. What I can do, I ought to do. What I ought to do, by the grace of God, I will do. 'Lord What Wilt Thou Have Me Do?'"

Ethel R. Jacobs (1924)

Director of the division of public health nursing of the Indiana State Board of Health. In 1963, was given the Indiana Public Health Association Award for Distinguished Service.

Julia Miller (1925)

She was Dean of the Arkansas University School of Nursing. In 1957 she was chosen nurse of the year by the Arkansas State Nurses Association. In 1958 she went to India where she organized a school of nursing at the university, Indor, India. Over the years, there were a number of St. Barnabas graduates who served as foreign missionaries, but her contribution appears to have been the earliest among them. St. Andrews Alumnae also had at least one missionary nurse among their ranks, Eileen Bader (1945).

Appendix K

Alumnae Presidents
(Year of graduation in parentheses)

The St. Barnabas Alumnae Association was the first nursing school alumnae association in the city of Minneapolis. It was organized in 1901 at the urging of Harriette Hartry (listed as Harriet Hartig in some publications). Miss Hartry was the superintendent of nurses from 1899 to 1907 and superintendent of St. Barnabas Hospital from 1907 to 1935.

1901	Belle Langley (1898)
1902-1909	Minnie Patterson (1897)
1910	Alice Angst (1909)
1925	Ann Connell (1914)
1928-1929	Marie Haas Winslow (1926)
1933	Edith Steinke Hofer (1922)
1938	Marie Anderson Walden (1931)
1940	Mildred Freeberg McHale (1935)
1941	Lulu Casselman MacMurchy (1919)
1942	Helen Sorenson Williamson (1938)
1943	Beverly Fie Fahland (1938)
1947	Amelia Peterson Gunderson (1916)
1950-1951	Verna Jordan Long (1937)
1952	Sylvia Carlson Chadwick (1926)
1953	Evelyn Dressel Tollefson (1950)
1954-1955	Dolores Friedli Holl (1952)
1956	Grace Kornmann Terry (1951)
1957	Signe Naes (1956)
1958	Genevieve Kretchmar Featherstone (1941)

1959	Tina Harding Peck (1946)
1960-1961	Barbara Scott Werling (1957)
1962-1963	Joyce Carlson Massahos (1955)
1964-1965	Jane Medhus Lundgren (1958)
1966-1967	Dorothy Sheffield Pulido (1958)
1968-1969	Kathryne Heltzel Schrader (1958)
1970-1971	Frances Ott Bly (1966)
1971-1982	Joyce Carlson Massahos (1955)
1983 to present	Sheila Malmstrom Gahr (1957)

Additional officers as of July 2003
1955-1966 and 1971 to present Secretary, Beverly Bell Weber (1952)

1977 to present Treasurer, Margaret Bowyer Alexander (1960)

Appendix L

St. Barnabas Graduates Who Worked At the Hospital As RNs
(Listed by year of graduation)

1897
Ella Gibson Birum

1899
Eleanor Hamilton, Chief Anesthetist

1906
M. Dorothy Rhodes, Director of Nurses 1916 to 1938
Anna Armitage, Head Nurse Maternity

1909
Rebeka Johnson, Obstetrics Head Nurse
Katherine Reid, Operating Room Supervisor
Orilla Hennemuth, Assistant Operating Room Supervisor

1911
Christine Peterson, Acting Superintendent of Nurses 1938

1915
Bertha Ellingson, Assistant Anesthetist
Anna Nyquist, Assistant Anesthetist
Ella May Thompson, Head Nurse Fourth Floor

1916
Amelia Peterson Gunderson, Operating Room Supervisor, Anesthetist

Grace Mirick, Anesthetist

1917
Elva Thexton, Treatment Room in Martin Wing
Effie Newman, Night Supervisor
Helen Cribbe Dick, House Mother, Student Health Nurse, Treatment Room

1919
Lulu Saunders, Nursing School Instructor

1920
Zelma Moores Farnham, Operating Room Supervisor

1923
Ruth Anderson Reynolds, Assistant Head Nurse, Head Nurse, Supervisor Maternity

1926
Sylvia Carlson Chadwick, Float, Treatment Room, 5 Pavilion, Central Supply
Marie Haas Winslow, Float
Clara Myrland Philbrook, Maternity

1927
Mae Palmer Carlson, Central Service and Emergency Room

1928
Florence Watts Buck, Head Nurse 5 Pavilion and 3B
Gladys Burt Goodspeed

1929
Grace Kersten Bailey, Night Float

1931
Vinnie Schleuter, Head Nurse 2 Pavilion

1933
Helen Fremont Perusse, Float

1935
Lucy Wells, Night Supervisor

1936
Helen Krieg, Head Nurse 3 Whitney, Central Supply Room
Helen Parker Hayden, X-ray Technician, Instructor and Director of X-ray Technician Program

1938
Beverly Fie Fahland, Float

1940
Thora McCauley Kron, Evening Supervisor, Nursing School Instructor

1941
Genevieve Kretchmar Featherstone, Delivery Room

1942
Gertrude Braun Sears, Instructor, Acting Director of Nursing Education

1943
Betty Olson Born, Float

1945
Dora Daniels Sanders, Joined Minneapolis Police Force, Float on days off

1946
Kathryn Ness, Nursing School Instructor, Associate Director of School
Audry Schanil Brown, Central Service and Emergency Room
Josephine Holmberg Pletscher, Central Service and Emergency Room
Shirley Kilmartin Svendsen, 3 Whitney

Tina Harding Peck, Central Service and Emergency Room

1947

Carol Holle Paulson, Head Nurse Pediatrics
Joan Reiber Tupa, Operating Room, Oncology
Norma Vermeer Torvik, Operating Room
Carolyn Anderson Stucky, Float
Marlys Kilmartin Bailey, 2 Whitney
Genice Broin Gaasedelen, Operating Room
Marian Westman Nyberg, Pediatrics

1949

June Golden Dosen, Central Service and Emergency Room
Shirley Dolvin Peterson, Central Service and Emergency Room, Shift Supervisor
Irene Peper, Assistant Head Nurse 3 Whitney, Head Nurse 5A, Central Supply Room, back to 5A in 1962, Head Nurse Intensive Care Unit
Jean Lawson Jaye, Operating Room
Audrey Thompson, St. Andrews, Newborn Nursery, Delivery Room

1950

Evelyn Dressel Tollefson, 2 Pavilion, Assistant Head Nurse 2 Whitney and Instructor in Nursing School
Marcia Eckert, Night Supervisor
Verna Hansen Jones, Operating Room
Evelyn Hoffmeyer, Premature Nursery

1951

Grace Kornmann Terry, Clinical Instructor, Director of Nursing School
Gilma Joy Prestemon, Assistant Head Nurse and Head Nurse 2 Pavilion, 4A
Delores Johnson Roberts, Head Nurse Post Anesthesia Recovery
Margery Stone Bischoff, Labor and Delivery
Jane Tollefson Falk, Float
Dorothy Peterson Grill, 5 Pavilion and Float
Dorothy Jensen Allard, 4 Martin and Float

Norma Hedland Cremisino Logsdin
Doris Pentz Visser
Marilyn Olson Wegner, Maternity
Mildred Carstens Johnson, Central Service and Emergency Room
Carol Rugland Meade
Elizabeth Fessler, 2 Pavilion
Dorothy Hoyles Bolstad, 3 Whitney
Naoma Thompson Huckabay

1952
Betsy Sperbeck Williams, Emergency Room, Health Director
Geraldine Passarella Lawton Bolla
Coreen Needham Olson, 4 Martin
Nancy Nyline Pugh
Marjorie Asklund
Beverly Gacek Hilt Johnson, Evening Supervisor
Mary Fran Nelson Bottoms Maternity
Del Rita Dombeck Grills, 3 Whitney
Margaret Johnson Cloyd Assistant Night Supervisor
Mary Thompson Sherf
Charlotte Hess Saari
Mary Stiles Sorenson
Beverly Bell Weber, 2 Pavilion, 5 Pavilion

1953
Eleanor Krogstad Gausman, 2 Pavilion
Ruth Koester Darnell, Assistant Evening Supervisor
Avis Hernwall, Central Service and Emergency Room
Jean Gustafson Singh, Administrative Assistant, Nursing School
Janet Constenius, Fourth Marin, 5B
Marilyn Siewert Westenberg, Operating Room
Elizabeth Olson La Fontsee, Maternity
Joyce Watts Dudley, Pediatrics

1954
Marilyn Huntley DelPlaine, Assistant Evening Supervisor

Bonita Losness Morse, Float
Janet Lundborg Long
Marian Hakarin Marshall, Central Service and Emergency Room, 5 Pavilion, Post Anesthesia Recovery, Float
Kathleen Spohnholtz Rosin, Labor and Delivery
Mae Knudsen Horns, Pediatrics

1955
Lorraine Burdorf Smith, 2 Pavilion
Margaret MacDonald Renn, Pediatrics
Janice Jacobson Dimke, 5 Pavilion
Joyce Carlson Massahos, Maternity and Newborn Nursery
Shirley Kelling Hagerty, 3 Whitney and 4 Martin

1956
Janet Kumpala Hahn, Pediatrics
Mary Holmes Babscock, Newborn Nursery

1957
Rita Diercks Jurgens, 2 Whitney, 3B, 5B
Carmen Bergman Kjellsvig, Head Nurse Pediatrics
Sheila Malmstrom Gahr, 5B, Head Nurse Intensive Care
Virginia Severin Dahlman, 3B

1958
Betty Lou Reynolds, Emergency Room
Florence Dochow, 2 Whitney, 3B Assistant Head Nurse
Barbara Marquardt Sigurdson, 2 Whitney
Dorothy Sheffield Moe
Sandra Barnes Fisher
Karen Bjornsen Hirman
Shelvie Bowen Christian
Deanna Carter Folsum
Valerie Covell
Evelynne Graves Thompson
Mary Beth Kline Schipke

Carolyn Kuiters Lindsay
Dora Lattery Trotter
Jane Medhus Lundgren
Phyllis Stelter Richman
Nancy Stowe Galler
Marlene Thimgan Wasson, Pediatrics
Sally Ann Thomas
Adelle Widdifield VanOstrand
Kathy Heltzel Schrader

1959
Diane Fadden Lindvall, Assisted Clinical Instructor on 5B, 4A
Shirley Connelly
Beverly Giles Cooper
Audrey Bowen Anderson
Beverly Giles Cooper, 3B
Katherine Elias Lowe, Operating Room
Karen Haertel Musser, Pediatrics
Barbara Furst Cox, 4A
Dorothy Telschow Hagadone 4B

1960
Fern E. Krikku, Delivery Room
Mary Ekblad Brown, Operating Room
Yvonne Barstow Allen, 5B, 4A, Newborn Nursery, Maternity
Karen Peterson Bessler, Operating Room

1961
Marilyn Tonsager Rydland, 2A
Judith Larson Hybsa, Assistant Head Nurse 4B
Mary Ann Graff Clemmer, Medical-Surgical
Judith Warner Penske, Operating Room
Doris Gaddis Haglund, Pediatrics, Labor and Delivery, Night Supervisor
Mary Ellen Andrew Baxter, Nursing School Faculty

1962
Diane Deuser, 4A
Diane Thorp Hudgins, 4A
Patricia Stone Falk Kane, Assistant Head Nurse 4B
Delores Carlson Flo, 3B
Linda Temple Duffy, Emergency Room
Carol Kruse McInnes, Operating Room
Nancy Peterson Larsen, Operating Room

1963
Marian Steffy Ulrich, Nursing School Faculty
Janis Berglin Rhodes, 3B, Intensive Care Unit
Mary Greenslit Pryor, 2A
Patricia Petty Wennerlund, Pediatrics
Nancy Coleman, Pediatrics
Susan Kuklish McCaffrey, 2A
Susan Wherry Plumhoff, Operating Room
Kathryn Winsel, Operating Room
Betty Fossen Johnson, Pediatrics
Jean Kodesh, 5B
Lynne Eastwood Olson, 5B
Sharon Krampitz Clausen, 3B

1964
Susan Klein Ackley, 4B
Judith Gerber Rosenberger, 3B
Twila Evink May, 5B
Jean Pontius Hansen, 4A, 5A

1965
Marilyn Beeth Hirsch, Pediatrics
Joan Branjord, 5B, 3B
Cheryl DeMoe Hoskin, 2A
Janeen Hainrich Vassar, 5B
Faye Ruda, 5B, 5A
Sally Stinger Werling, 3B

Judy Larson, 3B
Elaine Schmidt Johnson, 3B
Margaret Sunde, 4B
Jenny Taylor Peterson, 2A
Jacquelyn Dawson Hull, 5A
Pam Loza Bakken, Pediatrics
Bonnie Hermanson, 4B
Marilyn Beeth Hirsch, Pediatrics
Muriel Hegg, Mental Health Unit
Sandra Kay Hall, 5B

1966
Kathryn Nordby Alm, Pediatrics
Jan Olson Danger, Delivery Room
Terry Watson Kellenberger, 4B
Mary Baden Pierce, 5B
Kay Flom Erickson, 5B, 4A
Linda Knutson Erlandson, 4A
Erene Gross, Intensive Care Unit

1967
Elizabeth Henderson Eiselein, Delivery Room
Corrine Gustafson Berry, 5B
Eileen Mercier Nystrom, 4B

1968
Arlene Ostergaard Fuller, Medical-Surgical and Maternity

1972
Linda Grover Busby, 4B
Rosemary Sadler Olson, Intensive Care Unit
Mary Meyers Bacha, Maternity
Teresa Erichsrud

Appendix M

Nursing Student Award Winners

BOARD OF TRUSTEES SCHOLARSHIP FOR ADVANCED EDUCATION
(Senior award)

1951 Mildred Carstens
1952 Gretchen Cotterman
1960 Jeanne Wrabek
1963 Carol Ellis
1964 Lois Buhl
1965 Cheryl DeMoe
1965 Muriel Hegg
1966 Jan Danger
1967 Nancy Plowman
1968 Carol Ostmoe
1970 Mary Strand
1972 Rosemary Sadler

MEDICAL STAFF AWARDS
(All were Senior awards)

Excellence in Obstetric Nursing

1952 Dorothy Meyer
1955 Joy Lessard
1958 Deanna Carter
1959 Shirley Connelly
1960 Fern Krikku
1963 Sally Mulligan
1964 Gloria Larson

Excellence in Pediatric Nursing

1958 Marlene Thimgan
1959 Katherine Elias
1960 Marian Anderson Locke
1963 Margaret Lindquist
1964 Alma Sandbo
1965 Sharon Juntunen
1966 Delores Vietzke
1967 Corrine Gustafson
1968 Marylou Pederson
1970 Judith Anderson Lawson
1972 Laurene Bruget
1973 Roger Jacobson

Overall Excellence in Nursing

1952 Beverly Gacek
1955 Muriel Minge

1963 Sharon Krampitz
1964 Lois Buhl
1965 Joan Branjord
1966 Kay Alm
1967 Diane Carlson
1968 Sarah Stenzel
1970 Barbara Gulbro
1972 Julie Kleven
1973 Colleen Murphy

Highest Scholastic Average, Three Years

1951 Mildred Carstens
1952 Gretchen Cotterman
1959 Melissa Robinson
1960 Mary Ekblad
1963 Janet Troop
1964 Naomi Schweiger
1965 Judith Kovar
1966 Kay Alm
1967 Nancy Larson, Janis Leppen
1968 Sarah Stenzel
1970 Dursita Anderson
1972 Linda Grover
1973 Catherine Gustafson

AWARDS GIVEN BY THE AUXILIARY
(Two were senior awards, one was a freshman award)

Excellence in Psychiatric Nursing

1972 Joan Klow
1973 Colleen Murphy

Highest Scholastic Average, First Year

1953 Shirley Kelling
1958 Mary Ekblad
1959 Patricia Bauer
1961 Janet Troop
1962 Twila Evink
1963 Milka May
1964 Katherine Nordby
1965 Pamela Kruger
1966 Terry Anderson, Sarah Stenzel, Mary Gilbertson (three-way tie)
1967 Susan Andersen, Jean Arndt, Becky Bangert (three-way tie)
1968 Kathy Britz
1970 Jerianne Alick
1971 Connie Baumgartner

Citizenship Award

1955 Janice Johnson
1958 Betty Lou Reynolds
1963 Sharon Krampitz
1964 Elizabeth Dawn Rolandson
1965 Mary Jo Bixby
1966 Sharon Jopp
1967 Janice Nelson
1968 Nancy Bartlett
1970 Joyce Savre
1972 Rosemary Sadler
1973 Colleen Murphy

Schleicher Award: Best Bedside Nurse

(Junior award)
1953 Mae Knudsen

1954 Sharon Jones
1957 All 26 members of the class
1958 Jacqueline Youderian
1959 Jean Wrabek and Audrey Younker
1961 Jean Kodesh
1962 Margaret Lindquist
1963 Terrie Pfleider
1964 Sandra Hall
1965 Kay Carlsen
1966 Janis Leppen
1967 Sarah Stenzel
1968 Mary Taylor
1970 Geraldine Gustner
1972 Colleen Murphy

Junior Student Who Consistently Utilized Opportunities for Advancement in Nursing

1958 Susan Bramsen

AWARD GIVEN BY ALUMNAE ASSOCIATION (Senior award)

Excellence in Medical-Surgical Nursing

1958 Vila Dahlke
1959 Dianne Fadden
1960 Marlene Bjerkeset
1972 Julie Kleven
1973 Catherine Gustafson

Students Who Maintained B Average or Higher for Entire Three Years

1963
Sharon Clabots
Nancy Coleman
Arlene Drabek
Carol Ellis
Sharon Krampitz
Susan Kuklish
Rosalynn Libra
Margaret Lindquist
Dianne Muetzel
Sally Mulligan
Mary Nelson
Joanne Palmgren
Margaret Parks
Judith Pittack
Sally Stephenson
Sandra Tillisch
Susan Wherry

1965
Pamela Bakken
Joan Branjord
Sandra Erickson
Dianne Guentz
Janeen Hainrich
Sandra Hall
Muriel Hegg
Bonnie Hermanson

Bonnie Johnson
Sharon Juntunen
Milka May
Jacqueline McElvey
Mary Quist
Sally Stinger
Janice Weiss

1966
Kay Carlsen
Donna Collett
Sybil Deutsch
Kay Flom
Judith Gallea
Terry Kellenberger
Linda Knutson
Sharon Leuddecke
Eileen Olson
Julie Reinseth
Barbara Rolland

Award for Most Progress in the First Year

1953 Izelle Benoy

Appendix N

Family Members Who Graduated From St. Barnabas

The Haas sisters (all graduated in 1926, though they were not triplets)
Leona
Marcella (McConville)
Marie (Winslow)

The Kilmartins
Shirley (Svendsen) 1946
Marlyce (Bailey) 1947

The Muetzels
Wilma (Schmidt) 1949
Verlaine (Sandberg) 1960
Dianne (Mork) 1963

The Watts (mother and two daughters)
Florence Robinson Watts 1928
Joanne (Torres) 1951
Joyce (Dudley) 1953

The Dochows
Mary (Sabe) 1955
Florence 1958

The Bowens
Shelvie (Christiansen) 1958
Audrey (Anderson) 1959

The Kornmanns (they were cousins, not sisters)
Grace (Terry) 1951
Judith (Prehar) 1966

In reviewing the Roster of St. Barnabas graduates, several other groups were identified who appear to have been sisters, though there is no verification of that fact. They were:

The Thextons
Edna (McKibbon) 1913
Elva 1917
Myrtle (Ludwig) 1917

The Uggans—(both graduated in 1922)
Agnes (Ware)
Julia (Vogt)

The McPeeks
Maud (Trageser) 1902
DeEtte (Olson) 1906
Sarah Grace (Cole) 1912

The McKays
Edith May (Bickel) 1912
Catherine (Sawyer) 1915

The Blankenhorns
Florence (Hansen) 1926
Jennie 1929
Julie (Waddell) 1929

The Drewelows (both graduated in 1929)
Alberta (Nolan)
Anne (Ingle)

The Doblers (both graduated in 1935)
Martha (Peterson)
Ruth (Woody)

The Dickersons
Valma (Warros) 1932
Marlys (Schaaf) 1936

The Hansons (two of them graduated in 1938 and the third one in 1940)
Frances (Barnes)
Jeanette (Benson)
Grace (Covey) 1940

The Jesses
Edna (Ware) 1942
Peggy (Pike) 1944

The Olsons (both graduated in 1945)
Isabelle (Mattson)
Maxine (Mitchell)

The Andersons (both graduated in 1947)
Martha (Stuckey)
Mary (Kent)

The Savres
Arla (Drill) 1955
Joyce 1970

There were other names, common for Minnesota, with multiple members, but these were considered probably not related to one another. There were Millers, Andersons, Johnsons and Petersons.

Appendix O

Transfer Students

The following students transferred to St. Barnabas Hospital School of Nursing at various times over the years and for various reasons. The year indicated is the year the student graduated from St. Barnabas.

1950 Geraldine Nelson from St. Andrew's Hospital School of Nursing
1951 Frances Warde from St. Andrew's Hospital School of Nursing
1954 Louise Moberg from a school in the Dakotas
1954 Bonita Losness Morse
1955 Kathryn Hunter from Swedish Hospital School of Nursing
1960 Susan Palmer from a California nursing school
1963 Adrienne St. John Hurley from a Duluth nursing school

Appendix P

St. Barnabas School of Radiologic Technology Roster

This program was begun in 1950. It was two years in length, after which students took examinations to become Registered Radiologic Technicians. Fifty-six students graduated from the program in the years prior to 1961, the first year for which we could identify class members. Following are the graduates for the years after 1961.

1961
Arla Thorkelsson
Pat Sager
Pat Doran
Arlene Smith
Roberta Thill
Dorothy Thompson
Kathy Chase

1963
Carol Nelson
Ingrida Klavins
Sharon Peterson
Betty Gakle (joined St. Barnabas X-ray staff following graduation)
Margaret Erickson

1964
Nancy Sandeen
John Gaffney
Cindy Knapp
Brenda Peltz
Susan Millet
Carol Fay
Beverly Hegberg
Gloria Kranak

1965 (two members of this class joined the St. Barnabas X-ray staff)
Ruth Buchmueller
Joan Mazurko
Judy Harmeyer
Betty Maher
Diane Matteson
Kathleen McCune
Gary Sunsten

1966
Ken Chinnock
Zeta Clark

Diane Beske
Sandra Johnson
Ludmilla Harmasz
Darlene Lacina
Paulette Tisdall

1967
Karen Paquin
Marjorie Welch
Diane Smith
Kathy Ready (joined St. Barnabas X-ray staff following graduation)
Kaye Robinson (joined St. Barnabas X-ay staff following graduation)
Naomi Orum (joined St. Barnabas X-ray staff following graduation)
Lavern Miller
Patty Jo Patka

1968
Sandra Anderson (joined St. Barnabas X-ray staff following graduation)
L. Douglas Davis
Eloise Fjordbak
Carol Martinson
Margaret McNaghten
Sharon Ordorff
Patricia Thompson Readmond
Ann Weaver
Donna Wiese

1973
Sharyl Holstad
Connie Klaers
Barbara Mattox
Melissa Mortenson
Olivia Nosie
Debora Schimmele

Index

Y

Z

Order Form

To get your autographed copy of *With Faith and a Marketbasket*, simply photocopy this page, add the necessary information, and mail it with your check or money order, payable to Grace Terry to:

Grace Terry
1539 South 5th Street
McAlester OK 74501

Author: Grace Terry
ISBN: 1-930374-14-3
With Faith and a Marketbasket $29.95 each Qty. ________

Total: ____________________

Shipping: $4.00 first book, $2.00 each additional book ____________

Total enclosed: ____________________

Name: ____

Address: ____

City: ______________________________ State: _____ Zip: __________

Phone: (____) ____________ Email:______________________________

You can also order this book securely from DeForest Press at www.DeForestPress.com, or by calling toll-free 1-877-441-9733.